CRANIOSACRAL
BIODYNAMICS

CRANIOSACRAL BIODYNAMICS

VOLUME TWO

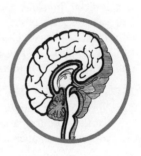

FRANKLYN SILLS

Illustrations by Dominique Degrangés

North Atlantic Books
Berkeley, California

Published by
North Atlantic Books
P.O. Box 12327
Berkeley, California 94712

Printed in the United States of America

Illustrations by Dominique Degrangés
Cover design by Paula Morrison
Book design by Jan Camp

Craniosacral Biodynamics is sponsored by the Society for the Study of Native Arts and Sciences, a nonprofit educational corporation whose goals are to develop an educational and crosscultural perspective linking various scientific, social, and artistic fields; to nurture a holistic view of arts, sciences, humanities, and healing; and to publish and distribute literature on the relationship of mind, body, and nature.

North Atlantic Books' publications are available through most bookstores. For further information, call 800-337-2665 or visit our website at www.northatlanticbooks.com.

Substantial discounts on bulk quantities are available to corporations, professional associations, and other organizations. For details and discount information, contact our special sales department.

Library of Congress Cataloging-in-Publication Data

Sills, Franklyn, 1947–
    Craniosacral biodynamics / by Franklyn Sills.
        p. cm.
    Includes bibliographical references and index.
        V. 1.—V. 2.
    ISBN 1-55643-390-5 (alk. paper)
    1. Craniosacral therapy. I. Title.
    RZ399.C73 S57 2001
    651.8'9—dc21

                                                    00-067885
                                                    CIP

        1 2 3 4 5 6 7 8 9 DATA 09 08 07 06 05 04

Contents

Preface to the Second Volume

This second volume is meant to support foundational training in Craniosacral Biodynamics. It explores the healing principles discussed in Volume One within a more specific context. In this volume we will look at the major tissue structures that organize around the primal midline. The intention is to learn to relate to these within a wide perceptual field and a craniosacral biodynamic orientation. Learning to create a relationship to major tissue structures is a step that cannot be omitted in training. I cannot stress this too strongly. If this step is omitted, clinical work tends to lose precision and focus. Once these relationships are second nature, you be able to support the action of potency in very specific ways within an open and intuitive biodynamic approach.

I am generally not discussing specific conditions in this volume, as these are best explored in supervised and educational situations. My focus in this book is on overall perceptual and clinical skills and the ambience of biodynamic craniosacral practice. I hope that you find this volume helpful and that it is a resource both for learning and in clinical practice.

STARTING POINTS

I have had many years of experience in the health field. I believe that my initial interest in the work of Randolph Stone, D.O., opened my field of awareness beyond the basics of structure and function. The extraordinary world of human energy, life force—

whatever you want to call it—came to the forefront. I perceptually discovered a whole new realm of organization that was not necessarily based on conditional processes. I discovered that there was a universal underpinning to the human system that could be appreciated by the practitioner. The ever-changing patterns and forms of the human condition were found to be held within a much larger and deeper matrix. An introduction to the work of William Garner Sutherland, D.O., deepened my appreciation of the subtlety of this and also showed me that an osteopathic understanding of structural and functional issues was essential and led to a greater precision in work and understanding. This all yielded a deeper appreciation of the elegance and flawlessness of the underpinnings of the human system and allowed me to develop a greater clinical effectiveness. With a deepening knowledge of the depths of the human system, and a growing appreciation of the Health that centers its experience, a related efficiency arises within the nitty-gritty of daily clinical practice. The key to this is an ongoing inquiry into the nature of perception and the ability to respond to what is perceived.

In my early clinical practice, I found myself spending a lot of time chasing compensatory patterns, but it became obvious that this was not an effective or efficient way to proceed. Much of the energetic, fluidic, and tissue motions I was following were simply forms generated by deeper forces within the system. The tension balance I was seeking was within these compensations. Sometimes this led me to the heart of the issue within the system and sometimes not. Sometimes the *unerring potency* came through and sometimes not. Sometimes symptoms would get better and sometimes not. This variability of results led to a deeper listening process on my part. I discovered what Sutherland, Stone, and others had been saying all along: that healing occurs at the fulcrum within stillness. I stopped chasing forms and listened to what organized those forms. I better appreciated the forces at work and the Stillness that centers it all. So the essence of the healing process became accessing a neutral, dynamic state of equilibrium and wholeness as the starting point for clinical process. I feel that this led me to the gateway of the Health of the system, the primary respiration it expresses, and the healing processes as they unfold. Work became less about my choices and my activity and more about listening and maintaining space. The offering of space and stillness in a negotiated manner became the heart of my clinical approach. This also led to a marked increase in the effectiveness of my clinical work.

listening & maintaining space
offering of space, & stillness

Acknowledgements

I want to wholeheartedly thank John Chitty for his editing work on this volume. I also want once again to thank Dominique Degranges for his illustration work and his easy and fluid communications. Both editor and illustrator are well versed in this field, and that has been a godsend for me. I want to thank my publisher, North Atlantic Books, and Richard Grossinger in particular, for their patience with this volume being completed well beyond the original due date. Lastly, once again, I'd like to express great gratitude to my family. My wife, Maura, a pioneer and teacher in her own field, has given me much space and encouragement to finish this work. Her warmth and love have been my foundation throughout. My little daughter Ella has given me the space at the end of every day to remember that bedtime is not just her time; it is our time. This has been a great resource for me. Finally, my older daughter Laurel, when she saw me anxiously speeding towards another self-imposed deadline, took me out to the cinema and helped me remember that life is also about fun, contact, and relationship.

1

Clinical Nuances

Volume One of *Craniosacral Biodynamics* established a foundation in basic theory and practitioner skills. In this volume we turn our attention to applying these general principles and skills in specific ways. We will survey the major body areas, including motility, structure, and anatomical relationships. Throughout this volume, practical applications will be offered. Some of these may seem mechanistic at first, but this is just a necessary part of the learning process. Once the skills are well-established and the anatomy is thoroughly understood, these exercises open into a more dynamic orientation to primary respiration, letting the clinical information arise from the inside out. Learning the anatomical and structural details is a necessary prerequisite to the later skill of listening and responding to the Inherent Treatment Plan.

We will begin this exploration by reviewing and expanding on the foundation laid down in Volume One. A discussion of some clinical issues sets the stage for the practical material covered in this volume and helps us avoid "missing the forest because of the trees."

In this chapter we will discuss:

- *Orienting.*
- *The Neutral.*
- *Levels of Neutral.*
- *The Dynamic Stillness.*

ORIENTING

One of the first clinical necessities is to learn to orient to the system in such a way that deeper levels of organization become more obvious. I have worked in training courses for over twenty years. As the years have passed, I have noticed many things about the student learning processes. One kind of difficulty that students encounter has to do with a loss of orientation. They may lose orientation to the patient's system and to the forces and inherent motions within it. They may feel that they can't sense anything, or will never be able to do the work. They may feel bewildered and vulnerable. In this state, students commonly call a tutor over and say that they are lost and confused. They have lost perception of what is going on within the patient's system and have lost contact with its dynamics. They may not be able to perceive primary respiration or may have lost an awareness of the patient's process. Their own processes of insecurity and anxiety may arise and get in the way of listening. When these kinds of things happen, it is not that they cannot sense anything. It is either that they are misinterpreting their perceptual experience or that they have lost orientation to the system. Even a state of seeming nothingness can be inquired into. In my attempts to assist students I have become very keen on the idea of orienting and helping them with orientation processes. What we are commonly dealing with is not an inability to perceive, but a loss of orientation. Thus, I felt that a discussion on *orienting* would be a good way to start this volume. If a loss of orientation occurs in your own process, or in a student's process that you are monitoring, here are a few orienting steps that may be of help:

- Orient to your own process.
- Orient to your practitioner fulcrums.
- Orient to the patient and their system; establish a relational field.
- Orient to the biosphere and the mid-tide.
- Orient to primary respiration.
- Settle into a holistic listening.

Although these steps may seem obvious, initially, each one has to be remembered and practiced consciously and clearly until they are second nature. Most of these were discussed in Volume One and are reviewed here in a slightly different way. Let's look at each of these orienting steps in turn.

Orient to Your Own Process.

- The first orienting step when you are lost or confused, is to orient to your own state. Where am I? What does this feel like? What is prominent within me? What sensations within me are prominent just now? What am I organizing around? What is between me and contacting this person? Do an internal check of your own state. Simply acknowledge what is there. Don't try to change anything. This simple acknowledgement is the key. Take a breath and slow things down. Do these sensations and mental states feel familiar? Notice your tendencies and get to know them. Work with the focusing process discussed in Volume One if that is helpful. See if you can clear space from what is arising within you that is in the way of contact.

Orient to Your Practitioner Fulcrums

- Once you are oriented to your own process, and have established some space, re-establish your practitioner fulcrums. "Practitioner fulcrums"

are your points of reference in space, to help you develop steadiness and consistency in your relationship with the client and neutrality in your perceptual process. First work with your midline fulcrum and then your inner fulcrum. Re-establish a practitioner neutral.

Orient to Contact with the Patient and Their System.

- Once you have settled into your fulcrums, especially your inner fulcrum, orient to your contact with the patient. Establish and negotiate your physical contact. Establish and negotiate your attention and viewing distance. Take your time with this and note the response of the patient's system to your presence.

Orient to the Relational Field, the Biosphere, and the Mid-tide.

- Once you are again oriented to contact, establish a relational field and orient to the patient's biosphere. The term *relational field* denotes the conjoined fields of both practitioner and patient. The biospheres of both join in a wider field of intercommunication. Your boundaries are still clear here. This is not a merged state, but a field of interconnectedness. Communication is exchanged within this relational field at many levels. The same inherent forces at work within the patient are at work within you. Extend a wide perceptual field. Let your awareness modulate with the boundaries of their biosphere. Let this be an intuitive process. As you extend your awareness to hold the whole of a person, there may be a sense of alignment to their biosphere, its midline, and its boundaries. Here your awareness holds the whole of the person, your hands have the sense that they are immersed in fluid, and your mind is relatively still as it abides within a state of active listening. Maintain an awareness of the whole fluid-tissue field as you do this.

Orient to Primary Respiration as Expressed in the Unified Field.

Orient to the fluid tide.

- An orientation to primary respiration is an initial entry into the Inherent Treatment Plan. First orient to the fluid tide. See if you can begin to sense the inhalation and exhalation cycles of primary respiration. Listen for a sense of welling up and widening and receding and narrowing. Do not worry if it is not being expressed within the patient's system just then; simply orient to the fluids. If the fluid tide is not being expressed, listen for the *quality* of information manifesting in its stillness.

Orient to the potency.

- The quality of potency can be sensed. Is there a dullness or flatness? Is there a sense of an underlying strength? Is potency building? Is it moving within the stillness? What is its quality?

    Now orient to the tissues. Orient to their motility and motion. As you listen to the fluid tide, include the tissues within your perceptual field. Sense your direct contact to whatever tissues you are palpating. Orient to the motion of the tissue field within the cycles of primary respiration. Notice the tensile motion of the tissues as a unified field of action. Notice the wholeness of potency, fluid motion, and the tissue field. If you sense no motion, trust that perception. This lack of motion has much to tell you. What is the quality of this stillness?

Settle Into a Holistic Listening.

- Listen to the whole of the body and the field around it. Do not lose the sense of the tissues as a field of action. The potency-fluid-tissue matrix is a unified field. See if there is a shift in the system to this sense of wholeness. Settle into a stillness of listening. This is not a passive state but an active, engaged listening within a wide and holistic perceptual field. Nothing within this field is of greater or lesser importance. Even the "little" things within this field are of significance. Listen to the whole without expectation. Let the whole tensile field speak to you, listen for the action of the potency within the fluids, listen for shifts and distortions of the tensile field around particular fulcrums, listen for wider and deeper forces to come into play.

I work with these orienting intentions as appropriate with my hands over a student's hands while they palpate a person's system. Another common loss of orientation can occur when a student orients to the tissues and loses a sense of the fluids and the organizing forces involved. A localized tissue pattern may clarify, and they may too quickly follow it or get confused by a myriad of patterns arising. I try to have the student widen their orientation from the local pattern to the whole tissue field. I simply have them slow down their intentions, encourage them to let go of knowing what is occurring, and slow their process of engagement down. I help them widen their field of awareness and listen to the phases of primary respiration. I help them include the fluids, and then the force within the fluids, as they listen to the tissues, tissue structures, and their motility and motion. Many times it is a case of widening their perceptual field and not narrowing to the particulars, but allowing the particulars to come to them within a much wider context. I may say something like, "Okay, you sense a tissue pattern, let that go for now. Widen your perceptual field to the whole tissue field and include the fluids and the fluid tide here. . . . Don't lose the sense of the tissues and orient to the fluids also. Great! Now sense the potency driving that. Stay with this until you really sense a unity here, the wholeness of the system."

Again, I do this with my hands over the student's hands; that helps to amplify their awareness of these intentions and perceptions. This may take some time, but once students are again oriented to primary respiration and to the three functions of potency, fluids, and tissues, their clinical skills can develop more clearly and with less confusion. They also begin to gain more confidence. If no motion is clearly expressed, I help them inquire into that. Is this a resourcing state or is this a state of stasis? What is the quality of this? The most important thing here is to begin to gain trust in our abilities to simply listen without self-judgment or internal needs.

ORIENTING TO THE WHOLE

In this orienting and listening process, we as practitioners need to have a relationship both to the Health within the system and to the present nature of conditioned form and the suffering it may hold. Within a craniosacral biodynamic framework, we do this within the context of an awareness of the whole. Rollin Becker, D.O., wrote elegantly about this important clinical skill.[1] Knowledge of the whole allows the practitioner to have a clear relationship to the ever-changing forms and patterns within a patient's system. In a clinical context we attempt to hold the whole of the human system within our field of awareness. We orient to the whole of the patient's body and body-mind system. We allow both the Health and the conditions being centered to be held within this perceptual field. We allow our minds to still and we settle into a receptive field of listening. This allows clarity to arise relative to the ever-changing patterns within their system.

The Inherent Treatment Plan unfolds as we hold this kind of holistic orientation. Things clarify and specifics come to the forefront. You cannot analyze or diagnose to know this. You certainly can't motion test for it. This is a function of the Breath of Life and its potency. You must learn to listen and to appropriately respond to its call. The nature of your attention is whole, as is your field of awareness. You hold the whole of the patient's system within your perceptual field as its particulars clarify.

BEHIND THE CURTAIN

I realize that the longer I practice this work, and the more clinical experience I accumulate, the less I know. Sutherland used to say that all you know goes "behind the curtain."[2] This is not a curtain of ignorance, but is more about a deepening appreciation of the mystery of life. I can never "know" this mystery. I can only let go and enter into a relationship with it. Even ideas I have written about in these volumes simply go behind the curtain into a place of unknowing. This is the heart of my clinical practice. Likewise, I can never know the needs of another person and their system. Nor can I know another's system as well as that person can know themselves. Nor can I diagnose, analyze, or understand what needs to happen in another's healing process. I have seen this over and over again. It is very humbling.

Yet within the darkness of unknowing, clarity arises. The Intelligence takes over and I am shown the way to proceed. Somehow practitioners must come to a place within themselves that allows them to hear and respond to the unfolding intentions of the Breath of Life. I find that the crux of this is a growing ability to listen to the whole of a person's system with an open heart, without agenda. This is based upon a mind that is still and totally at rest within itself. Within this field of awareness, all of my diagnostic knowledge and procedures, and therapeutic techniques and interventions, literally go "behind the curtain" within the humbling process of simply listening to the whole of that person's living form and the Stillness and Health that center it. As the Inherent Treatment Plan unfolds, the potency of the Breath of Life leads the way. The particulars come to the forefront as a factor of the intentions of the Breath of Life, not as a response to my interventions or analysis.

THE NEUTRAL
AND QUALITIES OF THE NEUTRAL

The neutral is an important concept to grasp within this work, and I would like to review it before we enter into the bulk of this volume. It can be a strange term when first met. It does not denote a state that is bland or void of activity. It points to a state within which balance and equilibrium are accessed. The healing process within a patient does not really begin until a neutral is established within their system. The neutral becomes a focus for the Intelligence and the action of potency within the system. When it is established, it is as though a new fulcrum coalesces, within which potency can concentrate and focus. When the practitioner can access and orient to the Inherent Treatment Plan, the neutral accessed is a precise expression of the healing intentions of the Breath of Life and its potency within that person's system. The neutral is a nonlinear concept. A neutral state is accessed totally in present time. It has depth and breadth. It is important to stress that the neutral we orient to in a craniosacral biodynamic context is a systemic state. It will seem as though the whole body-mind is unified. This is a state of dynamic equilibrium, a neutral within all of the factors present. This dynamically balanced state acts as a gateway to the deeper forces and healing intentions of the Breath of Life. It can take us into unknown territory.

In Volume One, we explored a number of types of neutral states, and I would like to review those concepts here. The first neutral we explored was the *practitioner neutral*. This is an inner state of stillness accessed by the practitioner which becomes a still ground for the patient's process. Your practitioner neutral becomes an initial orienting ground for the patient's system and for the action of the Breath of Life.

INHERENT TREATMENT PLAN

The next neutral explored was the point of balanced membranous tension. This was called a precise neutral by Magoun.[3] The idea here is to access a precise point of balance in the tension factors found within the membranes and tissues. This neutral is a local phenomenon. It is a tension balance point within the local strains and tensions in the pattern being palpated. The practitioner can be very active in an attempt to access this point.

The next neutral we explored was called the *state of balance*. We differentiated this from the point of balanced membranous tension. The state of balance, unlike the point of balanced membranous tension, is a systemic neutral. In the state of balance there is a shift from local tensions to the unified dynamics of potency, fluid, and tissues. It is a dynamic equilibrium within the potencies and forces that organize the fluid-tissue field and the tensions present. It is

accessed not just within local tissue tensions, but within the body as a whole. As the system settles into the state of balance, the unity of potency, fluids, and tissues is sensed and the neutral occurs everywhere in the system, all at once. This neutral orients to the specific fulcrum being attended to. This is the starting point for the actual healing processes in the session. It is a gateway to the deeper healing principles within the human system. It is within this systemic neutral that inherent forces come into play. We used Becker's three-phase awareness of the healing process as a structure for exploring this state. It seems to give students a real entry to healing processes. It is an excellent starting point.

A HOLISTIC SHIFT

[handwritten margin note: Becker's 3 phase awareness?]

I would like to discuss another kind of systemic process that naturally arises as a starting point for session work. I alluded to it when discussing the Inherent Treatment Plan in Volume One. Becker encouraged practitioners to wait in a receptive and still state until "something happens." In a transcript of Becker's verbal teachings called "Mechanism to Mechanism, How to Get Started,"[4] this "something" was directly sensed as a shift within the body from seeming fragmentation to a sense of wholeness. This is a literal shift within the system from its patterning and pathology to primary respiration. Not a stillpoint or state of balance, it is a dramatic shift in orientation from the conditions present to the Health that centers those conditions. Potency, fluid, and tissues are then really sensed to be a unified field of action. The system may be sensed to be unified and whole. You may also feel that your hands are floating within or merging with this unified field. You have to be patient and not follow or engage the conditioned patterns present until this shift in orientation manifests. The inhalation and exhalation phases of primary respiration may then clarify, and this is really the starting point for session work.

You may have already noticed that when you first contact a person's system, one of the things that is communicated is the history and patterning present.

You might sense various strain patterns, compressions, conditioned patterns of motion, etc. Alternatively you may sense a system-wide stasis that seems to dampen down any motion. These are conditional patterns of compensation organized by the deeper forces at work within the system. Initially, these patterns and states may be more obvious than the inhalation and exhalation phases of primary respiration. Sometimes a huge amount of history may be communicated to you in a relatively short time. It is important here to remain receptive and not follow any of this. Just let it be and simply orient to the inhalation and exhalation phases of primary respiration. After a while, perhaps after ten minutes or so of listening, you may notice a settling and a sense that the system is expressing its wholeness.

In the past I have encouraged students to wait for this sense of unity and wholeness, but I did not give it a specific name. Becker oriented practitioners to "something happens." Jealous calls this state the "patient's neutral."[5] I have been simply calling it a *holistic shift.*"

The holistic shift and the state of balance are not the same. The state of balance is a systemic neutral, a dynamic equilibrium, oriented to a *particular* inertial fulcrum, while the holistic shift is a literal shift in orientation from conditions and patterning to resources and Health.

When students have enough awareness of anatomy, primary respiration, and conditioned patterns, we have them orient to this holistic state as a starting point for healing processes. We usually introduce this concept in the second half of our training program. This is the beginning of a step-by-step palpation journey into the Inherent Treatment Plan and is taught along with all of the structural and tissue relationships outlined in this volume.

Sometimes a patient does not seem to be able to express this kind of holistic shift. I have found that this is generally due to high levels of inertia and to processes of shock and dissociation within the system.[6] It is here that trauma skills may be essential and the processing of autonomic nervous system cycling is critical. Dissociation is an expression of a real mind-body split and is a protective process. Please remember when working with dissociation that these patients are protecting themselves from very difficult sensations and feelings. In that context, dissociation must be honored and carefully worked with. It is very useful to initiate a verbal, felt-sense inquiry into the nature of the dissociative process. Within the cranial context, gentle EV4s can aid the reassociative process. This may be the main focus for a number of sessions. Once there is a shift back to embodiment, then you will find that holistic neutrals as described above naturally arise.

Likewise, when first palpating the patient's system you may sense a depth of inertia and stagnation. Here again the holistic shift may be difficult to attain. Inherent resources may be difficult to orient to. Resourcing processes like stillpoints and CV4s, and encouraging a felt-sense of resourced feeling tones and sensations can be very helpful here. There may then be a shift to inherent resources and the Inherent Treatment Plan will then manifest.

THE HOLISTIC SHIFT AND THE INHERENT TREATMENT PLAN

The holistic shift heralds the unfolding of the Inherent Treatment Plan. As you contact the patient's system, simply orient to the inhalation and exhalation phases of primary respiration. Various patterns may be shown. Acknowledge these, but do not follow or engage them. Let them go. Simply orient to primary respiration. Over a period of time, usually around five to ten minutes, you will sense a shift within the system to wholeness, and primary respiration will commonly clarify. If this does not occur, then systemic processes like CV4 and EV4 will help.

Once a holistic shift is sensed, the practitioner again simply orients to the phases of primary respiration. It is important not to do anything here. Simply listen and see what unfolds. Tidal motions will be more obvious and the potency-fluid-tissue field will seem to be unified and whole. This heralds a shift in orientation, from the conditions and patterns present to primary respiration and its inherent potency and resources. Listen within this unified state. Note the quality of the unified field and listen in a receptive state.

With patience, the Inherent Treatment Plan will begin to unfold from this starting point. As this occurs, the system may orient to a specific fulcrum. You may sense a shift in potency within fluids and a distortion of the tissue field around a particular fulcrum. You may sense the three-phase process that Becker pointed to: (1) Seeking, (2) Settling and Stilling, and (3) Reorganization and Realignment. As the tissue motions generated by the inertial fulcrum still, you may still sense an underlying primary respiration. Orient to this and listen for the action of potency within the state of balance.

Other phenomena may also arise after a holistic shift is sensed. These concepts were introduced in Volume One. As the system deepens into a unified field, you may sense potency shifting through the fluids to particular areas within the system. Potency may shift to one area and then another. It is important as this occurs to maintain a wide perceptual field and to not crowd the system with your presence or interest. Session work then focuses on this shifting of the potency through the fluids and on the support you can give to the process.

Alternatively, once a holistic shift manifests, wider phenomena may enter your perceptual field. A wider and deeper shifting of potency may be sensed. As you widen your field of awareness, you may become aware of the wider ordering matrix and the Long Tide. Wind-like motions may be sensed around the body. Inertial fulcrums may be sensed as vortex-like forms within the biosphere. You may sense something coming into the patient's body from outside-in. A sense of a wind-like, almost electric quality of shifting may be sensed to occur within the body. This shifting may be sensed to move relatively quickly from one fulcrum to another. Related fulcrums may be processed in a precise order.

I first had this experience as patient. I was in the skilled hands of a colleague who works through Stillness. There was a very deep neutral accessed within my system. Within a depth of Stillness, "something" began to shift through my system. This was very different from what I had experienced before, the shifting of potency through the fluids. That kind of shifting occurs like a force within the fluids and is definitely integrated with tissue and form. This new kind of shifting had a wind-like quality to it. The nature of its shifting was more like air and fire. It seemed to come from outside the body and work very specifically and then leave. Becker notes that this is the nature of the action of the Long Tide as it expresses a healing intention within the system.[7]

Holistic States and Neutrals

The holistic shift

- A dramatic shift in orientation within the system from conditional forces and seeming fragmentation to wholeness. The unified nature of potency, fluids, and tissues is directly sensed. A real starting point for session work.

The point of balanced membranous tension

- A localized neutral accessed within the tension factors present in the tissues. The practitioner may be very active in obtaining this "precise neutral."

The state of balance

- A systemic neutral accessed within the whole field; a stillness and settling within the forces present that relate to specific inertial fulcrums and issues.

DYNAMIC STILLNESS

There is an even deeper starting point for session work. This occurs when the practitioner holds a wide and still perceptual field, orients to space and spaciousness, and enters a deep stillness within their own inner processes. With patience, a stillness will come to the forefront. Becker called it a *dynamic and alive stillness*. It is not a localized phenomenon, but is sensed within and around both practitioner and patient and beyond. This Dynamic Stillness is an even deeper starting point for session work. Intentions seem to come into play from deep origins as an interchange takes place between Stillness and form. It may seem as though Health unfolds within a Stillness that seems to permeate everything. Its precision is directly experienced. Here any thoughts, intentions, or needs of the practitioner will get in the way of the process. The practitioner's thoughts may even be experienced as an inertial force to be centered.

Becker wrote a wonderful letter to Anne Wales, D.O., entitled, "Using the Stillness."[8] Please read it, for it is beautiful and directly points to awareness of Stillness and rhythmic interchange. He talks about a direct perception of an interchange between Stillness and the conditions present within the body-mind. He called it "rhythmic balanced interchange." Stillness is seen to be the ground of emergence and direct support of all form. Healing processes at this level are perceived to be based upon an interchange between the Dynamic Stillness and form. The inertial forces present are perceived to dissipate into the Stillness as more energy rhythmically manifests from it. In other words, form and energy return to the Stillness from which they originally arose. This rich and dynamic process unfolds itself to our perception within Stillness. It is this Stillness that supports the lives of both patient and practitioner. As we have seen, the more you listen to the human system within a still and wide field of awareness, the more you sense unanticipated phenomena and are touched by the mystery of life. Space and Stillness begin to come to the foreground. Enfolded and ordered within space are the infinite interchanging patterns of life. These patterns are in constant motion.[9] As you palpate a patient's system, rhythmic balanced interchange begins to clarify within the greater space that is Stillness.

I feel that this level of work becomes available and its precision clear only if you can also negotiate the levels of work discussed in these volumes. In other words, you have to know the human system as best as you can. You need to know anatomy and physiology; you need to be able to relate to individual tissue structures and their motions. You have to be able to recognize compressions and inertial fulcrums. Then you have to let it all go. It all goes behind the curtain! This is the challenging part for many of us. Within the ambience of unknowing, as we let go of what we know and of the need to do anything, the stillness of our listening allows us to open to the potential of the present moment.

LEVELS OF NEGOTIATION

As our work matures, we begin to appreciate the subtleties of our contact with a patient's system. This gives rise to a deepening sense of the negotiation process. At any level of contact with a patient's system, a negotiation process ensues in which the practitioner must learn to contact that patient's system without enlisting its defensive processes. If the system experiences you as an intruding force, then its potency will act to manage your presence in some way. As this occurs, you may sense lateral fluctuations and expressions of potency that may, at first, seem to be expressions of the inherent patterns within that person's system. What you are actually sensing is the system's response to your presence. If you follow these patterns and assume that they are intrinsic to the patient's system, you will end up chasing shadows. This does not help the patient and may even activate symptoms needlessly.

As this understanding dawns upon the practitioner, a growing appreciation of the negotiation process arises. At first this may be most clearly sensed in relationship to the tissues. If you physically or mentally grab onto tissue structures, or generate too strong a contact, or force your work upon the system, a growing sense of futility arises. The tissues may lock up against your contact and work may become more and more forceful with less and less clear results. Alternatively, the patient's system may lead you on a merry chase. Symptoms may activate and may move around the patient's system. You may encourage the activation of symptoms and emotions without appreciating the possibility of re-traumatization. You may find yourself going around in circles that do no one any good. However, a growing regard for the subtlety of physical contact should arise, and a clearer sense of negotiation with the tissue structures will ensue. Then, over time, this process clarifies in relationship to the fluids and to the potency that underlies the intrinsic motions within the system. An appreciation of intimacy and relationship continually deepens and the process of contact and negotiation becomes more clear and subtle.

Within the CRI level (tidal cycles of about 3–10 seconds), the negotiation of physical contact and management of emotional responses should clarify for the practitioner. As you interface with the results of suffering, a negotiation must occur with the nature of that suffering. A resonance with that person's suffering may ensue and the possibility of settling into the deeper tidal forces and rhythms may then occur. Basically, within a perception of the CRI, the practitioner must acknowledge and negotiate with the suffering that is expressed at that level of action. This does not mean that you engage it in any way. You simply witness and acknowledge its nature and help orient the system to its deeper resources.

Within the mid-tide (tidal cycles of about 20–25 seconds), a deepening of the negotiation process then takes place. The practitioner senses how the patient's potency responds to external forces, including the practitioner's touch or attention. Here it is not just a negotiation with tissues and tissue patterns. It is literally a negotiation with the potency that centers and organizes those tissues. It is not just about physical contact, but also the negotiation of your attention, intentions, and listening distance. If your attention moves too close, or if it is intrusive or invasive, a protective response will be elicited within the tidal potency. The potency will respond to your presence and will attempt to center your intrusion in some way. Again, this can be confusing both to the practitioner and to the patient. Safety and trust issues will be elicited and fluctuant phenomena will be generated in response to your presence.

Within the Long Tide a further deepening of the subtlety of negotiation may occur. Within this field of awareness, we may have the direct experience that we are not separate. All of life's processes are whole and totally interconnected in a vast matrix of relationship. Within the Long Tide level of perception, boundaries are subtly softened and the co-arising nature of all of life may be sensed. *My* primary respiration is not separate from *yours*; my organizing field is not separate from yours. We are mutually arising fields of creativity, not separate from the vastness we co-inhabit. The neat boundaries of subject and object break down as mutuality is more directly experienced. Here the subtlety of any response on the practitioner's part may generate a protective intention within the matrix centering the whole process. An intrusive thought or a grasping intention on any level may be sensed within the matrix as an intrusion, and a field-level protective response may be elicited. Within this realm of practice, the practitioner learns to trust the intentions of the Breath of Life and healing occurs via a mutuality of presence, appropriate and congruent intimacy, and a deep resonance with the unfolding process. The more I practice, the clearer it becomes that healing occurs in Stillness, not in motion. Stone used to say that healing occurs at the neutral of the conditions present, not at the poles of its expression. The healing process really begins when all tensions are reconciled around a neutral.

ORIENTATION TO THE INHERENT TREATMENT PLAN

In this section, I would like to briefly review some themes discussed at the end of Volume One. In an open clinical setting the intention is to be receptive and to wait for the Inherent Treatment Plan to unfold. If it cannot engage, it is usually because some systemic process, like fluid inertia, shock states, or dissociation may be present. We would then orient to processes such as stillpoints, CV4, and EV4 as appropriate. Once a holistic shift can occur, then it is a matter of waiting for the priorities of the Breath of Life to come to the forefront. We might listen for an expression of potency in some form, for a particular inertial fulcrum to be highlighted, or for a healing process of some kind to initiate. For instance, we may sense a shifting of potency within the fluids or the field around a patient, or we may have a sense that the whole tensile fluid-tissue field distorts around a particular fulcrum. If a state of balance cannot be attained in relationship to a particular fulcrum, or if it lacks depth, then various clinical conversations such as disengagement or fluid skills can be initiated. These are ways to engage the system in a process of inquiry. Once a state of balance is attained, then it is a question of entering into deeper and deeper states of stillness and dynamic equilibrium. The following is a chart I use near the end of foundation trainings. It may be a useful orienting form as we begin this volume and its exploration of specific structural and functional issues (Fig. 1.1).

1. Rollin Becker, *The Stillness of Life* (Stillness Press, 2000).
2. Ibid., 240.
3. See Harold Magoun, D.O., *Osteopathy in the Cranial Field* (The Journal Printing Company, 1951).
4. A lecture recorded by Ken Graham, D.O., Tulsa OK, March 1988.
5. James Jealous, *The Biomechanics of Osteopathy: The Patient's Neutral,* 2000. For copies, contact Tari Sargent, 196 Weeks Mills Road, Farmington, Maine 04938.
6. Ibid.
7. Rollin Becker, *Life In Motion* (Rudra Press, 1997).
8. Becker, *Stillness,* p. 66.
9. Ibid., 186–187.

*wait for priorities of the Breath of Life

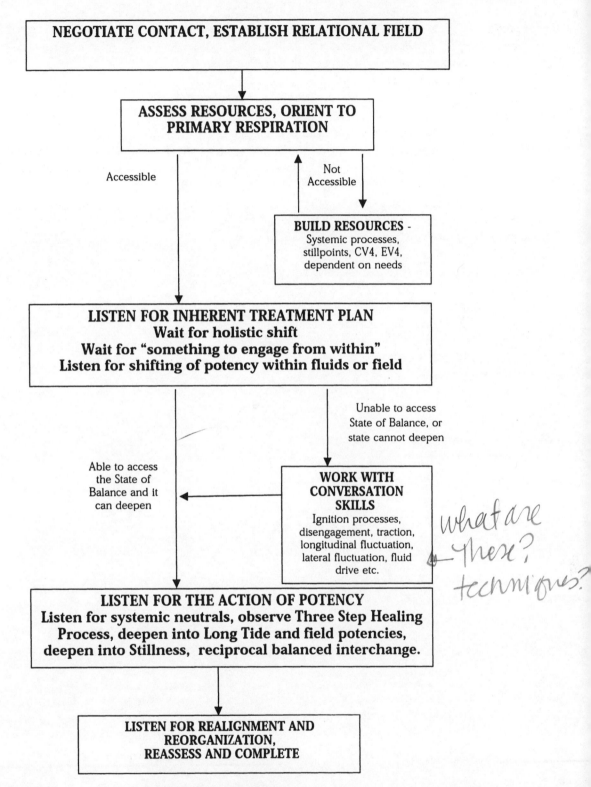

NEGOTIATE CONTACT, ESTABLISH RELATIONAL FIELD

ASSESS RESOURCES, ORIENT TO PRIMARY RESPIRATION

Accessible

Not Accessible

BUILD RESOURCES -
Systemic processes, stillpoints, CV4, EV4, dependent on needs

LISTEN FOR INHERENT TREATMENT PLAN
Wait for holistic shift
Wait for "something to engage from within"
Listen for shifting of potency within fluids or field

Unable to access State of Balance, or state cannot deepen

Able to access the State of Balance and it can deepen

WORK WITH CONVERSATION SKILLS
Ignition processes, disengagement, traction, longitudinal fluctuation, lateral fluctuation, fluid drive etc.

what are these? techniques?

LISTEN FOR THE ACTION OF POTENCY
Listen for systemic neutrals, observe Three Step Healing Process, deepen into Long Tide and field potencies, deepen into Stillness, reciprocal balanced interchange.

LISTEN FOR REALIGNMENT AND REORGANIZATION, REASSESS AND COMPLETE

1.1 Treatment Orientation

2 Formative Forces and Midlines

In this chapter we will develop important concepts about formative forces and the midlines they generate, with a practical focus on the *primal midline*. The primal midline is the ordering axis for embryological development, and an appreciation of its expression yields a wealth of clinical information. The ability to perceive midline phenomena is a key clinical skill and allows for a more precise understanding of structural relationships and of processes of healing and reorganization. Midline phenomena include *suspended automatically shifting fulcrums* and the energetic midlines from which they are derived. As discussed in Volume One, when inertial issues are resolved, potencies, fluids, and tissues naturally realign and reorient to the midline functions of the body.

In this chapter we will:

- *Discuss formative forces and midline phenomena.*
- *Further discuss the primal and dorsal midlines.*
- *Explore some perceptual and clinical exercises related to its expression.*
- *Review suspended automatically shifting fulcrums.*

FORMATIVE FORCES

The universe is whole, and we human beings are not separate from that wholeness. As seen in the work of physicist David Bohm, the universe is considered to be a holographic unity. It is whole, and all of its parts reflect this whole. Within this understanding, all forms generated within the universe are considered to be local phenomena within huge fields of action. Thus, the formation of a galaxy is not separate from the universe in which it is formed. Likewise, the formation of the human system is not separate from the universe within which it is created. Forms within the universe, whether galaxies, human beings or trees, are generated as an expression of vast forces at work within a holistic framework. Separateness, fragmentation, and disconnection are all illusions. As we have seen, no matter how seemingly fragmented the human system is, it is never un-whole. Wholeness is never lost, and the Health within the human system, which is a manifestation of this unity, is also never lost.

As we discussed in Volume One, Viktor Schauberger considered these formative forces to be an expression of an Original Motion.[1] This motion was considered by him to be the most formative, generative force found within the universe. In the cranial concept, we call this motion the *Long Tide*. Schauberger saw this force in action throughout the whole of the natural world. He wrote of vast spiraling forces that come into play during creation. This can be seen

health is a manifestation of wholeness.

13

in the generation of all forms within the world, and even within the creation of a galaxy. Vast spiraling forces come into play as a galaxy forms. Energy and matter seem to spiral in vast centripetal and centrifugal winds to generate its form. He likened this to the generation of a tornado in the atmosphere. In a similar way, Randolph Stone wrote of the formative centripetal and centrifugal forces that generate the human energy system, traditionally called the chakra system. Schauberger looked at creation as an on-going process. He considered all of life to be orchestrated by a Creative Intelligence at work within all processes: it can be called God, Dao, Brahma, or simply the Creative Intelligence. Within the cranial field we refer to the agent of this Intelligence as the *Breath of Life.*

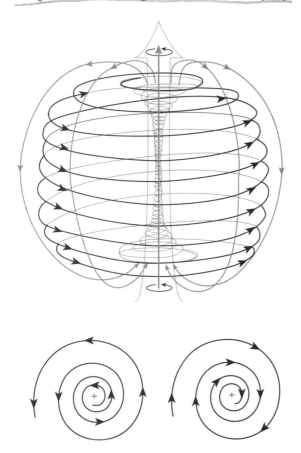

2.1 Schauberger conceived original motion to be an expression of dynamic equilibrium between centripetal and centrifugal forces

Great organizing winds, the formative forces of creation, are called into play via its action as form is generated and ordered (Fig. 2.1).

THE BREATH OF LIFE ORGANIZES FORM

The Breath of Life organizes form by enfolding and organizing space. It lays down organizing fulcrums and axes of orientation that organize cellular and tissue form and generate rhythmic motion. This can be seen in the developmental motions within the embryo and in the motion of potency, fluids, and tissues within the adult. I was struck by a recent theory in new physics called the *braneworld theory*.[2] "Brane" stands for "membrane." In this theory, space is conceived to be folded upon itself. The universe is conceived to be a membrane-like layer of enfolded space. Our familiar three-dimensional world is located within one such membrane. Other membranes, representing other universes, other dimensions, and even other realities, may be enfolded within our own space time. Three-dimensional space may be enfolded within six dimensional space and so on. Each dimension is like a membrane that is enfolded within the others. This harkens back to Bohm's holographic universe concept. The image of enfolded space struck me as confirming my perception of the action of the Breath of Life. Space is folded, and organizing fulcrums and axes are generated within the folds of space. Think of space as the medium within which form is organized. Think of natural fulcrums and midline axes as orienting forms within this media. It is to these reference points that all forms orient.

I recently came across a fascinating book, *When Time Breaks Down,* by Arthur Winfree.[3] I was especially impressed by some of his computer-generated images. Winfree, a medical science researcher, looked at organizing factors within chemical, biochemical, and bioelectrical phenomena. I was struck by the similarities between his research work, Mae Wan Ho's work, Schauberger's concepts, and Sutherland's perceptual understandings. Winfree states that chemical, biochemical, and bioelectrical phenomena seem to be organized around midlines and discrete *organizing centers* that move along them. He also called these *phase singularities,* moving points of stillness that organize rhythmic phases of electrochemical or bioelectric motion and order. These organizing centers, or fulcrums, have momentary existence and move in a pulsating fashion along the midline axis. In other words, they automatically shift along this axis. Wave forms, called scroll waves, are generated from the midline. These wave forms underpin the organization of the chemical reaction. Does this sound familiar? This has clear connections to the ideas of fulcrums, midline axes, longitudinal and transverse fluctuations of potency and tidal wave forms found in a craniosacral biodynamic understanding. A fulcrum is a localized state of stillness and power that organizes form and motion. Indeed, Winfree's term *organizing center* is a great name for a fulcrum!

Furthermore, these organizing centers are found to be three-dimensional, connected along vortex-like axes of orientation. Individual organizing centers are joined in a continuous axis around which form organizes. Again, this is a direct corollary to the concept of automatically shifting fulcrums and midline phenomena. The organizing centers, and the fields of action

they generate, have the vortex-like forms similar to those discussed by Schauberger when he spoke of the "Original Motion." The organization around the organizing axis and its phase singularities is seen to be that of a *torus* in shape. A torus is a hollow doughnut whose center acts as an organizing axis (Fig. 2.2).

The torus is essentially three-dimensional space enfolded into a stable form that is constantly being generated in the present in cycles of centrifugal expansion out from the core and centripetal contraction back in to the center. Again, as we have seen, the Breath of Life organizes form by organizing space! In figure 2.3, based on Winfree's book, you may actually get a sense of an enfolding process. Here the medium within which the chemical reaction is occurring literally becomes enfolded to organize the form of the chemical compound generated. It is like space is enfolded in order to generate form.

Some physicists claim that the torus is the shape of the universe, with the hole of the doughnut representing the organizing center that was established at the time of the "big bang." As previously discussed, the action of the Long Tide, and the organizing centers and axes it generates, gives rise to spiral motions

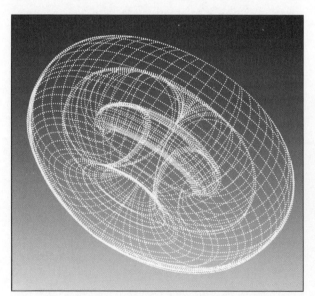

2.2 The torus in three-dimensional space, after Winfree's computer-generated model

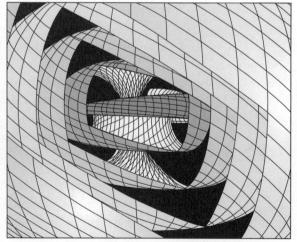

2.3 Space is enfolded in order to generate form, after Winfree

15

and torus-like organization. All of the rhythmic motions generated around phase singularities orient to the central axis. The spiral waveforms that organize around the organizing centers and their axes are called *scroll rings*. These form fields of action around the organizing axes. The field that organizes around an axis is not separate from the axis. Organizing centers, axes, and the forms generated around them are all one phenomenon. The vortex-like core is not separate from the resulting dynamic form. Likewise, within the cranial concept, the midline is not separate from the form organized around it (Fig. 2.4).

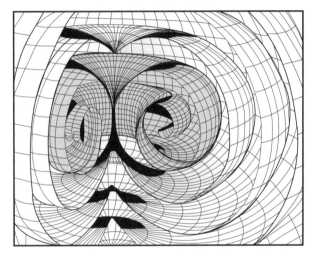

2.4   Wavefronts are generated and organized in relationship to phase singularities along the midline axis, after Winfree

Organizing forms like this have been found in chemical and biochemical reactions, in bioelectric processes, in the cardiac rhythm, and even within the spiral organization of DNA. This is also congruent with the findings discussed in Mae Wan Ho's book, *The Rainbow and the Worm, the Physics of Organisms.*[4] We discussed her work in some detail in Volume One. Ho describes discoveries from the field of biophysics. In studies on quantum effects in single cell and invertebrate animals, she found and demonstrated that these animals are organized within quantum-level fields of light with an orienting midline. Ho also describes how the fluids of the body, especially those within connective tissues, seem to be the media for

the transmission of quantum-level waveforms and information exchanges at near the speed of light.

Ho's references to quantum effects will become useful as our discussions progress. The word "quantum" refers to a subatomic-sized wave/particle that demonstrates behaviors vastly different from our conventional experience of the world as described by Newtonian physics. Quantum effects, or quantum physics, can be a useful metaphor, and possibly a solid explanation, of phenomena I have experienced in craniosacral biodynamics. Sutherland, when questioned as to what his work was about, was reported to have replied, "Study quantum mechanics!" and Becker called his palpation contact, "quantum touch."[5] Stone also suggested (in 1948) that future studies in atomic physics would confirm and explain his energy principles.[6]

I think that Ho's explorations into the *light matrix,* and the liquid crystalline nature of the body, mirrors Sutherland's perception of liquid light. In single-celled and invertebrate animals, these fields of light were found to respond to the environment before the fluids and tissues of the animal did. The quantum-level field response came first, then the physiology and form of the animal responded. Organizing centers, spiral forms, and axes of orientation are all part of the quantum field that seems to organize living systems. The understanding that organisms are organized within quantum fields of action has wide ranging implications for the healing professions. We are truly creatures of light![7]

In summary, as I wrote above, the Breath of Life organizes form by organizing space. It does this by laying down organizing centers and axes of orientation. As these arise, *space itself is enfolded* and physical form follows this template. The reason I am discussing this is to show that the concepts of organizing fulcrums and midline axes are not unique to my discussions of craniosacral biodynamics. It seems to be how form is universally organized, from the form and motion of a cell, to the spiraling, swirling dance of a galaxy. Fulcrums and orienting midlines, or axes, are a universal mechanism for the ordering of form, both within the human being, and for the universe as a whole.

THE ORGANIZING WINDS

From a craniosacral biodynamic viewpoint the Long Tide is considered to be the creative wind that generates form by generating field phenomena. It is the foundation of primary respiration within living beings. In my experience, these field phenomena have a very similar form to those described by Winfree, Schauberger, and Stone. The Long Tide is a slow, rhythmic, tide-like motion that seems to permeate everything. It is airy, yet potent. It is Schauberger's "Original Motion." He described this motion in terms of centripetal and centrifugal spiraling forces. A stable bioelectric field is generated when a dynamic equilibrium within these spiraling forces is attained. This bioelectric form can be considered to be a subtle quantum-level template for the human system that is made of light. Remember Sutherland's description of liquid light. This concept is not just a metaphor; it is based on direct perceptual experience. The Breath of Life generates this Original Motion—the Long Tide—and the Long Tide generates a stable bioelectric field. This field or matrix holds what Stone called the "pattern energy." It is a level of subtle energetic form that is the template for the unfoldment and organization of the human system.

This is not an arbitrary or mechanical energy. It is a play of consciousness and a function of the Creative Intelligence that imbues all of creation. Thus, the Breath of Life can be considered to be a manifestation of a divine intention to create. Like the Holy Spirit in Christianity, It connects and informs all beings and is the creative intention in action. The Breath of Life organizes space via the field phenomena described above. Organizing centers and axes are laid down within space. This is a local phenomenon within a huge field of action.

The Tibetans call the Long Tide, and its localized spiraling forces, the *Winds of the Vital Forces*. They consider these to be the unconditioned organizing forces that maintain the integrity and organization of human form. As we have seen, spiraling centrifugal and centripetal forces, generated by the "winds" of the Long Tide, coalesce into a localized stable bioelectric field of potency. This occurs via a dynamic

equilibrium within these seemi... This is similar to the concept o... nese medicine and philosophy, ... ity Therapy. This human bio... subsequently organized by the fulcrums and ... orientation found within it, the organizing centers and ... phase singularities described above. As the bioelectric field is generated, uprising forces are also generated within its core. Schauberger likened this to the uprising force generated within a tornado as its winds spiral inward. The midline generated becomes a manifest organizing axis for the generation of form within the embryo. The notochord and neural tube are formed in relationship to its action (Fig. 2.5).

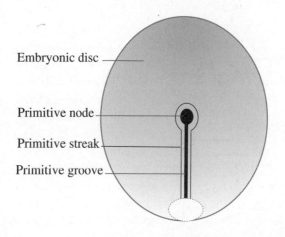

Embryonic disc

Primitive node

Primitive streak

Primitive groove

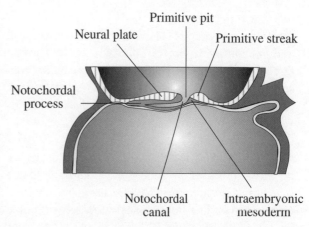

Primitive pit

Neural plate

Primitive streak

Notochordal process

Notochordal canal

Intraembryonic mesoderm

2.5 Primitive streak and notochord

Sutherland also spoke of spiraling forces within the human system. He likened the motion of the potency within the fluids to the action of spirals within spirals. He noted the spiraling action of the Tide and the Stillness at the heart of this action. It is fascinating how the spiral form is found everywhere in nature. At the heart of the cell nucleus, our DNA is expressed as a triple helical spiral form. The proteins that make up collagen fibers are also triple helical structures. The organization of life, even at this molecular level, is based on the spiral. It seems that life is an expression of spirals within spirals, all in constant change and constant formation.

H₂O witching idea! (handwritten)

MIDLINE DESCRIPTIONS FROM EASTERN TRADITIONS

The concept of a human energy field, and a midline-orienting axis within it, has roots in traditional medical systems such as the Chinese, Tibetan, and Indian systems. Oriental medicine sees the organization of the human body-mind to be based on these principles of energy. The foundation of tissue function, and of health and disease, is seen to be based on interactions that occur within an embodied energy field.

In the Chinese tradition the balance of *chi,* and of other energy factors such as *jing,* are used both diagnostically and in treatment processes. *Jing* is a subtle form of life force that is found within the fluids of the system. It is sometimes called "essence." It is especially active within cerebrospinal and generative fluids. Its function is to generate motive force within the system and to maintain its organization as a whole. This is a direct corollary to the "potency within the fluids" concept in craniosacral biodynamics. Chinese philosophy calls the energy midline the *central channel* and its vortices, or organizing centers, are called *Dan Tian.* In the Chinese system, this midline is located just anterior to the vertebral column from the center of the perineal floor to the vertex of the cranium. It is one of the esoteric channels of Chinese medicine. It is basically a straight line from an energy center within the third ventricle, the upper Dan Tian, to the coccyx. *Shen,*

which can be likened to consciousness and spirit, is said to reside within upper Dan Tian.

Similarly, in the Indian and Tibetan systems, the body's organization is seen to be based on an energy matrix called the chakra system. This is seen to be organized around a midline function called *sushumna* and around vortices that function as energy fulcrums called chakras. As in the Chinese system, *sushumna* also descends from the third ventricle as a straight line in front of the vertebral column to the coccyx. In the yogic system, *sushumna* is likened to a shaft of pure and intense light. Randolph Stone called it the *ultra-sonic core.*[8] The chakras found along its axis can be thought of as organizing fulcrums, pulsating vortices that organize form, function and motility. It is possible to learn to synchronize your perceptual field with these light-energy forms (Fig. 2.6).

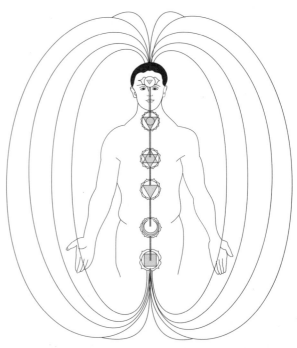

2.6 The yogic quantum midline with phase singularities called chakras

The chakra system is said to ignite within the conceptus at the time of conception. Stone discussed this

✓chakra

and worked with ignition processes in his Polarity Therapy. A primal fulcrum or chakra called the *ajana chakra* is laid down within the fertilized ovum. This is located in the third ventricle of the fully formed individual. From this organizing center, *sushumna* descends, and the rest of the chakra system forms from the "bottom up." This quantum shaft of Intelligence remains a straight and true orienting axis throughout life, forever orienting our system to its source. In the yogic system, elemental forces known as ether, air, fire, water, and earth are seen to be generated from this core. It is along this axis that potency, or *prana* in Eastern terminology, ignites within the fluids of the embryo and the cerebrospinal fluid of the fully formed infant. I will refer to this formative midline as the *quantum midline* or *central channel*.

Think of the human ordering field as a matrix of light with an orienting shaft of light in its center. As seen in Ho's studies with single cell and invertebrate animals, all animals researched were organized within a quantum-level bioelectric field. She also noted that within this field, there is a quantum midline around which the organisms are polarized from anterior to posterior. So the reality of an energetic organizing midline, a shaft of light, is being discovered in purely scientific circles. It represents the orienting core of a human being. This core maintains and expresses the wholeness of the reference beam of the human hologram. In craniosacral biodynamics, it is the Long Tide that is considered to be the organizing wind which generates this matrix of light with its quantum midline. When they perceive the action of the Long Tide, practitioners and patients alike commonly talk about experiences of radiance and light.

Within the embryo, as the Long Tide generates the ordering matrix with its quantum midline, an *anterior notochord midline* and a *posterior fluid midline* within the neural tube are also generated. The notochord midline becomes the orienting axis for the development of form and the motility of tissues, while the posterior midline becomes the orienting axis for the fluid field and fluid fluctuation. I call the anterior midline the *primal midline* and the posterior midline *the fluid midline*.

In the fully-formed body, the primal midline is expressed as an uprising force within the centers of the vertebral bodies and the midline of the cranial base. This is the same uprising midline described by Schauberger and others. The fluid midline is located within the neural tube of the embryo. In the adult it is found in the central canal of the spinal cord and the ventricle system of the brain.

THE MIDLINES AND EMBRYOLOGICAL FORMATION

The primal midline is the major axis for the development and organization of form within the embryo. It is expressed as an uprising force within the midline of the embryonic disc. The primitive streak and notochord form within the embryonic disc as a response to its action. When clinicians perceive the primal midline, they are in direct relationship to a fundamental embryological principle that constantly organizes the human form. Clinical work oriented to embryological forces helps realign structure and function to these most basic ordering energies.

As the notochord forms, ectoderm cells follow. The embryonic disc thickens in the midline and the neural groove and neural plate begin to form dorsal to the notochord. This process of formation is essentially about the organization of *space*. The Breath of Life functions to enfold and organize space, and form follows. The neural tube organizes around the space generated by the intentions of the Breath of Life. Cellular form flows into the space generated and organized by its potency. As differentiation continues, cell growth is uneven and the neural plate folds to form the neural tube (Fig. 2.7). The neural tube is the primitive nervous system. Within its spaces, a second midline is generated. This *fluid midline* becomes the organizing midline for the expression of potency within the cerebrospinal fluid. From this midline, the intentions of the Breath of Life clearly manifest as an organizing potency within the fluids. Cerebrospinal fluid is considered to be the initial physiological recipient of the Breath of Life. This is an intelligent biodynamic force that generates the fluid tide and orders the structure

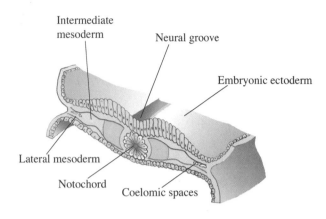

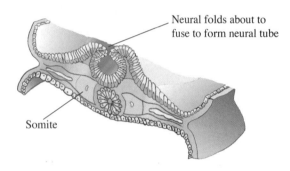

2.7 The Neural Tube at about 18 days (above)
and 20 days (below)

and organization of cells and tissues.

Thus, there are two important midlines around which the cellular and fluid worlds naturally organize: the ventral, *primal midline* around which the cellular and tissue world will organize and the dorsal, *fluid midline* around which the cerebrospinal fluid tide is organized (Fig. 2.8). The fluid midline is not separate from the primal midline. It is a derivative of its organizing function. Fluids, cells, and tissues will naturally orient to the primal midline as the definitive organizing axis of the physical body. Both of these midlines, in turn, orient to the quantum midline described above.

We are creatures of light and are constantly oriented to the light, whether we perceive it or not. The

Breath of Life is the motivating and organizing principle of the human body. Its currency is space, light, and radiance, and all manifest things orient to its creative intentions. The potency it generates organizes the fluid and tissue world and is its driving force. All fluid and tissue motility is an expression of its action. All fluid and tissue organization must always refer back to the midlines as the main organizing axes for structure and function. These midlines are like the reference beam of a hologram.

Awareness of the midlines enables practitioners to establish clear clinical baselines founded on a perceptual relationship with the health of the system. In session work, awareness of these midlines greatly clarifies session work and helps practitioners sense how a system is healing itself. When inertial issues are resolved, the tissues and fluids of the system naturally reorient to these midlines. An awareness of midlines gives the practitioner a clear sense of this reorganization and realignment process.

THE PRIMAL MIDLINE

As we have discussed above, the primal midline is the embryological organizing axis for the generation and coherency of form. Schauberger likens the formation of this midline to the vast vortex-like uprising force generated within the center of a tornado. Like a great wave, it moves through the centerline of the embryonic disc. The primal midline becomes the organizing midline around which structure and function develop. The primitive streak and notochord develop in relationship to this midline (see Fig. 2.5). The bodies of the vertebra form around the notochord, and the nucleus of its intervertebral discs are directly derived from it. The primal midline manifests within the center of the vertebral bodies and cranial base. The cellular and tissue world naturally orient to this midline function from the moment of conception to the day we die.

Stone called the action of the primal midline, the "fountain spray of life."[11] It can be perceived to arise from the coccyx, ascend through the center of the vertebral bodies, follow the cranial base through the body of the sphenoid, and manifest as the fountain spray of life at the ethmoid bone. In *The Wireless Anatomy of Man,* Stone writes,

> The centerline through the body is the location of the path of the ultra-sonic energy substance as the primary life current and core of being. . . . It is the primary energy that builds and sustains all others. It flows through the sixth ventricle of the brain and spinal cord when these are formed out of its mind pattern energy field.[11] It becomes the primitive streak and the notochord in the embryo. . . . This core is the center of attraction and emanation of all currents from the brain to the extremities. It is the internal gravity of the individual . . . distinct from the gravity of the earth.[11]

In referring to the "center line through the body" Stone is pointing us towards the quantum midline

within the ordering matrix. It is the "ultra-sonic" core, a core of high vibrational quality that is the "primary life current of being." The other midlines are derived from it. It generates the notochord and expresses its potency within the fluids of the ventricles. Stone considered the quantum midline to have a primary orienting and ordering function within the human system. It is an expression of a primary energy that builds and sustains all other energies and forms within the human system. It is expressed as a pattern energy field that organizes the form and function of the human body-mind. Here we are talking about field phenomenon, the province of the Long Tide. The organizing field of the human system is an expression of the play of Intelligence. It is not an accident, it is not an artifact; it is an expression of an intentional act of conscious creation. Stone maintained that it is the mind pattern energy field, a field of intentional

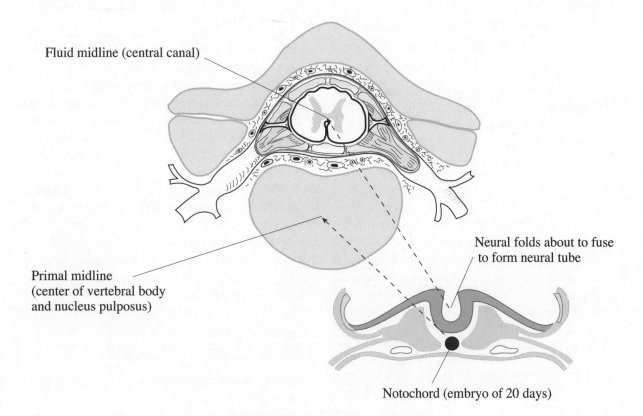

Fluid midline (central canal)

Primal midline
(center of vertebral body
and nucleus pulposus)

Neural folds about to fuse
to form neural tube

Notochord (embryo of 20 days)

2.8 The primal and the fluid midlines

creation and organization, that orchestrates the formation of the spaces within which the central nervous system forms. The notochord, the central canal of the spinal cord, and the ventricles of the brain are manifestations of this organizing process.[12]

This is so important to understand. We live within the midst of continual creation. Moment to moment we are engaged in the creative process. Embryological order is with us from the moment of conception until the day we die. Tuning into this depth of unfoldment is a truly humbling process. This points to a powerful shift in clinical understanding. The clinician can literally perceive these processes at work. When one initially experiences it, a great joy may arise, joy in the remembering of something never lost, but perhaps forgotten.

The Midlines:

- The *Long Tide* generates a quantum-level ordering matrix. This matrix is the blueprint for the form and organization of the human system.

- A *quantum midline,* or central channel, is generated within this matrix. It can be perceived as a shaft of light within the center of the body. It orients and aligns the being with the source of its creation. All other midlines, such as the primal and fluid midlines, are derived from its action.

- The *primal midline* is the axis around which structure and function orient. This axis can be palpated as a subtle midline arising force that seems to disappear at the ethmoid into the biosphere, or energetic field, around the person being palpated.

- The *fluid midline* is the organizing axis for the fluid tide and the motility of fluids in general. It is located within the neural tube of the embryo and the ventricle system of the fully formed person.

TUNING INTO THE MIDLINES

Practitioner awareness of these midlines has clear clinical value. As inertial fulcrums within the body are resolved, the cellular and tissue world will naturally reorient to midline functions. Furthermore, the practitioner's awareness of midline phenomena can, through resonance, help the patient's system realign to its ordering matrix. As the cellular and tissue worlds reorient to midline phenomena, their *original intention* is remembered. Cells remember their original function and tissue structures and systems reorient to natural organizing centers and midline axes. Tuning into the midlines is also a useful way of accessing the healing priorities of the system. You may perceive the potency of the Breath of Life moving within the midline and then expressing itself within the body wherever it is appropriate. Awareness of midlines is one way of sensing the Inherent Treatment Plan as it unfolds in the human system.

In the next clinical application, you will tune into the primal midline. The intentions of the Breath of Life are expressed within this midline as a core organizing principle for form, structure, and motility. As you tune into its energy, you may sense an arising of an airy yet powerful potency. This awareness may lead you to particular inertial fulcrums and particular healing processes. It is also important to note that there may be so much inertia within a person's system that the midline phenomena may be obscured and not easily accessed by the practitioner. This is not uncommon. Remember this in the following exercise and do not be discouraged if the uprising force within the primal midline is not perceptible at first. Like the perception of the Long Tide, a clear manifestation of the midline can herald a deep healing process.

Clinical Application: Perceiving the Primal and Fluid Midlines

Tuning into the primal midline entails another shift in your perceptual field. The quality of experience as you perceive this midline is "airy" as opposed to "watery," as in the fluid tide. It is simply a matter of holding a wide perceptual field and listening to the midline within the vertebral bodies. Don't look for it, don't narrow your attention to it, simply listen.

As you tune into this midline, you may begin to sense an airy, yet powerful, rising of life force up the midline. Stone likened the quality of this midline to *air and fire*. This is the potency of the Breath of Life rising as a midline ordering principle. You may sense waves of this life force rising up the midline. You may be able to track its expression from the coccyx, through the spine, cranial base and ethmoid bone. You may sense the primal midline as though it is an empty air shaft in which hot air is always rising. As you catch the "air in the shaft," you may sense that you are carried upward as potency ascends within the midline. Hold all of this in a gentle awareness and don't try to sense anything. Don't look for anything. Simply place your attention in the midline and let it take you.

Once you perceive this, it is useful to sense the difference between the primal midline and the more dorsal fluid midline. After you have sensed the more anterior primal midline, both participants can shift their attention posterior to the fluid midline. Both participants place their awareness within the dural and neural tubes of the person being palpated. As practitioner, again hold a wide perceptual field. You may now come into relationship with the dorsal midline and the expression of the fluid tide. Notice how this feels different from the ventral midline. You may sense the more watery tidal motion of the fluid tide. This midline may be sensed to be more embodied, more suggestive of *water and earth*. This awareness will help you know which midline you are palpating in clinical practice. In this clinical application, you will be tuning into these phenomena via the sacrum.

Clinical Application: Sensing the Midlines

1. Place the patient in the supine position. Hold the sacrum in the sacral hold previously learned (Volume One). Use your caudad hand (the hand closest to the patient's feet) to do this. Establish your practitioner fulcrums and hold the bio-

sphere within your perceptual field. Settle into this first. Then slowly widen your perceptual field toward the horizon. Gently listen to wider and wider fields of action. Do not lose awareness of the person, their tissues, and a sense of their midline. Hold the sacrum spaciously. Do not mentally or physically grab onto it. Imagine that your hand is under the table giving the sacrum a lot of space. Even though there is weight on your hand, see if you can float on the tissues of the sacrum.

2. Maintaining a wide perceptual field, gently bring your attention to the primal midline. Orient yourself to the midline from the coccyx through the center of the vertebral bodies and cranial base. Do not narrow your perceptual field as you do this. Have patience; don't immediately try to sense anything. Still holding a wide perceptual field, simply become aware of the midline and let it come to you. This may take a number of minutes. Don't rush; see if you can let go of any anxiety about perceiving something. It will come to you eventually. You may sense the midline as an uprising force within the centerline of the vertebral bodies. I have heard practitioners describe it as a wind within the midline, as a geyser, and even as a volcano. It may be sensed as airy, yet powerful, sometimes like a gentle breeze, other times more like a tornado. You may sense it as a hot air shaft where the air is always ascending. As you catch this with your awareness, it is like hitching a ride on this air stream. It seems to arise at the coccyx and disappear into space at the ethmoid bone. The structural axis of the body, from the coccyx, through the vertebrae and cranial base, form in relationship to it. Structure and function coalesce in relationship to it.

3. Once you have a sense of the primal midline, shift your awareness to the more dorsal, fluid midline. Within a wide perceptual field, simply orient to the neural tube and the cerebrospinal fluid. Let the fluids come into your field of awareness. Again, see if the fluid tide comes into

your awareness. The fluid tide has a more embodied feel to it, more like water and earth, instead of air and fire. It will also express itself within the 2.5 cycles per minute phases of the mid-tide.

4. There is another simple perceptual exercise that seems to help people orient to the primal midline and its uprising force. Again palpate the patient's sacrum as described earlier. Establish a very wide perceptual field. Let your field of awareness extend toward the horizon. Do not lose orientation as you do this. Maintain your fulcrums and do not go into dissociation. Extend your perceptual field to where it is comfortable. See if the Long Tide and its deeper, slower rhythm come into awareness. See if its organizing winds clarify. You may simply sense this as a radiance. Then, very, very slowly and gently narrow your perceptual field toward the biosphere. As you do this, you may "catch" the Long Tide as it enters the biosphere and be literally taken up the midline, almost as if you are riding on a great wind.

Clinical Application: Sacral-Ethmoid Hold

The contact for this application is derived from the work of Randolph Stone. Stone was very attuned to the energy dynamics within a human being and emphasized the importance of midline phenomena. The intention of the following contact is to help you tune into the midline and to help a patient's system reorient to it as an ordering principle. Many times, if resources are available in a patient, simply tuning into the primal midline can reorient the system to it and initiate healing processes. Its use is also helpful at the end of sessions to help integrate and complete session work.

1. Place the patient on their left side, with their knees slightly bent. You might place pillows under the head and also between their knees for comfort. Sit facing their back. Place your right hand over their sacrum with your fingers pointing cau-

dad. Your middle finger is placed over the coccyx. Having established that contact, place your other hand over their ethmoid bone. To do this, bring your other hand over the top of their head, and gently, with negotiation, place your index and middle fingers over the center of their forehead to the bridge of their nose. Your wrist and lower arm gently wrap around the top of the head without actually touching. Establish an elbow support for this contact. Some practitioners prefer to have their index and middle fingers in a "V" shape straddling the ethmoid area (Fig. 2.9).

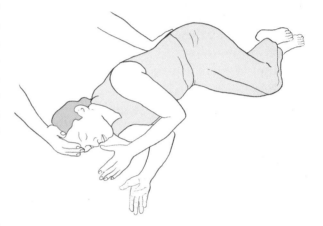

2.9 Sacral-ethmoid hold

2. In this position, first orient to their biosphere and then to the primal midline within the biosphere. Settle into a receptive state and slowly widen your perceptual field towards the horizon to a distance that is comfortable. Do not lose a sense of the patient's midline as you gently do this. Now simply rest in your listening and see if a sense of the primal midline clarifies for you. See where this awareness takes your session work.

Suspended Automatically Shifting Fulcrums

Next, let's review the concept of suspended automatically shifting fulcrums in light of the midline discussion. These fulcrums organize the motion and action of the tensile fields of the body. They are oriented to the midlines discussed above. Within the midtide, tissues can be perceived to be a unified tensile field of action. We saw (in Volume One) that the inherent motion of the tissue field as a whole was organized around automatically shifting fulcrums such as Sutherland's fulcrum at the junction of the falx and tentorium. Automatically shifting fulcrums are suspended within their fields of action and are free to move. In their most formative nature, they are points of condensed potency within the ordering matrix laid down by the action of the Long Tide. These fulcrums, like the midline, are also part of the wider bioelectric field. Automatically shifting fulcrums move along the midline with the inhalation-exhalation cycles of the Tide.

Imagine a unified field of potency. Imagine that within this field a condensation of potency forms along its midline. This site of condensed potency is not separate from the field. As this site of condensation arises, the whole field is pulled toward it and tensile patterns are generated. Imagine that this site of condensation is a still place within this field. Imagine that, as the Tide expresses respiratory cycles of inhalation and exhalation, this still center shifts along the midline. As this occurs, the whole field shifts with it (Fig. 2.10). Fulcrums, as we have seen in Winfree's terms, are organizing centers around which form and motion are organized. Winfree has also noted that these natural fulcrums shift along the midline, and that the scroll waves generated orient to them.

So we see that the field organizes its motion relative to the fulcrums generated within it. If you look again at figures 2.2 and 2.3, based on the images from Winfree's book, you may perhaps see organizing centers and the midline they are part of. You may get the sense that somehow space is enfolded and form is generated. Within craniosacral biodynamics, this form is the human bioelectric ordering matrix. You may also see that this matrix is not separate from the wider space within which it organizes and that its organizing centers and midline are, in turn, not separate from the form of the matrix itself. Thus, suspended automatically shifting fulcrums are organized along midline axes and are not separate from each other or from the field within which they arise. They are unified in their nature, form, and function. In osteopathic language, they are a *unit of function*.

All of the inherent motions within the body, including potency, fluids, or tissues, are organized by suspended automatically shifting fulcrums. Each field of action has a natural fulcrum around which it is organized and by which it is moved. A fulcrum gives the whole field of action a focus that maintains order and coherent relationship. Fulcrums both organize the

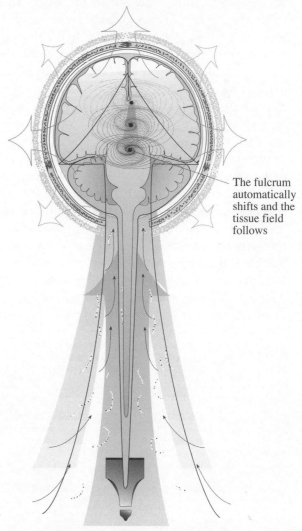

The fulcrum automatically shifts and the tissue field follows

2.10 Automatically shifting fulcrums

field and are the points around which it moves. Natural fulcrums are expressed embryologically and maintain order throughout life. All reciprocal tension motion is organized and generated by the action of these fulcrums. If fulcrums were not present, all would be chaos. They define the natural tensions and boundaries of every field of action.

To Follow

In the chapters that follow, an awareness of the midlines, and their related suspended automatically shifting fulcrums, will be integral to the work. This awareness will help to clarify clinical practice. In our previous exercises, we have listened to the fluctuation of cerebrospinal fluid within the dorsal midline and perceived the expression of potency within this midline. We explored an awareness of the more ventral midline, the primal midline. An awareness of midlines allows us to more clearly sense how the system is organized, its inertial issues, and how it has reorganized after processing inertial forces. The chapters in the rest of this volume are organized as an exploration of the midline from the "bottom up." We will first learn to relate to the *core link,* the dural tube, and then begin an exploration of the pelvis, the vertebrae, the occipital triad, the cranial base, and facial and TMJ dynamics, all in relationship to these midlines. We will be applying the clinical skills already developed to these relationships.

1. See Volume One, Chapter 5 for a discussion of the work of Viktor Schauberger. See *Living Energies* by Callum Coates (Gateway Press, 1996).

2. Alison Boyle, "The Edge of Infinity," New Scientist 29 (September, 2001).

3. Arthur Winfree, *When Time Breaks Down: The Three-Dimensional Dynamics of Electrochemical Waves and Cardiac Arrhythmias* (Princeton University Press, 1987). Figures 2.1, 2.2, and 2.3 are based on images from this book and redrawn by Dominique Degranges.

4. Mae-Wan Ho, *The Rainbow and the Worm: The Physics of Organisms* (World Scientific Publishing Co., 1993). See Volume One for a more detailed discussion of some of the concepts in this book.

5. Becker, *Stillness.*

6. Randolph Stone, *Polarity Therapy* (CRCS Publications, 1986).

7. Ho, op. cit., Vol. I.

8. Stone, op. cit., Vol. I, Book II, p.10.

9. Randolph Stone, *Polarity Therapy Volume One, Book Two, The Wireless Anatomy of Man* (CRCS Press, 1986, 1987).

10. The "sixth ventricle" of the brain and spinal cord can be thought of as the "space" created by the *primary life current,* the *primal space* which form manifests and coalesces around. The ventricles of the brain and spinal cord can also be counted as six: the two lateral ventricles, the third ventricle, the aqueduct of Sylvius, the fourth ventricle, and the central canal of the spinal cord.

11. Stone, op. cit., Vol. I, Book II.

12. Randolph Stone, *Polarity Therapy Volume One, Book One; Volume Two, Book Five* (CRCS Press, 1986, 1987).

3

The Motility Of The Central Nervous System

In this chapter, we will begin to explore one of the traditional aspects of the Primary Respiratory Mechanism, the motility of the central nervous system. In previous explorations (in Volume One), we have become familiar with the motility and motion dynamics of the bones, membranes, and fluids that surround, support and bathe the central nervous system. All tissues and cells of the human body express motility within the inhalation and exhalation cycles of primary respiration. The cranial bowl with its bones, membranes, and fluids is moving along with its contents, the central nervous system. As the bones, membranes, and fluids express motility and motion, so does the brain and central nervous system as a whole. The human system expresses a totally integrated dynamic, and every part is in relationship to all other parts. It is a holographic, nonlinear system. The body is never fragmented. Its unity may be obscured, but this wholeness is inherent within each and every moment.

In this chapter we will:
- *Describe the motility and motion of the CNS.*
- *Take the "Tour of the Minnow."*
- *Explore CNS motility through palpation.*
- *Explore inertial fulcrums within CNS dynamics.*
- *Explore ignition processes.*

An understanding and perceptual awareness of the dynamics of the central nervous system (CNS) is absolutely necessary in craniosacral biodynamics. The ability to perceive CNS motility has huge clinical value for both diagnosis and treatment. The inertial patterns found within the central nervous system have a direct relationship to the dynamics of cranial bones, the reciprocal tension membrane, fluid dynamics and vertebral relationships. Similarly, membranous-articular strains, inertial issues within cranial bones, and any inertial issue involving the vertebral axis of the body, including the pelvis, will directly affect the motility of the central nervous system. The dynamics of the motility of the central nervous system can have a direct effect on the physiological functioning of any system, any organ and any tissue in the human body.

CEREBROSPINAL FLUID FLOW

Let's now look at how cerebrospinal fluid (CSF) flows around the ventricular system. I recently saw an impressive time-lapse magnetic resonance imaging (MRI) technique that showed the flow of cerebrospinal fluid around the ventricular system in a variety of subjects. The majority of cerebrospinal fluid is produced in the lateral ventricles. These large ventricles are lined with choroid plexus tissue that continually filters blood plasma to produce cerebrospinal fluid. Choroid plexus tissue is also located at the top of the third ventricle and within the fourth ventricle. The cerebrospinal fluid circulates from the lateral ventricles through the Foramen of Monro, into the third ventricle. The newly formed cerebrospinal fluid is literally dumped into the anterior-superior aspect of the third ventricle from both lateral ventricles. Here it expresses a circulation around the third ventricle that moves with a clockwise motion when viewed from the right side of the head. It thus circulates from the Foramen of Monro inferiorly to the floor of the third ventricle, then posteriorly and superiorly up the rear aspect of the ventricle and then anteriorly and inferiorly down its front aspect. This circular motion can be palpated via the *vault hold* as we bring our attention into this area.

From the third ventricle, the cerebrospinal fluid flows inferiorly through the Aqueduct of Sylvius. This aqueduct is sometimes narrowed due to birth trauma, such as the use of vacuum extraction during the birthing process, or other experiences. From here CSF flows into the fourth ventricle, a pyramid-shaped space. The cerebrospinal fluid is held up by the pyramidal shape, creating a turbulence. In the MRI video, this turbulence was quite dramatic. Sutherland notes that there is a radiance of potency from the fluids within the fourth ventricle.[1] The radiance literally bathes all of the nuclei in the brain stem. This may be an expression of a direct relationship between the potency within the fluids and the regulation of autonomic function. Perhaps this is one reason that the flow is held up here, to create a concentration and radiance of potency. Below the fourth ventricle the fluid descends inferiorly through the central canal of the spinal cord (Fig. 3.1).

From the fourth ventricle the cerebrospinal fluid enters the cisterna magna via its median and lateral foramina. The cisterna magna is the largest waterbed in the cranium. It is continually renewed and charged with potency. Stone noted that this waterbed energetically balanced the inferior waterbed below, the lumbosacral cistern. Ideally these two pools of potency, the cisterna magna above and the lumbosacral waterbed below, are in energetic balance in the human system. Stone likened this relationship to a balanced six-pointed star (Fig. 3.2).

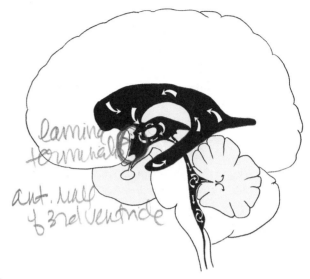

3.1   Flow of CFS within the ventricles

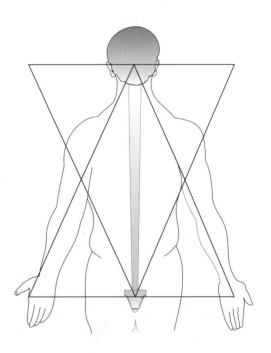

3.2   The balance of potency within the cisterna magna and lumbosacral cisterns

THE TOUR OF THE MINNOW

In his cranial courses, Sutherland would take students through what he called *The Tour of the Minnow*. This was a tour in imagination and inner sensing through the spaces around and within the brain. It was a visualization that he devised for his students to help them really sense the spaces and relationships of the brain from within. This tour gave students an opportunity to perceive within their own systems the radiance and mystery of the potency at work in the fluid spaces. It was a living tour through anatomy and the action of potency within the core of our body. During the tour, he commonly oriented students to the radiance of potency, or to the motion of structures, such as the rising and sinking of the SBJ. Two versions of the Tour have been transcribed in *Teachings in the Science of Osteopathy*.[2]

The bottom line here is that you need to know your anatomy. Look through an atlas to refresh your memory of the parts and spaces of the brain. Very good videos and CD-ROMs of the anatomy of the brain are now available. This tour will enable you to be in a clearer relationship to your patient's central nervous system, to the potency that moves it, and to the radiance within it. It will also orient you to the anatomy of the brain and thus positively influence your ability to help in the resolution of its inertial issues.

In the following, we will use a shortened form of this tour and will *swim* through the spaces of the ventricles. In his tour, Sutherland asked his students to be aware of both the anatomical and energetic aspects of the system. He talked about the Breath of Life, its healing potency, and its expression as liquid light in the same breath as the detailed anatomy of the central nervous system. These perceptual experiences are not separate, but all are an expression of the true unity of the human system. It is literally a breathtaking tour! You might want to speak this version of the tour, or one from Sutherland's book, into a recorder and then follow it as you play it back. Remember to review your anatomy first!

- First of all get into a comfortable sitting or lying position and take a few deep breaths. We are about to go on an inner tour where your imagination will swim inside the ventricle spaces within your brain. Sutherland asked people to imagine that they were a little minnow (a very small fish). This minnow had mysterious properties. It could get very small and squeeze into the smallest of places and it could radiate light so that you could see the nearby structures more clearly. Use whatever image helps you most. You may simply want to let your awareness travel through these spaces.

- We will start our tour within the cisterna magna. See if you can inwardly settle into your cisterna magna. Let yourself imagine/sense the anatomy around you as you settle within its space. Imagine and sense that you are the little minnow swimming in your cisterna magna. Let yourself have a sense of floating and swimming within it. Now, as you settle within this inner space, look above you, and you will see the inferior aspect of the cerebellum. Now look anterior and you will see an opening. This is the median foramen into the fourth ventricle. Swim up to this opening and squeeze through.

- You are now in the fourth ventricle. The little minnow looks up and sees a sloping wall above. This is the cerebellum. You also note a narrow tunnel that seems to go upward farther than you can see. This is the Aqueduct of Sylvius. You also notice a sloping floor below you that slides into another very narrow tunnel and seems to go downward forever. This is the central canal of the spinal column. The little fish waits and watches in the pyramidal shaped fourth ventricle. You take it all in.

- Within the fourth ventricle, you are buffeted about by a turbulence. The fluids in the fourth ventricle swirl about and bounce around before they leave the ventricle to enter the cisterna magna. In this swirling you notice something very powerful. You are surrounded by a radiance of light. Out of the turbulence there is light! This is the *liquid light* that Sutherland speaks about. It seems that the fluids are held up here, and that the potency held within them radiates to all of the physiological centers that surround the fourth ventricle. The light reflects off of everything, but does not mix with anything. It is like golden reflections off of clouds. You also notice something else here. There is a high-pitched buzzing sound emanating from these physiological centers. The area is alive with activity.

• The little fish decides to swim upward. You push yourself up the narrow Aqueduct of Sylvius. You are swimming against the current like a salmon returning home. Finally you find yourself in another space, the third ventricle. It is shaped like a flattened hollow inner tube of a tire with a solid center formed by the interthalamic adhesion. You let yourself be carried by the currents of cerebrospinal fluid up and around this tube. The current takes you around and around the tube. You are carried posteriorly and superiorly within this space, then through the top of the tube, down the front, posteriorly along its floor and back up its rear aspect again. You decide to explore this inner tube. You take a swim in this space. You swim again posteriorly and superiorly to the roof of the third ventricle. You then look behind you. You see a small funnel-shaped opening at the bottom of the rear of the ventricle. Ah! This must be the opening into the pineal gland. In many spiritual traditions, the pineal gland is considered to be the site of the soul. You swim up to it and stick your nose into its opening and see inside. What do you see? You may see the crystals that grow inside of the pineal gland; perhaps you may even see them glowing. Some brain researchers are looking at the brain as having radio sending and receiving capabilities. Perhaps these are the crystals in the radio set. All you know is the radiance coming from them. As you rest there, you notice the gland gently and rhythmically moving superiorly and inferiorly. Ah! you think, this must be

its expression of motility and motion, inhalation and exhalation. You take your nose out of the funnel and swim anteriorly through the upper part of the ventricle. You notice fluid motion coming inferiorly towards you from the top of the ventricle. Like a curtain, the structures hang down and fluid motion is sensed. This must be choroid plexus tissue, secreting new fluid.

• You then swim anteriorly and posteriorly down the front part of the third ventricle. You notice another funnel in the anterior aspect of the floor of the ventricle. Ah! This must be the opening into the pituitary gland at the floor of the third ventricle. You stick your nose in and try to swim down the pituitary stalk. You find it is a tight fit. Maybe your little minnow needs to shrink even smaller. Here, you must squeeze through the diaphragma sellae that straps the pituitary into the sella turcica of the sphenoid bone. You squeeze into the stalk of the pituitary gland and find, after all that effort, that you are tired and need a rest. You settle down and rest on the pituitary gland. Ah! What a relief! You notice a gentle rocking, first one way, then the other. You realize that the pituitary lies in the saddle of the sphenoid bone and is gently rocked by its motility. You are cradled in the arms of motility and gently rocked to sleep.

• After a rest, you awaken and swim upward to squeeze out of the pituitary stalk. You are again in the anterior-inferior aspect of the third ventricle. You look above and notice two more openings in the anterior-superior aspects of the third ventricle. You swim up to them. These must be the Foramina of Monro, each giving access into one of the lateral ventricles. You swim up to one and swim into one of the lateral ventricles. You first swim anteriorly into the anterior horn and soon swim into the end of its most anterior aspect as you bump into the frontal lobe of the cerebral cortex. You swim posteriorly through the body of the lateral ventricle and find that you are indeed in a relatively large space. There is choroid plexus tissue all along it, and much cerebrospinal fluid is produced here! You notice that, as you swim, you are descending posteriorly and that there are two horns, one that goes posterior and inferior, and one that curves inferior and anterior. You explore these. You swim posteriorly until you are in the area of the posterior horn. You swim into this until it ends in the occipital lobe, then you swim out and go inferior-anterior into the inferior horn within the temporal lobe. Just below is the hippocampus and just ahead is the amygdala, both very important centers. Let yourself swim around the lateral ventricle and get a sense of its shape and spatial arrangement.

• You now swim back into the third ventricle via the Foramen of Monro. You may want to repeat the tour of the lateral ventricle on the other side before continuing. Allow yourself to again be taken by the current of cerebrospinal fluid around the inner tube of the ventricle—first posterior-superior, and then anterior-inferior, around and around. You notice its turbine-like motion as you are taken by the fluids around the third ventricle. There is something important here, like a water turbine taking on energy or potency. Yes! It's the power of the Tide. You sense a radiance. You again need a rest. This time you rest on the floor of the third ventricle. You nestle down on the floor and notice an interesting thing happening here. There is a rhythmical rising and falling of the floor of the third ventricle. Ah! You realize that this must be the rise and fall of the sphenobasilar junction that is just under you. You listen to this motion for a while. You then swim to the rear of the floor and again start your descent through the Aqueduct of Sylvius. Here it is an easier descent because you are swimming with the current. You squeeze through and again find yourself in the fourth ventricle where you again experience the turbulence of the cerebrospinal fluid and the radiance of the potency within it. Then you swim out of the median foramen back into the cisterna magna.

Here you end your journey. Take a moment to rest here. Orient to your midline and very gently orient your senses to the outer world. Seeing, hearing and touching, you can reach out again into the world around you.

• I hope you found your tour interesting and also hope that you were able to stay with it both visually and with your attention. It is common to space out or fall asleep the first few times you do this. Again, I suggest that you put a version of the tour onto an audio tape or disk and follow it first with an anatomy atlas and then internally with your mind's eye. Persevere and this will turn out to be time well spent.

MOTILITY OF THE CENTRAL NERVOUS SYSTEM

The central nervous system, like all tissue systems, expresses motility and motion. This motion is organized around the spaces within its form, the ventricles of the brain and the central canal of the spinal cord. This organization has embryological roots. The CNS formed in relationship to the spaces within the neural tube (Fig. 3.3).[3] The central nervous system forms around the spaces generated within the dorsal midline of the embryo. In the adult, the motion of the central nervous system is also organized around the spaces within its form. This is important to understand. The ventricle system, including the central canal of the spinal cord, essentially organizes the motility of the tissues of the brain and spinal cord.

In the embryo, the most cephalad end point of the neural tube is called the lamina terminalis. This point later becomes the anterior wall of the third ventricle. The lamina terminalis of the neural tube is the fulcrum for the development of the central nervous system and continues to be the organizing fulcrum for CNS motility and motion throughout life. Like Sutherland's fulcrum, the lamina terminalis is a *suspended automatically shifting fulcrum*. As with all suspended automatically shifting fulcrums, think of this fulcrum as a concentration of potency that is ideally located

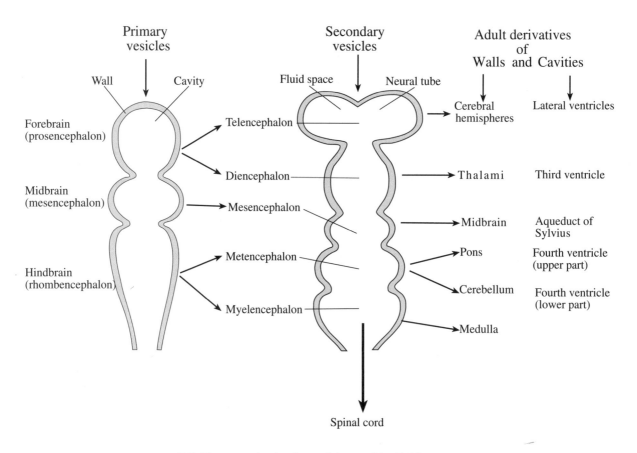

Primary vesicles

Wall | Cavity

Forebrain (prosencephalon)

Midbrain (mesencephalon)

Hindbrain (rhombencephalon)

Secondary vesicles

Fluid space | Neural tube

Telencephalon

Diencephalon

Mesencephalon

Metencephalon

Myelencephalon

Adult derivatives of Walls and Cavities

Cerebral hemispheres	Lateral ventricles
Thalami	Third ventricle
Midbrain	Aqueduct of Sylvius
Pons	Fourth ventricle (upper part)
Cerebellum	Fourth ventricle (lower part)
Medulla	

Spinal cord

3.3 The neural tube: its vesicles and its fluid space

at the lamina terminalis. The action of the lamina terminalis is, in turn, oriented to the primal midline (Fig. 3.4a and b).

Sutherland likened the motion of the central nervous system to that of a tadpole pulling in its tail. In the inhalation phase, the whole of the neural axis shortens towards the lamina terminalis of the third ventricle. The midline through the spinal canal and ventricle system rises and shortens cephalad towards the lamina terminalis. As this occurs, a rotation of the lateral ventricles is generated around a transverse axis through the Foramina of Monro (Fig. 3.5). The ventricle system generally widens side-to-side and the third ventricle widens in a "V" shape as its roof spreads wider apart (Fig. 3.6). As the ventricles shorten toward the lamina terminalis, the brain

becomes more compact in its anterior-to-posterior dimension. It narrows anterior to posterior and widens side-to-side. As this occurs, the spinal cord rises and shortens longitudinally.

Sutherland also compared the overall motion of the ventricles to a bird about to take flight. To get a sense of this motion, imagine a sparrow about to take off from a branch. Imagine that its body is the third ventricle, its tail is the fourth ventricle and the Aqueduct of Sylvius, and its wings are the lateral ventricles. As the sparrow starts to take off, the front of its body tips inferiorly, its tail rises and spreads, and its wings slightly spread apart. Imagine that this motion occurs around a transverse axis through the wings' attachments to its body (Fig. 3.7). Imagine that this bird is transparent and full of fluid and that, as it starts

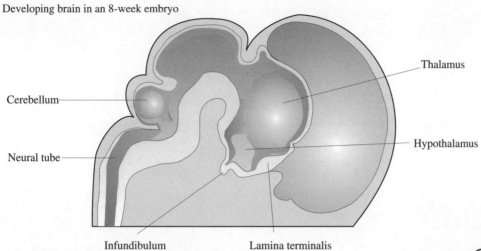

Developing brain in an 8-week embryo

Cerebellum

Neural tube

Thalamus

Hypothalamus

Infundibulum

Lamina terminalis

3.4a The lamina terminalis in the embryo

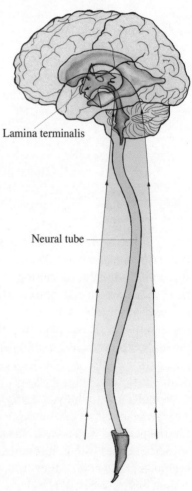

Lamina terminalis

Neural tube

3.5 The motility and motion of the central nervous system

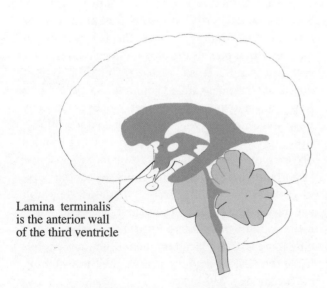

Lamina terminalis is the anterior wall of the third ventricle

3.4b The lamina terminalis in the adult

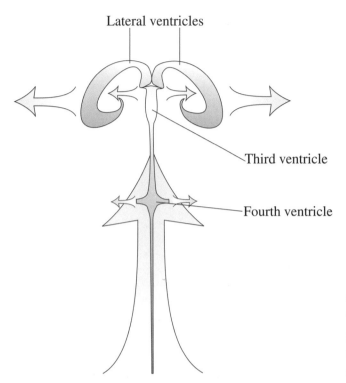

3.6 The ventricles widen in inhalation

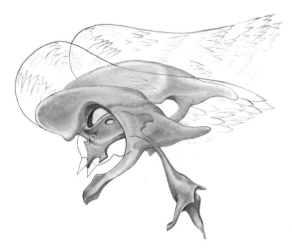

3.7 The bird takes flight (the inhalation phase)

ANATOMICAL CONSIDERATIONS

There are important anatomical considerations to take into account when exploring the central nervous system. The spinal cord is stabilized within the spinal canal by the denticulate ligaments that arise at each spinal segment. These ligaments are formed from pia mater that pierces the arachnoid layer of the meninges and attaches to the interior of the dura mater. Take these ligaments into account when addressing dural tube and spinal cord dynamics (Fig. 3.8). The spinal cord is also stabilized at its inferior aspect by the filum terminalis. This is a filament of pia mater that pierces the arachnoid layer at its inferior aspect at S2. It is invested with a thin layer of dura and continues caudad within the sacral canal to firmly attach to the coccyx. A practitioner can directly sense the central nervous system via contact with the filum terminalis from the coccyx. It also becomes obvious that any trauma to the coccyx can have important repercussions throughout the central nervous system, and that any restriction in sacral motion will have a direct effect on CNS motility. For instance, if the sacroiliac joints are fixed in any way, a dragging force will be placed on the motility and mobility of the CNS in general, and on the brain stem in particular (Fig. 3.9).

to take off, its body is also widening generally—then you have an analogy for the motion of the ventricle system in its inhalation motion. As this is all occurring, the brain stem and spinal cord are also rising and shortening towards the lamina terminalis and widening side-to-side. Remember that all of the tissues in the body express a basic motility of *widening side-to-side, narrowing front-to-back and shortening top-to-bottom* in the inhalation phase of primary respiration.

Mobility and motility patterns of the CNS can be a cause or an effect of other aspects of the system. Inertial patterns within the CNS are often reflections of inertial issues within the cranial base, dural membranes, and the cranial bowl generally. Conversely, cranial patterns may reflect those within the central nervous system.

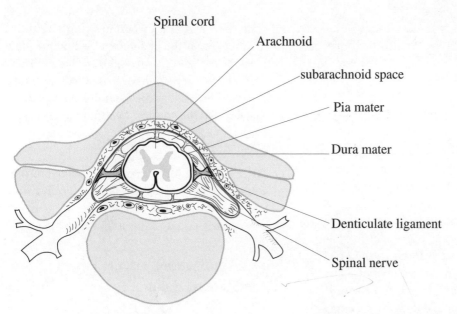

Spinal cord
Arachnoid
subarachnoid space
Pia mater
Dura mater
Denticulate ligament
Spinal nerve

3.8   The denticulate ligaments

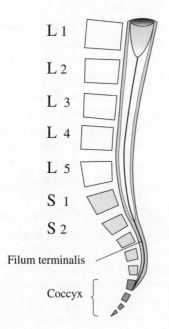

L 1
L 2
L 3
L 4
L 5
S 1
S 2
Filum terminalis
Coccyx

3.9   Filum terminalis attaches to the coccyx

Clinical Application: Palpating the Motility of the Central Nervous System

In the following clinical application we will explore the motility and motion of the central nervous system. The cortex has a quality of a dense sponge and it widens and narrows as the ventricles express motion. You may also sense that the lateral ventricles widen as they rotate around a transverse axis through the Foramen of Monro. The central nervous system should ideally express its motility in a balanced and harmonious way in relationship to the lamina terminalis. We will initially use the *vault hold* to tune into the central nervous system. In this hold, we orient to the action of the central nervous system within the mid-tide (2.5 cycles per minute) level of action. I find that CNS motility is clearest within this level of tidal unfoldment.

1. Establish your practitioner fulcrums and negotiate your contact with the patient's system as usual. Use either Becker's or Sutherland's *vault hold* (see previous chapters in Volume One for descriptions of these holds). Let your hands be immersed within fluids. Hold the biosphere within your awareness and orient to the mid-tide. First

tune into the fluid tide and notice how potency manifests within the fluids. What is the sense of the fluid drive within the system? How does the potency manifest within the system?

2. Now as you listen to the fluid tide, include the neural tissue within your field of awareness. Simply orient to neural tissue within your wide perceptual field. You must know your anatomy to do this. This is always an interesting process. We must know our anatomy and then, when actually listening to a human system, we must put it aside. Images of anatomy will never fully convey the truth of the system. But if we didn't have the images accurately, we would not hear the living anatomy's communications. So be sure that you have clear anatomical images of the brain and spinal cord, but put them aside and hold the *living system* within your hands when you are actually palpating. Float on the tissues with your hands immersed in fluids as you maintain a light contact in the *vault hold.* Then let the nervous system come to you. Let your hands float within fluid and let the motion of the brain and spinal cord come to you. Don't look for anything; simply rest within the fluids and let the spaces and tissues of the CNS come to you.

3. Let the ventricles within the brain take you into their motion. Is there a sense of shortening towards the lamina terminalis? Can you sense a rotational motion around an axis through the Foramen of Monro? How balanced is this motion? Give yourself the luxury of listening and let yourself be moved by the system. Do not look for anything; do not mentally grab onto the tissues as you listen. Maintain your wide field of awareness. Do not narrow your perceptual field down as you allow the neural tissue to come to you.

4. As you follow motility and motion, you may notice a number of things. Firstly, in inhalation, you may sense a general rising towards the lamina terminalis. You may also notice the lateral ventricles widening and rotating around a transverse axis as they curl in a ram's horn-like manner. See if the image of a bird taking flight helps. Seek the bird as it begins to take off. These motions are expressions of neural motility within the cranium. Remember that it is the ventricles that express this motion, and that the brain simply widens and narrows like a dense sponge.

5. After listening for a number of cycles, finish by contacting the sacrum. Perhaps integrative work such as a stillpoint would be helpful if any process arose that seems unfinished.

Clinical Application: Inertial Issues and the State of Balance

In the above exercise, as you followed CNS motility and motion, you may have noticed that it was expressing its motility in an eccentric way. You may have noticed any sort of motion or lack of motion. As you noticed an inertial pattern, did you also notice the fulcrum organizing it? Knowledge of neural anatomy is critical here. It is possible to be very accurate as to the location of an inertial fulcrum within the central nervous system. This might relate to a past accident or trauma of some kind, or to facilitation of nuclei within the brain. We will discuss facilitation in some detail later. The motility and motion of the CNS may be organized around a fulcrum located anywhere in the system. Patterns may relate to a classic cranial base pattern, an inertial suture, or an inertial issue located elsewhere in the body. Remember that inertial issues within the pelvis may literally tether the CNS as it attempts to express its motility. Let's recycle the listening process outlined above and include an awareness of any inertial issues that may arise.

1. Using the vault hold, negotiate your contact with the patient's system and orient to the mid-tide. Listen to the motion of the CNS within the phases of primary respiration. Give the system space. Wait. Listen. Give the system time to express its priorities. You may sense the system settling into

a sense of unity. Tissues will feel like a unified field and primary respiration will clarify.

2. Listen and wait for an inertial pattern to clarify. As this occurs, follow its expression. Again give space to the potency, fluids, and tissue. Follow the motion dynamic within the phases of primary respiration and listen for Becker's three-phase healing process to arise. If needed, very subtly help the tissue and/or fluid elements to settle into a state of balance. Very gently and subtly slow things down with your intention and internal pacing. As you sense the motion within the inertial pattern, slow the fluid and tissue motion down until there is a settling into a state of balance. Do not mentally or physically grab on to any of the three functions of potency, fluids, and tissues as you intend this. If you do, you may lock up the system. Maintain your wide perceptual field. Do not lose a sense of the whole as you do this. Listen for the unfolding of the healing process and for expressions of Health as previously explored in Volume One.

3. When motion is again re-established, listen for the third stage of Becker's process: the reorganization of the potency, fluid, and tissue fields. Does the motion of the CNS seem to be more aligned with its natural fulcrum at the lamina terminalis? Does the motion of the ventricles seem more balanced in inhalation and exhalation? Wait for the period of reorganization to complete. You may sense a surge within the fluid tide as this occurs and/or a consistent expression of a new pattern of organization in relationship to the midline and the lamina terminalis. Finish with integration work at the sacrum.

Fluid Direction Approaches

Next we will again work with the *Tour of the Minnow* and add a process of direction of fluid and potency. Directing potency within the cerebrospinal fluid to a specific fulcrum can be very effective clinically. These fulcrums may even include facilitated

nerve nuclei and force vector entrapments.

With the patient in the supine position, contact the system via the *vault hold* (preferably *Sutherland's hold*). Orient to the mid-tide. Allow the motility and motion of the central nervous system to come to you. Do not narrow your perceptual field as you do this. Sense your hands as being immersed in fluid, and moved by the motility and motion of the brain.

1. Listen to the inhalation and exhalation phases of primary respiration. Orient first to the fluid tide and then to the tissues of the central nervous system. Once a holistic shift occurs, wait for "something to engage from within." As a pattern clarifies, ask the question, "What organizes this?" via your proprioceptive and kinesthetic senses within your hands. Again be aware of Becker's three-phase awareness. See if the CNS settles into a state of balance around the organizing fulcrum. This is a systemic neutral, a settling within the whole system. Listen for expressions of Health, such as changes within the potency, a clear fluid drive, the processing of inertial forces, etc. Again sense for reorganization of the ventricles within the brain and of neural tissues toward their natural fulcrum, the lamina terminalis.

2. Now let's again take the Tour of the Minnow through the ventricle system. Start at the cisterna magna and work your way through the fourth, third, and lateral ventricles. As you do this, you may sense areas of narrowness, resistance, or density. When you encounter these, one approach is to direct fluids and potency to or through the area. Common areas of fluid backpressure and inertial forces include the Aqueduct of Sylvius (narrowing or congestion), areas within the third ventricle (densities or congestion), the Foramen of Monro (narrowing or congestion) and patterns through and within the lateral ventricles. These will be the results of inertial forces and potencies at work within the cranium. All of these may reflect cranial base patterns, to be discussed in Chapter 8.

3. For example, let's say that as you are "swimming" superiorly in the Aqueduct of Sylvius, you sense a narrowing of its walls. Perhaps this was perceived as a backpressure within the fluids, or as an inertial pattern that organizes around the aqueduct in some way. Alternatively, the tension within the aqueduct may be organized around a fulcrum located elsewhere within the cranium. In the time-lapse video of CSF motion through the ventricle system, the differences in the openness of the Aqueduct of Sylvius in different people and different age groups are remarkable. From a *vault hold,* direct fluid and potency through the aqueduct with your thumbs, which are somewhere on the superior aspect of the cranium. Imagine/sense that you are directing CSF and its potency from the third ventricle inferiorly through the aqueduct. Use a gentle touch and intention to do this without narrowing your perceptual field. Clarity of intention and knowledge of anatomy is essential here.

4. See if you can sense an expression of the potency within the fluid through the aqueduct. You may sense pulsation, heat and fluid release within the ventricle system. Wait for a sense that the CSF is clearing through the aqueduct. This approach can be used with any perceived inertial fulcrum within the central nervous system. Another common location for congestion is the Foramen of Monro. Each foramen is a passageway from its related lateral ventricle. If you sense resistance through the foramen, then direct fluid with your thumbs towards the Foramen of Monro and wait for therapeutic responses.

As you become more familiar with the dynamics of the central nervous system, you can combine your approaches. You can facilitate a state of balance and, within the stillness, you can direct fluid and potency to the perceived fulcrum.

THE THIRD VENTRICLE AND THE PRIMARY BIOENERGY CENTER

As part of this discussion of the central nervous system, I would like to include some thoughts on its relationship to a *primary bioenergy center,* a primary fulcrum for the potentization of cerebrospinal fluid. This idea links the CNS to traditional concepts of human bioenergy. As you may know, there are many traditional frameworks for understanding the subtle aspects of the human energy system. Indeed, there are whole medical systems based on a bioenergy perspective. The traditional Ayurvedic (Indian), Chinese, and Tibetan medical systems are examples of these. In the West, Stone's Polarity Therapy is another example. In these classical medical and spiritual systems, the third ventricle, the most central space within the cranium, is considered to be the location of an important primary bioenergy center. As discussed in our previous chapter on midlines, within the yogic tradition, it is the location of the *ajana chakra.* In the Chinese tradition this center is called the *upper Dan Tian* (field of elixir) or the *true niwan* (fulcrum or gateway of the enlightened state). In the Chinese system it is also perceived to be the site of *shen,* or spirit. In many other spiritual traditions it is also thought to be the site of the soul or spirit dwelling within the body (Fig. 3.10).

In the Indian system the *ajana* chakra is the fulcrum for the unfoldment of the human bioenergy system as a whole. It is considered to be the primary fulcrum that forms at the time of conception and from which the embodied human energy system, known as the chakra system, is derived. It is also the center from which a most primary breath, or *prana,* is transferred to the cerebrospinal fluid. In some Chinese systems, the same thing is said of the upper Dan Tian. Thus, in many classical medical and spiritual traditions, there is a perception that this primary center radiates a life force that imbues cerebrospinal fluid with the subtlest life essence. This echoes Sutherland's understanding that the cerebrospinal fluid is the initial recipient of the Breath of Life factor.

Potency ignites within the cerebrospinal fluid at birth. This ignition is perceived to occur especially within the third ventricle. I have not personally sensed this at a birth, but I know colleagues who have been at births and have had the privilege of perceiving this. I have personally worked with many children and adults whose fluids within the third ventricle did indeed ignite with potency as part of the session work. This is obviously an important center for cranial practitioners to understand.

In bringing these ideas up, I am entering what is for some a realm of fantasy or imagination. I ask you to simply be open to these ideas and not to prejudge them based on prior beliefs. Let your perception and your still and open listening be your guide. These concepts, whether within craniosacral biodynamics or spiritual traditions, were generated via a direct observation of the human system at a most primary level of order. Here I am using these concepts to provide a context that is meant to relate traditional medical and spiritual concepts to the work of Sutherland. I believe that when he spoke of the Breath of Life and its potency, he was pointing to a living Intelligence that imbues all form. This Intelligence manifests as a living and embodied life force coursing through the fluids of each and every person. It is not just an idea; it can be a perceptual reality. Its truth is echoed in many traditions.

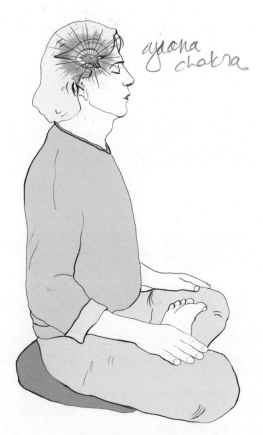

ajna chakra

3.10 The primary energy center within the third ventricle

THE DYNAMICS OF THE THIRD VENTRICLE, IGNITION, AND POTENCY

Sutherland wrote of a mysterious spark that ignites within the cerebrospinal fluid. It allows the Intelligence of the Breath of Life to manifest as a living embodied force or potency and the third ventricle is pivotal in this process. There are two major ignitions of potency, one at conception and another at birth. The first ignition occurs as the Long Tide acts to generate the ordering matrix, an Intelligent bioelectric form, within the single cell of the conceptus. An orienting midline is laid down and the blueprint ignites within the fluids of the embryo to become an embodied force. It is this embodiment of the ordering matrix into form that orchestrates the development and order of both structure and function. This embodiment of potency within the fluids becomes a driving force within the conceptus and embryo. This life force orchestrates cellular and tissue differentiation and development. It is a direct manifestation of the ordering matrix within the fluids and form of the embryo and is with us as an ordering and orienting force throughout life.

I first came across this idea of ignition through the work of Randolph Stone. Stone likened it to the fire of consciousness and Intelligence literally igniting within the conceptus. At this time, the classic chakra system, the subtle human ordering matrix, manifests within the embryo. Stone stressed the fiery nature of this process. Many years ago, I had a psychotherapy client who was exploring his process at great depth. He was about sixty-five years old and had been in many forms of therapy before. In one session he spontaneously experienced his conception process. He experienced this as incredibly fiery and painful. He directly perceived lines of life force being generated as a precise pattern and form within himself. They were laid down in a fiery and meticulous way. He later drew these and amazingly, they were a combination of the "feminine" and "masculine" patterns that Stone showed in his books.[4] I have also palpated these force lines within patients and know that they relate to the process of ignition at conception.

A second ignition occurs at birth. Ignition at birth generates a new fulcrum reflecting the infant's physical independence from its mother. The baby must now orient to a new world as a separate physical being. At the time of birth, when the baby takes its first breath and the umbilical cord stops pulsing, there is a further ignition of potency within cerebrospinal fluid centered in the third ventricle. During this second ignition process, potency literally ignites in a stronger way within the fluids as the baby becomes a physically independent being. It is a direct expression of that infant's empowerment to be here. Thus, empowerment is our birthright. This is a powerful truth for many people, and many of my patients, to sense. Ignition within the third ventricle occurs in each and every moment of our lives. It is a manifestation of our ongoing empowerment to be here, to incarnate and to move through life.

Stone also discussed the ignition at birth as the *light of consciousness* manifesting in form. It is the final process of embodiment as the infant separates from its mother. It is about the motive power, the fire of life, being directed outward towards its new world. The infant's consciousness and perceptual processes are now fully oriented externally. Stone linked birth ignition within the third ventricle with the *ajana* chakra (upper Dan Tian in the Chinese system). At this time he also noted a major ignition of energy at

the umbilicus and the *fire chakra* that it connects to. In his private practice, he noted that the ignition process, and the dissemination of fiery or motive energy throughout the body, can be dampened down. It is not uncommon for difficult births, umbilical shock, and anesthesia to dampen this second ignition down. Later in life, shocking experiences and fluid inertia and density can also reduce the ignition process. In a healthy system the practitioner may sense potency cycling around the third ventricle in a dynamo-like or pulsatory manner. In a system that is congested and inertial, you may sense a sluggishness in this motion around the third ventricle. Stone worked with ignition issues via the umbilicus and coccyx, the end point of the quantum midline, the central channel or *sushumna* of the yogic system.

When I have experienced ignition within a patient's system, I have seen a number of phenomena come into play. A rapid expansion, like a spark, arises within the third ventricle. Energy pulses downward along the *sushumna,* and the heart and umbilical centers light up. Stone noted that at birth a current of life force is pulsed outward from the umbilicus to enliven the infant's mind-body system with fire, or motive energies. Before this time, energy pulses inward from the umbilical cord into the infant's system. This is a major shift in orientation for the infant, from direct connection and continuity with its mother, where energy is pulsing inward, to an independent physical relationship to the world, where energy pulses outward. I have noted this shift in energy at the navel many times as a patient's system reignites with this fiery, motive energy.

I have also noted connections to the Chinese meridian system during this ignition process (Fig. 3.11). There seems to be a connection during this second ignition from the midline to both the *du mai* meridian, that moves superiorly from the coccyx, up the centerline of the rear of the body and head to the tip of the tongue and the *ren mai,* that moves from the tongue inferiorly through the centerline of the anterior of the body back to the coccyx. In the Chinese system, *du mai* relates to *yang,* or masculine energies, while the *ren mai* relates to Yin, or feminine energies. Thus, during birth ignition there is a direct connection to these meridians as both the masculine and feminine natures of the baby are "fired up" and oriented to the outer world. The *du mai* and *ren mai* help maintain a balance of these forces within us and are directly connected to the central quantum midline at the top of the head and at the coccyx. The Chinese call this central midline the *chung mai,* the vitality or central channel. It is said to maintain vitality and regulate the *qi* in the whole body-mind system. These three channels directly relate to the ignition process and the potentization of fluids with *jing,* or essence. They are considered to be mystical channels and are not normally needled in classic acupuncture. In the clinical applications below, I will refer to the quantum midline in front of the vertebral column as the *central channel*.

As cerebrospinal fluid ignites with potency, there is a direct relationship within the third ventricle to some very important structures. The third ventricle is surrounded by the thalamus, the hypothalamus, the basal ganglion, the corpus callosum, and the fornix. The pineal and pituitary glands directly connect to its space. The lateral ventricles also relate to very important structures, including the hippocampus, amygdala, and the temporal lobe of the cortex. The limbic system is organized around this central space. All of these structures are critical to processing information throughout the body-mind system. Responses to internal and external sensory input, links to the cerebral cortex and the autonomic system, physical coordination, autonomic activity, and emotional responses are all mediated here. All of these structures are nestled around the third ventricle and its energetic dynamics.

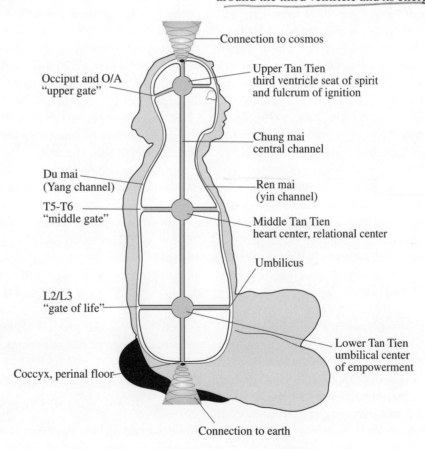

3.11 Ignition system and meridians

We have been working with ignition issues for about fifteen years at the Karuna Institute, and some of the processes we have explored are outlined below.

Introduction to Ignition Processes

If ignition occurs with full force at birth, potency will be expressed within the cerebrospinal fluid as a clear ordering and self-regulating force. The light of Intelligence will be ignited within the system and motive, fiery energy will become available to the newly born infant. Her perceptual processes will be directed outward and she will able to orient to her mother and to her outer environment. If ignition does not occur thoroughly, the cerebrospinal fluid will not become fully potentized, and stasis and lethargy may result over time. The fire of consciousness may be dulled, and developmental processes may be slowed. The fluid system may become sluggish, and a reduced fluid tide may be perceived. In this instance, the inherent resources of the person will become less available for life functions. I have worked with many infants and children with developmental issues that were helped by the ignition process and a general reconnection to inherent resources.

Many circumstances can dampen the ignition process. If the infant experiences a traumatic birth, and/or if anesthesia is used during the birth process, ignition within the third ventricle can be impeded. If the infant's umbilical cord is cut too soon, a shock can be introduced that can also dampen down ignition. In these circumstances, potency will only partially ignite within the cerebrospinal fluid. This is a common issue that can persist throughout life if it is not addressed, resulting in lowered vitality and a less efficient response to stress. Some practitioners claim that the ignition process is inhibited in ninety percent of births. Over the years, I have certainly seen this as a major issue in a majority of infant and adult systems.

The clinical applications below have been found to be very useful in facilitating the expression of potency when anesthesia trauma is active within the system. If anesthesia was used during the birthing process, it may also be part of birth trauma schemas.

The infant will directly experience the anesthesia given to the mother and their system may go into anesthesia stasis. A protective hypotonic state coupled with parasympathetic shock effects, may then become evident. These effects of birth process can stay with us our whole life. Anesthesia effects can also derive from surgical operations, dental work, or other trauma.

Ignition issues may be linked to many other phenomena, I have also observed that many cases of chronic fatigue can be tracked back to birth trauma, poor ignition of potency within the third ventricle, general fluid congestion, and chronic parasympathetic states. In these cases, it is important to resolve the birthing forces still present.

The presence of unresolved birthing forces is a common origin for cranial base and structural issues. Part of this work may entail facilitating the ignition process within the third ventricle. I will cover cranial base patterns later in this volume and will also introduce material on birth trauma and resultant traumatic patterning. Attending to the venous sinus system can also be helpful, at least in the short term, until major forces and inertial patterns have been resolved. Venous sinus issues and related fluid stasis are intimately related to the osseous-membranous system and are also covered in later chapters.

Remember that the issues that generate poor ignition and lowered vitality must also be addressed. An awareness of the action of potency and of the fluid motion around the third ventricle can give the practitioner useful information about the ability of the system to express the potency of the Breath of Life at a core level. I am including these sections on ignition in this chapter on the central nervous system, as awareness of its motility and the third ventricle is an essential part of this process. We usually teach this work in the later phases of training.

Clinical Application: Ignition Via the Umbilicus and Coccyx

Stone worked with "fiery energies" within the system via the umbilicus and coccyx. I will describe an approach used at the Karuna Institute derived from his work. The first step is to get a sense of some of the basic ignition dynamics. I will describe these as far as I can from my own experience. Ignition arises within the third ventricle like a mini-spark or pulsation. This drives down the central channel (the midline in front of the vertebrae from the third ventricle to coccyx) towards the coccyx and the heart and umbilical centers (chakras) seem to light up. Potency then seems to build and amplify within the fluids and the fluid tide surges. You may also sense the ventricles taking flight within an amplified inhalation surge.

With this in mind, let's explore some of Stone's ideas. Stone oriented his ignition-fire work to the umbilicus and coccyx, and the following clinical application will help you explore these relationships. In this work, you will make contact with the patient's navel. This can be a very sensitive area, especially if there was umbilical shock experienced at birth. This commonly occurs if the cord is cut too soon. It is important to carefully negotiate your contact with the patient and to work very slowly. Verbal communication is important, and all of the trauma skills outlined in Volume One may also come into play. Before you begin the procedure, clearly explain what you are going to do. Explain that you will be contacting their umbilicus and clearly negotiate this. Give the patient the power to say "no," or "enough," at any time. Be sure that they come to the session wearing a lightweight shirt or T-shirt. Many patients will allow you to make a direct contact to their umbilicus under their clothing if this is properly negotiated.

It is important to learn to perceive the quality of ignition and drive within a patient's system. A *vault hold* is a good starting point. In this position, orient to the biosphere and mid-tide. Note the strength of the fluid tide. Is there a sense of power and drive coming through? Once you sense its quality, orient to the motility of the central nervous system. In the inhalation phase is there a good sense of the ventricles "taking flight" like a bird? Do you sense a clear dynamo-like action of potency around the third ventricle? Does the potency seem to ignite within the fluids? These will all give you a sense of the quality of ignition within the third ventricle and fluid system

generally. You can also assess these from a *sacral hold*. If the potency within the fluids seems dampened down, then an ignition process may be useful. I will describe the ignition process derived from Stone's work in two steps.

Step One

1. With the patient still in the supine position, stand or sit at the right side of the patient's body. With the index and middle fingers of your left hand, place a V-spread transversely under the spine spreading across the disc space between L2 and L3. Your middle finger is on L3 and your index finger is on L2. This space is the location of the "gate of life" in the Chinese system and connects to the umbilical chakra in the yogic system. It also connects to the central channel or quantum midline (see Fig. 3.11).

2. Have the patient show you where their umbilicus is under their clothing. Place your right hand about two feet (two-thirds of a meter) above the patient's umbilicus. Maintain a wide perceptual field and do not narrow to the umbilicus or spine. Really hold the whole of their biosphere within your field of awareness. Be receptive and let the relationships and motions come to you. See if you can sense an outward motion of energy or force arising from the umbilicus. It will commonly have a spiral, centrifugal quality. This is the centrifugal pulsation that arises when the infant takes its first breath and the umbilicus stops pulsing. Note the quality of this. Ideally it will seem strong and pulsatory and will literally convey a fiery quality. See if the patient can sense your presence as a sensation, or felt experience in their umbilical area. Experiment with the distance your hand hovers over the umbilicus. You may have to be further away or much closer to sense this and for the patient to sense your hovering hand as a felt experience.

3. If there is low ignition, you may feel little motion or pulsation. If there has been umbilical shock, you may actually sense an implosion of energy

quality of ignition

43

as though your palpating hand or fingers are being pulled inward towards the person's central channel.

4. Very slowly allow your hand to float towards the umbilicus until your middle finger makes physical contact. Stone perceived that this finger resonates with fiery energies, and so its use is appropriate here. Let the patient know that you are about to contact their umbilicus before you make a gentle initial contact. Allow your finger to sense the dynamics there. If you sense you are being pulled in, allow your contact to deepen. If you sense a spiral-like motion, allow your finger to follow it in the direction it takes you. Keep a wide perceptual field and include L2-L3 and the space between them in your awareness (Fig. 3.12).

5. See if you can help access a state of balance within this contact. Once you sense a neutral, very gently direct potency from your finger at the umbilicus towards the central channel. Listen for the response at the spinal V-spread. When ignition is engaged, you will begin to perceive a pulsation at your V-spread and an expansion at the umbilicus. You may also sense that the umbilical center, or chakra, *lights up* between your palpating hands, and a strong inhalation-phase surge of the fluid tide. You may sense that your finger in the patient's umbilicus is pushed outward (anterior towards the ceiling). As your finger is pushed outward, follow this motion and allow your hand to lift off the body. Again sense the quality of the pulsation of life force anterior above the body. Does this seem stronger and more engaged?

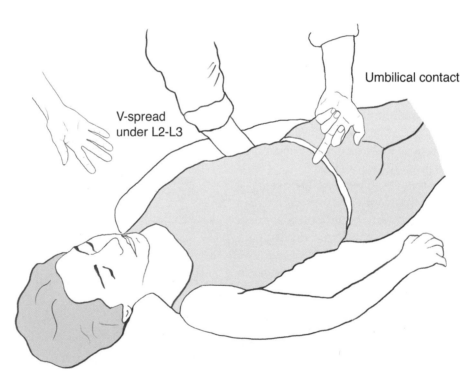

V-spread under L2-L3

Umbilical contact

3.12 Contact with umbilicus and L2, L3 for ignition

Step Two

1. Sit on the right side of the patient's supine body about diaphragm level, facing the pelvis and legs. Place your left hand under the sacrum with your fingers pointing inferior. Your middle finger is curled under the patient's coccyx and makes a relatively firm contact with it. Your arm rests under the patient's spinal area. Allow the patient's body to center and balance on your arm-hand contact. You are now in contact with the most inferior pole of the central channel at the coccyx.

2. Once a contact is negotiated, again place your right hand above the umbilicus. Again sense the quality of the spiral pulsation from the umbilicus. If it still seems low in potency, or if you need to be close to the body to sense it, contact the umbilicus directly as before (remember to negotiate this contact as needed). See if you can sense the continuity of the central channel and its connection to the umbilicus and coccyx (Fig. 3.13).

3. Settle into the relationship and wait for a state of balance to arise. Sometimes this is all that is needed. If the umbilical pulsation and midline are not clear and vibrant in the expression of potency and ignition, then again direct potency from the umbilicus to the central channel. Proceed as above. Again wait for a sense of "lighting up" and strong pulsation from the umbilical area outward. You may also sense a surge in the central channel, a building of potency and a strong surge of the fluid tide in inhalation. Again, does the system seem more vibrant with fire and vitality?

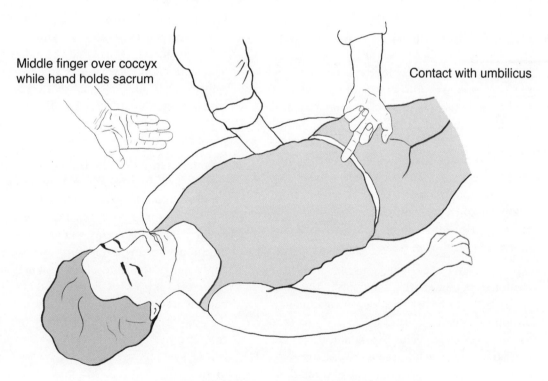

Middle finger over coccyx while hand holds sacrum

Contact with umbilicus

3.13 Umbilical–coccyx contact for ignition

45

Clinical Application:
Crank-Starting the Dynamo

This second approach is a simple fluid fluctuation process to aid ignition within the third ventricle. It is an alternative to the above and can be very effective if carefully used. We enter this process assuming that the issues discussed above are understood. In the application below, we will use our understanding of fluid fluctuation and fluid dynamics to help "crank-start" the dynamo within the third ventricle. An expanded clinical approach is then presented for use after this simpler process has become familiar. This process was developed at the Karuna Institute sometime around 1988. There are other processes available, but this is a good starting point.[4]

1. From the vault hold, negotiate contact with the patient's system and first orient to the mid-tide. Sense the motility and motion of the central nervous system, and then allow an awareness of the third ventricle to come into your perceptual field.

2. Start this process with an EV4 facilitated from the temporal bones or occiput (see Chapter 16 in Volume One, "Stillpoints Revisited"). Using the EV4 process, subtly facilitate a stillpoint within the inhalation phase of primary respiration. Listen for a surge of potency from below to above within the fluid midline. This alone will sometimes generate ignition in the third ventricle. If an ignition does occur, you will sense a build up of potency and a surge of potency from below, and then the ventricles, especially the lateral ventricles, will seem to "take off" like a bird lifting into flight from a tree branch.

3. After the EV4, see if you can sense a cyclical motion of potency within the fluids in the third ventricle. It may be perceived as a circular motion around the ventricle from its floor, up its rear aspect, over its superior aspect and down the anterior aspect. You may sense this as a dynamo-like quality between the palms of your hands. If the system is congested this motion may seem

very sluggish, or there may be very little sense of any motion at all. In a vital system it will seem lively and potent.

4. If the motion still seems very sluggish after an EV4, an additional process can help cerebrospinal fluid ignite with potency within the third ventricle. It is similar to the process of sensing lateral fluctuations of fluid and enhancing them by pushing against the pendulum swings of the fluctuations.

5. Again tune into the quality of potency and fluid motion within the third ventricle. Sense the motion as though it is in the palms of your hands. When you make contact with it, imagine that you are "push-starting" the motion of potency and fluid around the third ventricle. Initiate this just before the inhalation phase begins. Do this by imagining that you could push on the potency and fluids in a circular manner. If you are looking at the right side of the head, potency will pulsate in a clockwise direction, up the rear of the ventricle, anterior over the top, down the front, posterior along the bottom and up the rear, etc. You may imagine/sense that the palms of your hands are like large magnets and are energetically encouraging a circular motion of potency within the fluids in the third ventricle. Do not try to push potency into the ventricle as you do this; simply initiate a circular motion.

6. You may sense that the fluids start to pick up potency and the motion may then begin to have a more vibrant quality to it. At some point there may be a sense that the fluids ignite with potency. If ignition occurs, you may sense a surge of potency arising from below. To use Sutherland's image, the ventricle system may seem to "take off" like a bird entering flight. This may happen in stages. First one lateral ventricle rises, then another. When the bird truly takes off, it can be quite dramatic. It may seem like the whole system wakes up as potency surges through the midline. You may also sense the umbilical area "lighting up." The cycling of

potency around the third ventricle may then be sensed to be dramatically enhanced and the fluid drive augmented.

Further Clinical Issues

If the patient's system does not respond to the above work, then other inertial issues may need to be addressed. This is a function of the Inherent Treatment Plan. Do not be discouraged; just listen to the unfolding process. It may be important to help the build the patient's inherent resources first. Clinical focuses that might be appropriate in unresponsive patients may include:

- Facilitate stillpoints to encourage greater potentization of the fluid system with the ordering principle of the Breath of Life.

- Ensure that the outlets to venous drainage in the cranium are relatively clear. These include the thoracic inlet, the O/A junction and the jugular foramen.

- Ensure that the venous sinuses are relatively clear to reduce any backpressure that could affect the fluctuation of cerebrospinal fluid.

- Address cranial base patterns and compressive issues.

- Address intraosseous issues, especially of the occiput, sphenoid, and temporal bones.

- Be sure that the inferior pole at the sacrum can express its motility and motion (for example, address compressions compromising sacral mobility and motility) as these will affect the lumbosacral cistern, dural tube mobility, and central nervous system motility and will thus create backpressure within the fluid tide.

Spiritual Ignition

There is a further important process linked to ignition. This is the "igniting" of the spiritual journey back to the source. Many traditions speak about a reverse ignition process where potency rises up the midline, "spirit" ignites within the third ventricle and the soul, or being, orients to its source rather than to its outer world. Stone talked about this as an inward and upward journey back to the source of all form. I have experienced this process to some extent and know of others who also have. This upward ignition process is sometimes called the "kundalini" experience, where life force rapidly rises up the midline from the sacro-coccyx area to ignite a spiritual journey.

The Chinese discuss meditation processes that help raise the life force up the midline from center to center. Life force rises from the coccyx to the umbilical center, or lower Dan Tian, and an ignition again occurs within this center. Then a further rising and ignition occurs, first within the heart center and then within the third ventricle, or upper Dan Tian, the location of *shen* or spirit. Spirit ignites with a longing to return to its source and its orientation shifts from the outer world to the source of that world. The Chinese speak about this as a transmutation process in reverse. Meditation on the third ventricle and brow center are also common practices.

All of these are ideally practiced under the guidance of a teacher who knows this territory. If spiritual ignition occurs in an uncontained or too rapid fashion, disorientation and dissociation can result. In the Zen tradition it is called "Zen sickness." This can occur spontaneously, especially under extreme circumstances, or can happen due to intense practices such as yogic "fire breathing." I have treated a number of patients with this condition. Caution is emphasized here.

In essence, spiritual ignition is a matter of the heart. When self-view is truly relinquished, even momentarily, the heart may open and a longing for truth naturally ignites within our hearts. The whole ignition process along the central channel opens, and the heart-mind orients to its source.

The Central Nervous System and Sacral Dynamics

The inferior pole of the spine is intimately related to the dynamics of the motility of the central nervous system. If the sacrum is prevented from expressing its mobility and motility in some way, the motility of the central nervous system will be directly and strongly affected. This is due to a number of factors. Most importantly, the filum terminalis, that descends through the sacral canal, is directly attached to the sacrococcygeal complex. The filament is composed of pia mater that covers the central nervous system and is invested with a thin covering of dura. Its role is to stabilize the spinal cord at its inferior aspect (see Fig. 3.9). Secondly, the dural tube is strongly attached to S2 within the sacral canal. Inertia within sacral dynamics will be directly fed into the motility and mobility of the CNS via these connections.

In its inhalation phase, the sacrum subtly lifts superiorly and rotates around a transverse axis at S2, widening and uncoiling in its motility. This has the quality of an inner breath. If its superior rising is restricted by compressive issues within the surrounding joints, or by intraosseous distortions within the sacrum itself, then a direct dragging force may be fed into the central nervous system via the filum terminalis. Thus, inertial issues within sacral dynamics, such as compression within the lumbosacral junction and sacroiliac joints, and intraosseous distortions of the sacrum, will directly affect the motility of the central nervous system. It is imperative to assure that the dynamics of the sacrum and pelvis are free to express their own mobility and motility. We will explore these relationships later in this volume.

Clinical Application: Accessing the CNS Via the Filum Terminalis

In the following process, you will learn to directly access the central nervous system via the sacrum and the filum terminalis. This can be a useful way to relate to central nervous system issues and can also give you access to sympathetic stress responses. The Ganglion of Impar (the sacrococcygeal ganglion), the last sympathetic ganglion in the sympathetic chain, lies just anterior to the coccyx. As you meet the nervous system via the filum terminalis, you also have a direct relationship to the whole sympathetic chain. Stone

stressed the importance of forming a relationship to this ganglion in his clinical approaches to the autonomic nervous system (Fig. 3.14).

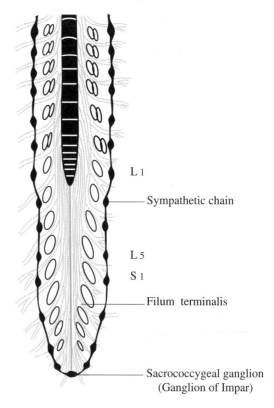

L 1

Sympathetic chain

L 5

S 1

Filum terminalis

Sacrococcygeal ganglion (Ganglion of Impar)

3.14   The Ganglion of Impar

1. Use the standard *sacral hold.* Orient to the mid-tide. Tune into the motion/motility of the sacrum. Then shift your attention to the filum terminalis at the coccyx. Let the filum terminalis come into your awareness. Do not narrow your perceptual field as you do this. Let the motion of the central nervous system come into your awareness from this vantage point. Don't look for it; just listen for it, be receptive and notice the ascending of the central nervous system in inhalation and its descending in exhalation. The first step might be to simply wait in a receptive state, sense

for a pattern to clarify, and work to access the state of balance.

2. As you listen to the system via this hold, let the nervous system come into your awareness. Then allow the Ganglion of Impar to more specifically clarify and enter your perceptual field. Sense its motility and motion within the phases of the Tide, as you would relate to any tissue structure. You may sense the whole sympathetic chain very subtly rising in inhalation and settling in exhalation. Follow its motion and facilitate the state of balance as you would anywhere within the system. This gives you a direct access into the dynamics of the autonomic system and the CNS as a whole.

3. You may also become aware of a clearing of related shock affects, especially sympathetic shock. You may sense this as a streaming of electric-like energy through the sympathetic chain, through the sacrum and coccyx, and even down the patient's legs. Allow shock affects to clear and reorganization to complete. Effectiveness with this depends on the quality of the space you are holding for the patient's process to unfold and complete. Alternately, a more direct conversation using traction can be initiated.

4. Engage the central nervous system in this conversation with a very gentle intention. Use an extremely subtle intention of caudad traction via the sacrum and coccyx. This will engage the filum terminalis and through it the central nervous system. If you use too much intention, you will engage the dural tube instead. As you do this, orient to the Ganglion of Impar. As you subtly intend traction, you can thus start a conversation with the sympathetic chain via this ganglion. Here, you are using the coccyx and the structures attached to it and anterior to it, as your handle for the central nervous system. As you do this, the CNS may begin to speak to you. It may show its patterns of inertia and distress. As usual, follow these into a state of balance. Listen for Becker's three-phase process. Be patient with all of this. Let the system complete whatever it needs

to. Listen for any reorganization and for the quality of both the motility of the CNS and of the fluid tide.

Clinical Highlight

Over the years, I have found that central nervous system issues will come up in almost all of the patients I see. CNS autonomic shock affects are very common and have many origins. When a person manifests a shock state, or has a new traumatic experience, it is common for layers of unresolved trauma to be activated.

The following case is a good example of this. A thirty-two-year-old patient came to see me after a car accident. She was sitting in the back seat with a friend when the driver lost control of the car and hit a tree head-on. The driver and her friend were hospitalized, but H. was released with only minor bruises. The repercussions of the accident, however, went far deeper than the bruising she received. H. began to experience anxiety attacks after the accident. These manifested as rapid breathing and intense feelings of fear. She also began having migraine headaches, insomnia and sacroiliac pain. Her headaches were familiar from childhood, but the insomnia, and sacroiliac pain were new symptoms.

Upon palpation, I found that her system was in a very activated state. There were torsional issues present from the accident and cervical-occipital compression due to whiplash. It was difficult to find a way into contact and relationship as her system was highly sensitive. In the first few sessions we worked mainly to help slow down her activation levels. She learned to slow her breathing down when a panic attack started. I also helped her orient to sensations and begin to access some sense of resourced sensations. This helped to uncouple the feeling of fear and panic from the sensations arising. We also worked with stillpoints via the sacrum and began to orient her system to its inherent potency. By the sixth session the Inherent Treatment Plan began to engage. The layering of her traumatic experiences began to uncouple, and potency began to work with one thing at a time.

The first area focused upon was her pelvic area and right sacroiliac joint. The torsional component of the accident had generated a protective contraction in the area, and an old intraosseous issue in the sacrum was activated. This had not previously manifested as pain, but the force of the accident intensified the original pattern. As her system oriented to these issues, some local tissue shock resolved. This was experienced by her as heat and tingling. I sensed an electric-like discharge through the fluids from the area. The sacral forces and related patterns resolved over a number of sessions, and then her system really began to uncouple layers of unresolved trauma.

Her potency then oriented to thoracic issues. A very deep sadness arose as this occurred, and she managed to allow this to resolve without being overwhelmed by the experience. This seemed to be a seminal moment in the treatment process. She said it was like a weight had been lifted. Memories of childhood were coupled with this. She remembered moving to a new house when she was eight and having to leave all her friends behind. This seemed like a theme in her life, and we spent some time simply exploring this and the related sensations in her body.

In the next few sessions, the work shifted to the cervical area and occiput. Although the contractions present seemed related to the accident, a childhood fall from a horse came to the forefront. This was coupled with memories of the accident and some feelings of anger. I supported the process of resolution both through states of balance and the direction of fluids to help process the force vectors present. After two sessions, the contraction resolved with a consequent lengthening throughout the midline. She remembered that her childhood headaches had began a year after that fall. During this time, her panic attacks subsided, but there was still a sensitivity to her system and some sleeplessness.

Next the cranium came to the forefront and a number of membranous-osseous issues were dealt with. Then the treatment plan shifted to an intraosseous occipital issue related to birth trauma and early childhood. This is when the nervous system came strongly to the forefront. The forces organizing the intraosseous issue had also generated fulcrums within the CNS. Her system clearly oriented to these fulcrums. As she entered a state of balance oriented to the motility of the CNS and related inertial fulcrums, she began to process autonomic shock affects. At first it was like she was flooded with electric-like pulsations that were dissipated throughout the cerebrospinal fluid. Then some nuclei in the brain stem began to discharge. I sensed that this was from the area where the locus ceruleus is located, an important pair of nuclei in the stress response.

As I subsequently held her sacrum, her system entered a deep state of balance and the whole sympathetic chain began to discharge its cycling. H. experienced waves of tingling down her back that felt very healing. I sensed the release of electric-like clearing down the chain through her pelvis and legs. When this completed, she entered a deep stillness and a strong rising of potency within her fluid midline manifested. As this occurred, her cerebrospinal fluid seemed to ignite. This occurred naturally within the stillness. It was like the last piece of her birth trauma had finally resolved. She said that she "felt better than ever." Sessions ended soon after that. In a follow up session about six months later her system was found to be stable with good fluid drive and access to resources.

This chapter is meant to be a basic introduction to extremely complex issues. We will discuss further aspects of CNS in later chapters on the cranial base and on neuroendocrine stress responses. The whole area of cranial nerve entrapment neuropathy has not been discussed and must also be considered. Issues of specific pathologies, such as cerebral accident and various neurological pathologies, have not been mentioned. This is just meant to be a starting point for your exploration. I hope you find this area deeply revealing and that you widen your appreciation of its clinical implications.

1. William Garner Sutherland, *Teachings in the Science of Osteopathy* (Rudra Press, 1990).

2. Ibid., 20, 227.

3. Fig. 3.3 is after Moore and Persaud, *Before We Were Born,* Fifth Edition (Fig. 19-19) (W.B Saunders Company, 1998).

4. See James Jealous, D.O., *The Biodynamics of Osteopathy: The Ignition System 1 and 2,* from a set of audio CDs. Contact Marnee Jealous Long, 6501 Blackfin Way, Apollo Beach, Florida, 33572, USA.

4

In this chapter we will:

- *Introduce the dynamics and major relationships of the dural tube.*
- *Learn to relate to its mobility.*
- *Learn to relate to inertial patterns.*
- *Introduce some trauma concepts.*
- *Learn to relate to major structures that interface with the dural tube.*

THE CORE LINK

The dural membrane defines the boundaries of the Primary Respiratory Mechanism (Fig. 4.1), and traditionally has been termed the *core link* of the body. In this chapter we will explore its relationship to midline dynamics and to craniosacral biodynamics generally. It connects the whole system, top-to-bottom and center to periphery. The dural tube is continuous with the inner layer of dura that surrounds the brain. It follows and surrounds the spinal cord as it leaves the cranium and extends all the way down into the sacral canal. It surrounds the brain and spine in one continuous envelope that expresses the unity of the entire system of bones, membranes, tissues, and fluids. The continuity of all these aspects in an interdependent holographic whole is one of the founding

nice!

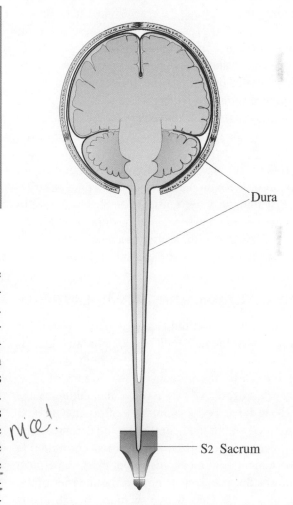

Dura

S2 Sacrum

4.1 The dura and the primary respiratory system

53

principles of craniosacral biodynamics, and the *core link* is a central medium for this unity. Forces and patterns anywhere in the system may be registered in the dural membrane, and membranous patterns in the core link can be reflected elsewhere.

Study of the sacrum and occiput reveals some interesting tensile dynamics. We can think of the sacrum and occiput as compression structures and the dural tube as a tension structure. The core link helps maintain and express the balance between the connected compression structures above and below (Fig. 4.2). For instance, looking from the bottom up, a balanced tension on either side of the sacral base would be an expression of balance within the occipital base, the tentorium and falx, and the cranial bones that connect to them. Inertial processes within a sacroiliac joint would thus have major repercussions for the whole reciprocal tension system. Another example would be that of inertial dynamics within the core link itself. The dural tube should be relatively free to glide within the vertebral canal. If there are adhesions anywhere along its length, the dynamic tension balance within the membranous-osseous system will be compromised.

If the reciprocal tension dynamics within the core link become conditioned and strained, then all structures within the whole tensile tissue field will have to compensate in some way. Since the dural tube directly links the occiput to the sacrum, occipital patterns will be directly reflected in the sacrum, and vice versa.

THE CORE LINK AND THE MIDLINES

Perception of the fluid tide is the foundation for awareness of the fluid midline. Longitudinal fluctuation is an expression of the motility of fluids as they are moved by the potency of the Breath of Life. Potency is expressed within the primal midline as an uprising force. A dorsal midline of potency is then generated within the neural tube, and cerebrospinal fluid becomes potentized with its force. The fluid tide then manifests as an expression of primary respiration. The dura defines the physical boundaries of the dorsal midline. Thus, within the dural membrane is found the fluid core of the body. It is within this core

that the neural tube forms and the cerebrospinal fluid tide is generated.

Practitioners can tune into the quality of the fluid tide in order to sense how the system can express its resources. If much potency is bound up in centering inertial issues, then the fluid tide may seem reduced in power or amplitude. As inertial issues are resolved within the system, you may sense a surge within this core as potency is freed and the fluids express a clearer and more potent fluctuation. You may also perceive the tissue elements realigning to the primal midline as inertial forces are processed by the system. An awareness of these midlines is essential for good clinical practice. Awareness of the midlines gives you clear indications of the resources of the system and how they can manifest, and of how the potencies, fluids, and tissues are reorganizing to their Original intention. It is very important in session work to give the system time to reorganize and to note how the fluids and tissues have reorganized. Indications to look for include a fuller and more potent fluid tide, a more balanced tissue motion in relationship to the primal midline and to natural fulcrums such as Sutherland's fulcrum.

ANATOMY OF THE CORE LINK

The dural tube can be considered a continuation of the inner meningeal layer of cranial dura and is comprised of only one layer. The outer, or periosteal layer of cranial dura is interrupted at the foramen magnum and, in the spinal column, the periosteum of the bone functions as this outer layer. The dural tube is thus continuous with the inner layer of dura that surrounds the brain. The dural tube extends from the foramen magnum, where it is firmly attached at its dural ring, into the sacral canal, where it is firmly attached at the second sacral segment. There are also attachments at the second and third cervical vertebrae and lower lumbar areas. Dural sleeves also follow nerve roots out of the spinal canal, and this provides continuity with all of the fascial relationships of the body (Fig. 4.3).

There is a layer of loose fatty tissue in the epidural space between the dura mater and the connective

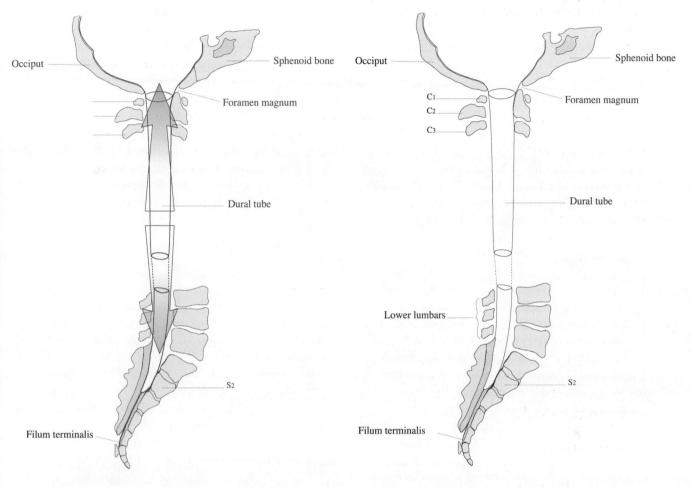

Occiput

Sphenoid bone

Foramen magnum

Dural tube

S2

Filum terminalis

Occiput

C1
C2
C3

Sphenoid bone

Foramen magnum

Dural tube

Lower lumbars

S2

Filum terminalis

4.2   The dural tube as a reciprocal tension structure

4.3   The attachments of the dural tube

tissues that line the inside of the vertebral canal. This fatty tissue acts as a lubricating layer, assisting in the ease of dural glide within the spinal canal. As you move your body and bend your spine, the dural tube should be able to glide relatively freely. As the body responds to experience and trauma, adhesions between the dural tube and the connective tissues of the vertebral canal may arise, especially near its intervertebral foramen, and this will affect the ease of dural glide within the spinal canal (Fig. 4.4). Connective tissue drag in other parts of the body may also be transferred into the dural tube via the continuity of dura and connective tissue. Vertebral fixations can also generate dural adhesions and restrictions to dural glide. Inertial fulcrums within the dynamics of the dural tube will also affect the expression of the fluid tide and its longitudinal fluctuation. Potency may become inertial within the core of the body in order to center the forces involved. Obviously this may have profound implications for the biodynamics of the whole system.

what can happen to the dural tube, & what does it mean.

55

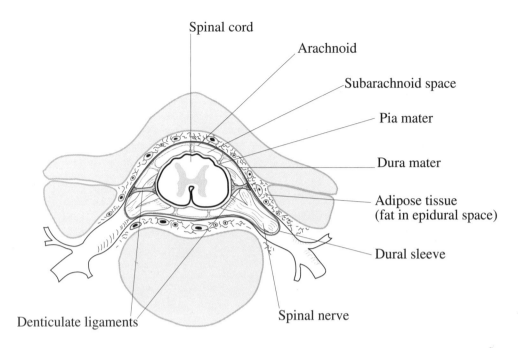

Spinal cord

Arachnoid

Subarachnoid space

Pia mater

Dura mater

Adipose tissue
(fat in epidural space)

Dural sleeve

Denticulate ligaments

Spinal nerve

4.4 Dural sleeves and fatty tissue

Finally, along the spinal cord are fine ligaments called denticulate ligaments that arise from the pia mater around the cord. These anchor the spinal cord to the arachnoid and dural layers. Twenty-one pairs of these ligaments arise laterally between spinal nerve roots. Their function is to stabilize the spinal cord within the dural tube (Fig. 4.4). I have seen dissections of the spinal canal in which these internal ligaments have been severely torsioned, generating adhesions between the meningeal layers. This was clearly because of torsioning of the dural tube as a whole. These patterns are commonly generated by a torsioned relationship between the occiput and sacrum, and can also relate to rotations between vertebrae. Adhesions within the meninges due to the denticulate ligaments being torsioned will have a profound effect on the dynamics of potencies, fluids, and tissues. The drive of the fluid tide may be affected as potency becomes inertial in order to center the forces at work within the core of the system.

These kinds of issues will also directly influence the motility and mobility of the central nervous sys-tem. At the most caudal end of the dural sac, within the sacral canal, the pia mater pierces the dura to form the filum terminalis that anchors the end of the spinal cord to the coccyx. It is covered with a thin invest-ment of dura as it forms the filum terminalis. Any teth-ering of the filum terminalis due to compressive forces within the sacroiliac joints or pelvis will have a strong effect on the central nervous system and on the fluid drive and biodynamics of the system generally.

MOTILITY AND MOBILITY OF THE DURAL TUBE/CORE LINK

The membranes are always under tension as they express their inhalation/exhalation motion, first in one phase and then in the other. In other words, they are a unified tensile field of action. The motion of the membranes ideally has a natural point of balance—Suther-land's fulcrum, at the anterior aspect of the straight sinus. The leaves of the reciprocal tension membrane can be thought of as being suspended from the straight sinus and Sutherland's fulcrum. For a review of the motion dynamics of the reciprocal tension membrane, see Volume One, Chapter 12. In the inhalation phase, the dural tube generally rises superiorly. Simultaneously, the spinal cord subtly shortens towards the lamina terminalis of the third ventricle, and the fluid tide ascends. None of these motions are separate. They are generated all at once by the action of potency within the fluids. All tissue motion is a unit of function—the system is whole and is never fragmented. We are simply describing parts of a unit of function for purposes of inquiry and learning (Fig. 4.5).

Clinical Application: Palpating the Dural Tube and Sensing Patterns of Motion

Perceiving the primal midline is a good starting point for exploring the dural tube. An awareness of the midline allows you to more clearly see how the system is responding to session work. If the motion and organization of potencies, fluids, and tissues reorganize nearer to the midline, and to the natural fulcrums that relate to it (such as Sutherland's fulcrum), then you have a clear indication of progress. Let's do a simple perceptual exercise to see if you can include the whole dynamic of bone and membrane within your field of perception.

1. The simplest way to begin to tune into dural motion is to place your hands on the sacrum and occiput of your patient in the side-lying position. In this position, place your cephalad hand over the occiput with your fingers pointing superiorly and your caudad hand over the sacrum, fingers pointing inferiorly. Orient to the biosphere and mid-tide (Fig. 4.6).

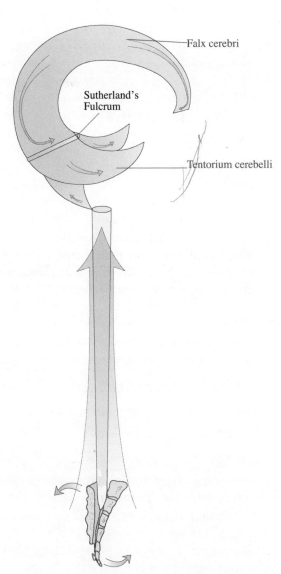

4.5 The reciprocal tension membrane and dural tube in inhalation

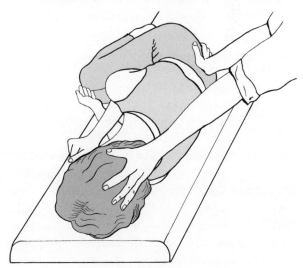

4.6 Sacrum and occiput hold in a side-lying position

2. First let your attention float on the bones being palpated. Let your hands be immersed within fluid. Sense the interrelated motions within the phases of primary respiration. In the inhalation phase, the squama of the occiput and the sacral base may be sensed to widen and rotate posteriorly into your palpating hands. This may feel like a filling within your hands. Fluids are ascending and the bones manifest an intraosseous expansion. Then include the dural tube in your perceptual field. Sense the occiput, sacrum, and dural tube as unified. In the inhalation phase, the dural tube will ideally rise, the sacrum will expand, its sacral base will rotate in a posterior-superior movement and the occipital squama will also expand and rotate inferiorly and posteriorly. The reverse will happen in the exhalation phase.

3. See if you can sense the motion of the dural tube rising and sinking in inhalation and exhalation. Just let your hands float on the tissues you are palpating and then shift your attention to the space between them. Let the system move you and its motion may become apparent.

As you do this, you may also notice various inertial patterns organized around particular fulcrums. You will begin to explore these shapes of experience in the sections below. You will also begin to relate to the specific structures and relationships that can affect the dynamics of the dural tube.

COMMON INERTIAL ISSUES RELATING TO THE DURAL TUBE

There are common somatic dysfunctions that will affect the dural tube and its ease of glide. Many of these unresolved forces may have traumatic origins. These include vertebral fixations, adhesions in the meninges and connective tissues within the spinal canal, local toxicity and edema, vertebral fixations, paravertebral tissue adhesions, and fascial resistances transferred to the area from other parts of the body. Please remember that all of these tissue changes are due to the presence of inertial potencies and experiential forces. Common sources of inertial issues include accidents, trauma, nerve facilitation, and visceral pathology. Traumatic forces, such as those encountered in car accidents or falls, may generate protective responses within dural tissues. This is most obvious in whiplash injuries where the cervical fascia and dura are strongly affected: connective tissues and membrane will express protective contraction. Force vector entrapment due to traumatic events can also affect dural mobility. Acute illnesses, such as meningitis or encephalitis, can also generate changes in the quality of dural tissue and adhesions in dural relationships. The following tissue patterns are effects of deeper forces at work. It is important to be able to relate to them in the context of those forces.

Vertebral Fixations

Fixation in vertebral dynamics can affect the mobility of the dural tube. Vertebral fixations and their related inertial patterns can be transferred to the dural tube via the dural sleeves that surround spinal nerves as they exit the vertebral canal. Thus, if vertebral mobility and function are compromised, dural function and mobility will also be compromised. Furthermore, vertebral fixations can directly affect the central nervous system. Their dynamics can be directly transferred to nerves as they leave the vertebral canal. Facilitation of nerves can result, as we will discuss later.

Fascial Adhesion and Contraction

The dynamics of the dural tube are continuous with all of the connective tissue relationships of the body. Any pattern of fascial strain can be transferred to the dural tube. Similarly, any inertial pattern within the dural tube can be transferred into the general connective tissue relationships of the body.

Dural Sleeves

It is not uncommon to sense adhesions between the dural tube and the connective tissues that line the spinal column. This is most common at, or near, the intervertebral foramina of the spinal column. As spinal nerves leave the spinal canal, they are invested with a sleeve of dura. These dural sleeves are continuous with the connective tissues that surround the spinal nerves and with paravertebral connective tissues. The dural tube is most vulnerable as its sleeves follow the nerve roots out of the vertebral column. The fatty tissue that separates the dura from the connective tissues lining the spinal canal thins out near the intervertebral canals. Somatic dysfunction in vertebral or paravertebral relationships can be fed into the dural tube at these locations. These patterns of vertebral fixation and paravertebral connective tissue contraction can be directly transferred to the dural tube. Adhesive fulcrums will be generated, and the dural tube's ability to glide freely will become compromised.

Transverse Relationships

Along the dural tube are found various transverse relationships that can directly affect its dynamics. Compression at either end of the dural tube will strongly influence its ease of glide. This includes the relationships of the *occipital triad* (occiput, atlas, and axis) at the superior pole, and the lumbosacral junction and sacroiliac joints at the inferior pole. These are very important areas to be aware of and to respond to clinically. Other transverse relationships include the thoracic inlet, the respiratory diaphragm, and the pelvic diaphragm (perineal floor). Contraction and adhesion found in any of these areas may compromise dural mobility and function.

Sacrum and Occiput

Think of the occiput, sacrum and dural tube as a unit of function. Any pattern of inertia within the dural tube will be directly transferred to the sacrum and occiput, and vice versa. The sacrum, occiput, and dural tube should ideally express their motility in an integrated and synchronous way. Inertial patterns from either side of this relationship will cause asynchronous motion. Mobil-

ity in occipital and sacral dynamics, and ease of dural glide within the spinal canal, are essential for a balanced and integrated motion.

Denticulate Ligaments

Resistances and adhesions between the layers of meninges in the spinal canal are most commonly found in relationship to the denticulate ligaments. The denticulate ligaments arise from pia mater all along the spinal cord, pierce the arachnoid layer, and anchor to the dura mater. They stabilize the spinal cord within the spinal canal. Any pattern of tension, compression or congestion in these relationships, and in vertebral or paravertebral tissues, will be transferred to the dural tube. These will also strongly influence the fluid dynamics within the subarachnoid space.

Tissue Changes

In all of these instances, the dural membrane may manifest local or global qualitative tissue changes. These may include loss of elasticity, a leathery feel to the tissues, densification of tissue, and even a sense of the dural tissues drying out and hardening. I have noted that extended usage of certain drugs can cause an extreme sense of dryness and loss of elasticity in dural tissues. This will strongly affect the biodynamics of the system, and the person involved may experience lowered constitutional vitality. I have also noted the effects of meningitis on dural tissues. Low grade inflammation and tissue densification can be a common result of infection.

Facilitated Segments

definition of facilitation

Vertebral fixations, dural adhesions, and visceral issues all may generate, and be generated by, nerve facilitation. In osteopathic terminology, the sensitization of a spinal nerve loop is called a *facilitated segment*. A facilitated segment is a segment of the spinal cord, including both sensory and motor nerves, that has become hypersensitive and has a lowered threshold of stimulation. Very small stimuli may cause the nerves involved to overreact and fire excessively. Vertebral fixations, dural adhesions, and visceral issues can all generate an overstimulation of a spinal nerve segment. This, in turn, will overstimulate the organs or muscles that relate to that segment, and a vicious cycle can be set up. The spinal nerve becomes hypersensitive and highly excitable. The hyperactivity in the spinal segment causes hyperactivity in the organs or muscles involved. The overstimulated organ or muscle sends back sensory stimuli to the spinal segment that keep the cycle going (Fig. 4.7). These can generate spinal fixation and dural adhesion. We will discuss this more in Chapter 18.

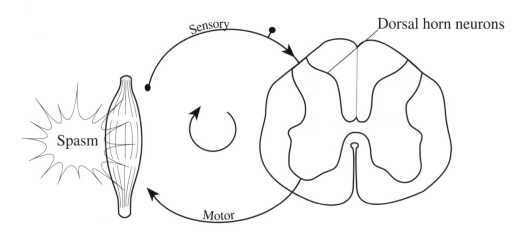

4.7 Hyper-sensitive nerve loop due to chronic vertebral compression, peripheral tissue damage, or inflammation

BIRTH TRAUMA

Birth trauma is another factor that influences dural tube mobility and the dural membrane generally. The whole of a person's birth history can be read in the dynamics of the dural membranes. I have had the pleasure of assisting William Emerson over the years in seminars dealing with prenatal and birth trauma. I was first amazed, and then deeply appreciative, of his ability to read the whole of a person's prenatal and birth history via the patterns held within the dural membranes.

During the birth process, the young system has to contend with extreme forces as it passes through the birth canal. Compressive forces during the birth process can introduce force vectors into the system. These forces can generate compression, torsion, and shear within the baby's tissue systems. This is especially true if the birth was experienced as traumatic and there was shock traumatization involved. In relationship to the dural tube, these inertial forces may set up patterns that may become habitual and restrict dural mobility in later life. These may include the compressive patterns discussed above and compression within the dural tube itself. It is not uncommon to find a dense and compressed dural tube whose etiology can be traced back to the compressive forces of birth. As practitioner, you may sense a shortened and dense dural tube whose compressive issues seem to be held within itself. The vertebral column may also hold axially compressive forces originating in the birth process. You may actually sense that potency has become inertial all through the core of the body in order to center unresolved axial compressive forces (Fig. 4.8).

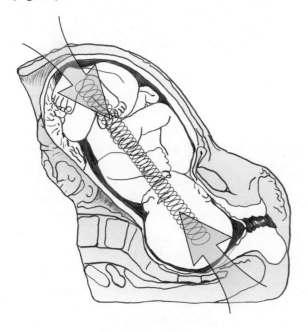

4.8 Axial birthing forces

The biokinetic forces involved may not be locally concentrated in particular inertial fulcrums; rather they are commonly spread throughout the core along the long axis. Whole areas of the spine may go into compression due to unresolved axial forces. Although these forces will generate localized fulcrums within vertebral and dural dynamics, we have to relate to these axial forces as a whole. Working with the intention of disengagement through the vertebral axis can help to liberate these forces. We will describe this in the next chapter, on vertebral dynamics.

Torsion and side-bending patterns within the sacrum or occiput, can originate in the birth process and these can give rise to twists and torsions within the dural tube itself. This will affect the dynamics of the denticulate ligaments, and meningeal adhesions can result. Whole body torsions that arise in the birth process can also be fed into the dural tube and affect the dynamics of the sacrum and occiput. All of this

depends on the length of time in labor, where and for how long the infant was stuck in any position, the relationship and connection between mother and baby, and whether any of this was experienced traumatically by the baby. We will go into this in much more detail in later chapters dealing with birth process.

Anesthesia during birth can induce what is known as "anesthesia shock." In this process, the fluid system may go into stasis. At birth the cerebrospinal fluid within the third ventricle ignites with potency. This occurs naturally at birth as the infant separates from its mother and must rely on its own resources. Shock traumatization and anesthesia can compromise this process. We will look at this issue in a later chapter. This will obviously impact the ability of the potencies, fluids, and tissues to express primary respiration and motility. The infant may also go into dissociative states that may continue throughout life unless they are addressed therapeutically. Because of all of these factors, the ability of the cerebrospinal fluid to express potency can be impeded. Indeed, the dynamics of the fluid tide itself may become compromised.

Shock traumatization will also affect the dural membranes, as they can go into chronic contraction as an effect of trauma. It must be remembered that it is the inertial forces involved that maintain all of these patterns within the system, and these must be addressed directly. It is within the state of balance and stillness that these forces can be initiated and processed.

Thus, there are many factors to consider when you are looking at the dynamics of the core link or dural tube. The most important thing is to listen and to be able to appropriately respond to what is communicated. All of the above dynamics will generate inertial issues. A reduced mobility of the dural tube and a reduction in the ease of its glide within the vertebral canal is a common result. This will become an inertial factor that may affect the whole of the system. It can generate inertial patterns anywhere within the system and can strongly influence the quality of mobility and motility throughout the body. As a result of the relationships of the core structures, everything attached to and within the dural membrane system will become less efficient in its expression of motion and motility. This includes the relationships of the cranial bones, the motility of the central nervous system, and the motion of the sacrum between the ilea. Dural tube inertia can strongly affect the relationship between the sacrum and the occiput and the ability of the sacrum to express balanced motion. Inertia within the dynamics of the core link can thus become an important fulcrum for the whole system. Reduced fluid drive, lowered expression of potency, and a general devitalization of the system can occur. The dynamics of potency and the fluctuation of cerebrospinal fluid will also be affected. This is probably the most important repercussion of core link inertial issues.

A Word of Caution

At this point we begin to explore specific tissues and relationships, and this will be our focus for most of the rest of this volume. Within all of the specifics in this and subsequent chapters, please remember that tissue effects such as compression, adhesion, strain, and resistance are not the issue. Tissue and fluid effects are compensations generated by the *action of forces* currently at work within the system. The clinical issues are the underlying forces that generate the effect and the potency that centers it. Wherever you have inertial effects, there are active forces at work in the present. The tissue and fluid changes are manifestations of these forces at work. It is important to have the clinical knowledge appropriate to the conditions being met. Then your knowledge will be used by the Breath of Life if you can hear its call. If the clinical knowledge and skill is not there, you cannot interface with this intention in precise and clear ways. You must have the clinical awareness and then put it aside. The Intelligence knows that you have this knowledge, and the Breath of Life will use you accordingly. Your knowledge and clinical skill generate safety and allow for clinical effectiveness. But remember that you are not doing the healing. The healing process is orchestrated by the Intentions of the Breath of Life, and it is your job to support and interface appropriately with these intentions.

In essence, with more clinical experience, you will find that you can largely leave fixations alone. They will take care of themselves when the forces at work are resolved. Even more deeply, they will be taken care of when the intention of the Breath of Life orients to the fulcrums involved. This is not the practitioner's decision to make; it is about humbly responding to the call of the Breath of Life and being a servant to its intentions, insofar as we can appreciate them. It is about serving and supporting and not getting in the way of the healing processes engaged from within. This is a function of the Inherent Treatment Plan and is not based upon the practitioner's mental processes or machinations. There are levels of work where our analysis and intervention will simply get in the way. Indeed, even our thoughts and intentions may get in the way at deeper levels of work. So the dictum "be still and know" is the imperative to follow as we orient to the Breath of Life and the unfoldment of the healing process. Having said all of this, it is crucial that we have the clinical skills that we need to be efficient and competent in this work.

Exploring Dural Relationships Via the Fluid System

In the following sections, we will begin an exploration into the dynamics and relationships of the dural tube. The first section focuses on the cerebrospinal fluid and its relationships within the dural tube. This will give information about the nature and quality of the spaces *within* the dural tube. Then we will sense dural dynamics by inducing a subtle traction into the dural membranes via the occiput. In both cases, we are initiating a conversation with the system, first through its fluids, and then through its membranes. This conversation will inform us about adhesions within the meninges and between the dural membrane and the spinal canal. It will also give information about any fascial pulls or resistances that are being transferred to the dural tube that may affect its ease of glide within the vertebral column.

Clinical Application: Fluid Direction

In this first process, we will begin to explore the dynamics of the dural tube via the cerebrospinal fluid within its spaces. The intention will be to start a conversation with the fluids and to respond to the communication received. We will be sensing and gaining information about the spaces between the dura and the spinal cord. You will be imagining that you are swimming down and through the dural spaces.

Another approach is to initiate a more direct conversation with the fluids within the dural tube by intending a direction of fluid from the heels of your hands caudad through the foramen magnum. This will initiate a conversation with the fluids. The resultant fluid response will tell you about the dynamics within the dural tube and show its patterns of inertia. When we place a subtle compression into fluids, their response will communicate to us the nature and quality of the inertial issues present.

1. With the patient in the supine position, place your hands in an occipital cradle. Orient to the biosphere and mid-tide. The patient's occiput should be comfortably supported by your hands. Your hands should be placed together under the patient's occiput with your fingers spread and pointing caudad. Be sure that you are not pressing on the occiput with the heels of your hands. Notice the quality of the fluid tide within the dorsal midline (Fig. 4.9).

2. From the occipital cradle, imagine that you are "swimming" within the cisterna magna. Starting at the foramen magnum, imagine that you can swim down the dural tube through the cerebrospinal fluid. Do this without narrowing your perceptual field. Perceive the spaces through which you are moving. You are beginning a conversation with the fluids and the spaces they inhabit. What are the spaces like here? How do you relate to them? Where is there backpressure within the fluid dynamics? As your awareness meets inertial fulcrums, you may sense resistance

to your swimming. Notice where your swimming is restricted. You may be able to sense the level of this resistance; perhaps this might be at a vertebral level, such as at T3 or L4. Perhaps it is at the level of a transverse relationship such as the respiratory diaphragm. Where does the dural tube become narrowed or thickened and your swimming become obstructed? You may sense an echoing back of fluids as you become aware of a more rigid resistance, such as a vertebral fixation, that is transferring its fixity to the meninges. Be open to the possibility that you can sense the information being communicated to you via the fluid system. After a number of practice sessions, you may be surprised at the accuracy of your perceptions.

3. Can you sense the different qualities of dural tissue as you swim down? Do you sense a densification of tissue, a drying out of tissue, a loss of elasticity or a leathery quality? You may also notice that your swimming has to take certain routes around the spinal column within the dural tube. As you meet torsions, shears, and other patterns within dural dynamics, you may sense that your awareness shifts in relationship to

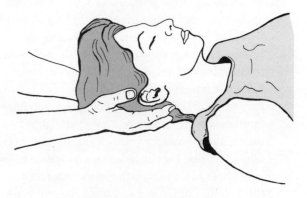

4.9 Occipital cradle hold

them. This may give you information as to the nature of these patterns and the shape of the spaces within the dural tube. Remember that torsion of the dural tube, and the vertebral and spinal columns, will generate torsion and possible adhesions within the relationships of the denticulate ligaments.

4. Some people get visual images such as colors and shapes as they swim through the spaces. If you do, try to sense a consistency in your images and reference them to the specific anatomy that you are exploring. What do the images or the colors mean? Build up your own vocabulary of how you gain information. As you become very familiar with the anatomy of the body, very clear anatomical images of the areas that you are exploring may become available to you. Have fun with this journey and you may be surprised at the accuracy of the information that arises.

5. As you swim down the spaces within the dural tube, you may encounter inertial fulcrums. One approach to the resolution of these fulcrums is to direct fluid and potency caudad from your occipital cradle toward the site of inertia. To do this, simply intend a movement of fluids via the heels of your hands from the cisterna magna, through the foramen magnum, toward the inertial site. You are directing potency through the spaces within the dural tube.

6. By intending a subtle compression into the fluids, you are initiating a conversation with them. If you initiate a conversation by directing fluids, you must listen to the story that is communicated to you. Note the responses of the cerebrospinal fluid to this intention. Note any echoing of fluid from the site. Listen to the echoing and fluid fluctuations that are communicated to you. What do they tell you? Wait for a sense of resolution. You may sense that the echoing stops and that there is a clearer sense of fluid fluctuation and motion through the area. When you sense the potencies, tissues, and fluids expanding and reorganizing, can you sense their new relationship to the mid-line and to Sutherland's fulcrum? Has the quality of the fluid tide changed?

THE PRINCIPLE OF TRACTION AND THE DURAL TUBE

In this section we will be using the principle of traction in relationship to the dural tube, or core link. When you introduce traction into membranes, they communicate their history to you. The suffering of that person and how it has become embodied in the tissues may be directly communicated. The traction must be offered in the spirit of conversation and inquiry, not as a demand to release anything.

In this exercise we are enquiring into the ease, or lack of ease, in the ability of the dural tube to glide within the vertebral canal. Engaging the membranes via a subtle intention of traction will help you sense the ease of glide between the dural tube and the structures it relates to. This will give you information about the nature of the adhesions between the dura and the structures around it.

Dural sleeves are in intimate relationship with local paravertebral tissues and are continuous with the connective tissues that cover nerves as they leave the spinal canal. Thus, inertial fulcrums located anywhere in the body may affect the dural tube and its ease of motion. A most important activity also occurs as the dural sleeves follow nerve roots out of the vertebral canal: small quantities of cerebrospinal fluid follow the dural sleeves out of the vertebral canal. Cerebrospinal fluid infuses the fluids of the body through these openings all along the vertebral column. It is an expression of the continuity of fluid dynamics within the body. Local tissue inertia can impede this exchange. Veteran practitioners maintain that this exchange occurs along all nerves and especially at synapses. It is a transmutation of potency from fluid to nerve and affects nerve function. It has also been discovered that cerebrospinal fluid leaves the dural canal via diffusion all along the length of the dural tube. This is an expression of the radiance of the potency of the Breath of Life all along its length. In the following section, we will explore the dynamics between the dural tube and the connective tissues of the vertebral column as well as local paravertebral relationships.

Clinical Application:
Traction of the Dural Tube

Continuing in the occipital cradle, shift your attention from the spaces within the dural tube to the relationship between the dural tissues and the vertebral canal and paravertebral tissues. In this process, you will engage the membranes in a cephalad traction via the occiput in order to initiate a conversation with them. You will sense your way caudad down the dural tissues. In the resulting conversation, the tissues may tell their story. As you engage the tissues in this conversation, you may sense patterns of inertia within their relationships and the inertial fulcrums that organize them. You may be able to sense specific sites of inertia, adhesion, and fixity that may be affecting the dynamics of the membranes. In the previous work with fluids, you were sensing within the spaces inside the dural tube. Here you are sensing the relationship of the dural tube to the connective tissues that line the vertebral canal.

1. Orient to the biosphere and mid-tide. Sense the quality of the fluid tide. This gives a baseline as to how the system can express its potency. At the occipital cradle, suggest a subtle cephalad traction through the dural tube via the occiput (Fig. 4.10). Remember that the connective tissue field is whole. As you intend your traction, hold a wide perceptual field. Bring the intention of traction to the field as a whole. The whole tissue field will respond to your intention all at once. As you suggest a superior traction, sense where the membranes seem inertial and cannot respond to your intention. Do not narrow your field of awareness to "find" the location; let it come to you as you hold the whole of the tissue field in your awareness. As you subtly intend a traction, the membranes will communicate their history to you, including any inertial fulcrums and patterns pres-

ent. These may include tissue effects of fixation and adhesion, patterns of torsion and side-bending, or other shapes and movements. The patterns may also include past traumas and the shock traumatization generated by them.

2. As you intend/suggest this cephalad traction, you may sense a boundary to your suggestion. It will feel like the dural tube cannot glide easily or is adhered at that level. Its ability to glide feels compromised. Remember that the boundary perceived is a site of inertial forces at work. These potencies and forces are generating an inertial fulcrum of some kind. See if you can sense the vertebral level of the perceived boundary. Do not lock the tissues up against this boundary. Listen for the space generated by your inquiry.

3. As space is accessed, help the potencies, fluids, and tissues access a state of balance. Once again, this is the key. It is within a systemic state of balance that the inertial potencies may be expressed and the relationship to the Breath of Life may be re-established. Wait within the stillness, and listen for expressions of Health. As potency is expressed, you may sense the biokinetic forces being processed and dissipated back to the environment. This may be perceived as heat or force

[handwritten notes:] ○ C.T. next to the dural tube. ○ space w/i the dural tube

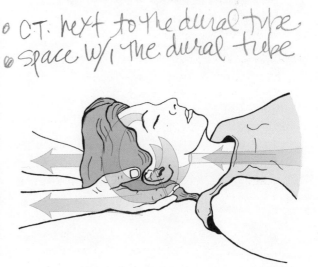

4.10   Traction of the dural tube via occipital hold

vector dissipation that is commonly sensed as a streaming of energy out of the body. You may then sense a softening, expansion, and resolution of the inertial forces and tissue effects involved. Potencies, fluids, and tissues are free to orient to their natural fulcrums. You may even sense a cerebrospinal fluid surge, and the dural tube may then be sensed to glide more easily. When you sense the potencies, tissues, and fluids expanding and reorganizing, can you sense their new relationship to the midline and to Sutherland's fulcrum? Has the quality of the fluid tide changed? Is it more forceful or potent?

If the inertia is intransigent and the inertial potencies cannot express themselves, you may also direct the fluid tide from your cradle hold through the foramen magnum. At the boundary of your intention of traction and within the state of balance, use the heels of your hands to direct fluids inferiorly toward the perceived inertial fulcrum. If inertial tissue effects such as tissue adhesion and compression have become very rigid and crystallized, you may sense the fluids echoing back to your sending hands. Wait for a sense of softening and ease within the inertial site. Again, you may sense a fluid surge through the area when the inertial forces resolve.

STRUCTURAL INTERRELATIONSHIPS

In the following chapters, we will introduce basic structural dynamics and related inertial issues that might affect the dural tube. I am not presenting this material in any kind of protocol. I am simply presenting the relationships of the body in a way that follows the embryological imperative, from the bottom up and from the center out. In clinical practice, protocols can get in the way of listening and allowing the Inherent Treatment Plan to unfold. Protocols have their uses in teaching and learning, but people are individuals, their healing needs are individual, and there are no rules here. The Breath of Life makes the decisions, not my limited human mentality.

In the following chapters, we will outline approaches to the major structural relationships within the human system. All of this must be incorporated into your palpation sense and become second nature. As the treatment plan expresses itself, you will hear the organization of the system and be able to respond accordingly. In this approach, you will not be learning new skills. You will simply be learning how to apply these skills within specific relationships. As you do this, a continual refinement of these skills will occur. Remember to have patience. Slowly, slowly is the way. Build up your knowledge and confidence and be open to the call of the Breath of Life and its potency.

5

Vertebral Dynamics

In this chapter, we will begin to explore the dynamics of the structures that develop around the primal, or notochord, midline. Whereas the dural tube surrounds the dorsal, or fluid, midline, the vertebral bodies form around the primal midline. As we introduce the various structural relationships of the body, the primal midline becomes an important reference point. Important clinical information may arise from an awareness of the dynamics of the primal midline and the suspended automatically shifting fulcrums that orient to it.

The vertebral column is directly organized around the primal midline as it forms embryologically in relationship to the notochord. As we have seen, the embryological imperative is expressed as a midline wave form within the embryonic disc. The notochord forms in relationship to this groundswell, and it then becomes the organizing axis for the fluid, cellular, and tissue world throughout life.

The basic biomechanics of the vertebrae will be introduced in this chapter. These must be experienced until they are second nature. The appropriate skill level will then naturally emerge as the inertial conditions within the patient's system arise in treatment sessions. Within a biodynamic context, tuning to the motility expressed within primary respiration, rather than orienting to biomechanical motion, will allow a more direct access to the Inherent Treatment Plan for that person. The Intelligence of the system will be sensed, and then you truly become a servant to the Breath of Life, rather than an orchestrator of technique.

> **In this chapter we will:**
> * *Explore the embryological imperative and its midline expression.*
> * *Review and deepen our appreciation of the dural tube and its relationship to vertebral dynamics.*
> * *Learn about basic vertebral mobility dynamics.*
> * *Learn to relate clinically to specific vertebral mobility and motility issues.*

VERTEBRAL DYNAMICS AND THE PRIMAL MIDLINE

In the following section you will apply your awareness of the primal midline to vertebral dynamics. This is a continuation of the work introduced in Chapter 2, "Formative Forces and Midlines." In this process you will monitor the midline and make a relationship to the inertial dynamics that have coalesced around it. Areas of tissue density or dryness, structural fixation, and fluid congestion are expressions of forces at work. These forces include the biokinetic forces that are maintaining the fixation and the potency of the Breath of Life that is centering them.

The intention here is to listen for the arising of the primal midline and to notice areas where its expression is not clear. As you tune into the uprising force within the midline, you may sense gaps or a lack of clarity in its expression. You are perceiving inertia, and condensations of potencies, fluids, and tissues that mask the expression of the arising force. The fountain spray of life is ever-present, but your awareness of it may be obscured by the presence of these core inertial issues. As traumatic forces enter the system, the potency of the Breath of Life becomes inertial to center and contain them. Fluids and tissues become inertial. Birth trauma is an example. The forces generated during the birthing process are very strong and can be focused along the spinal axis. The potency of the Breath of Life becomes inertial along this axis in order to center and contain the effects of the traumatic forces. If these forces are not processed during the time of the trauma, then they become inertial fulcrums that must be centered and contained.

Clinical Application: Accessing the Primal Midline and Vertebral Issues

In the following process we will make a relationship to an inertial vertebral area. While holding an awareness of the primal midline, we will then orient to the state of balance. As the primal midline comes into your awareness, it may be sensed as an uprising force within the centerline of the vertebral bodies. I have heard practitioners describe it as a wind within the midline, as a geyser, and even as a volcano. It may be sensed as airy yet powerful—sometimes as a gentle breeze, other times more like a tornado. It may appear as a hot air shaft in which air is always ascending. As you catch this with your awareness, it like hitching a ride on this air stream. It seems to arise at the coccyx and disappear into space at the ethmoid bone. Stone called it the fountain spray of life. The structural axis of the body forms in relationship to it, from the coccyx through the vertebrae and the cranial base. The primal midline is a function of the ordering matrix laid down by the action of the Long Tide. You can sense the Long Tide acting through this midline as a centering and organizing force. Sometimes, you may even have the sense that the deep, epigenetic force orchestrated by the Long Tide appears in the space

around you, enters the midline, and surges toward a fulcrum to initiate healing processes.

1. With the patient in the supine position hold the sacrum in the sacral hold with your caudad hand. Establish your practitioner fulcrums and hold the biosphere within your perceptual field. Settle into this first. Then slowly widen your perceptual field toward the horizon. Gently listen to wider and wider fields of action. Do not lose awareness of the person's tissues and the particulars within the field. Also establish elbow fulcrums and hold the sacrum spaciously. Do not physically or mentally grab onto it. Imagine that your hand is beneath the table giving the sacrum a lot of space. Even though there is weight on your hand, see if you can float below the tissues of the sacrum.

2. Maintaining a wide perceptual field, gently bring your attention to the biosphere and primal midline (Fig. 5.1). Orient yourself to the ordering field around the patient, and to the midline from

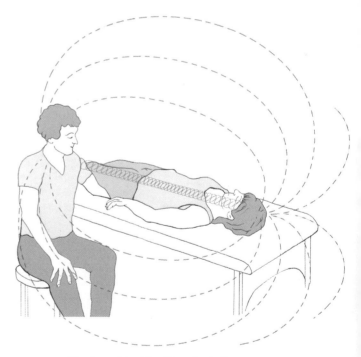

5.1 Sacral hold with orientation
to the ordering matrix

the coccyx through the center of the vertebral bodies and cranial base. Do not narrow your perceptual field as you do this. Simply orient to it within a wide field of awareness and let the felt-sense of the midline come to you. Don't look for it; listen for it. Have patience; don't immediately try to sense anything. This may take a number of minutes. Don't rush; see if you can let go of any anxiety about perceiving something.

3. Once you begin to sense the uprising force within the midline, notice how it is expressed. You may sense a smooth expression arising through the midline and vertebral bodies. You may also sense areas of backpressure or gaps in its expression. These indicate inertial potencies, fluids, and tissues. These generally manifest as compressive patterns, fixation, and congestion within the dynamics of the vertebrae. These inertial issues

in different areas of the spine may mask the midline expression of the Breath of Life and may make this uprising force difficult or even impossible to sense. This is especially the case if axial compression and related shock affects are being centered within and around vertebral tissue.

4. Wherever you sense a gap or backpressure, place your other hand under the spinous processes of that vertebral level and listen to its dynamics. Again, don't do anything. Listen. Sense the inertial dynamic at that vertebral level (Fig. 5.2). Listen to the inertial pattern through the tissues and help access the state of balance. While you do this, try to maintain awareness of the midline and of the larger whole. Try to maintain a wide perceptual field as you facilitate the state of balance. Let the state of balance be the gateway into the deeper forces at work within the field around

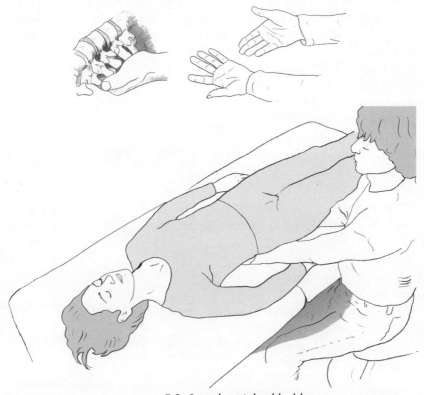

5.2 Sacral-vertebral hold

69

and within the patient. Within the state of balance listen for expressions of Health. Without losing your awareness of field phenomena and of the whole of the patient at the center of that field, open your awareness to fluids and potency. Can you sense an initiation of the inertial potencies within the inertial fulcrum? Do you sense a permeation of potency from the midline into that area? Can you sense a more general permeation of potency? As the inertia resolves within the fulcrum, notice how the midline is expressed. Is there a clearer expression of the midline through the area? Does the fountain spray clarify?

5. Once the inertial issue is resolved, can you sense the tissue elements realigning to the midline? This is their natural embryological centerline and organizing axis. Allow this to occur. It may take some minutes for the tissues to reorganize.

One way to approach clinical work is to allow your awareness of midline phenomena to lead you to the healing priorities of the system. Remember the dic-tum, *the treatment plan is inherent within the disturbance.* You are simply learning to orient to that plan. As you deepen your relationship with the action of the Breath of Life within the midline, you will be led to the inertial fulcrums that the Breath of Life has prioritized for healing. You may notice that it is not so much about what you do as practitioner, but more about how you are. It is an unfolding process that must be allowed space and time.

VERTEBRAL DISCS AND SUSPENDED AUTOMATICALLY SHIFTING FULCRUMS

All structure and function is naturally oriented to the primal midline and automatically shifting fulcrums. The motility and motion of the vertebra, and of the vertebral column as a whole, naturally orient to the midline. As we have seen, the vertebrae form in relationship to the notochord and the notochord forms directly in relationship to the primal midline (Fig. 5.3).[1] Some classic automatically shifting fulcrums are Sutherland's fulcrum, the sphenobasilar junction (SBJ) and the lamina terminalis. However, there are many

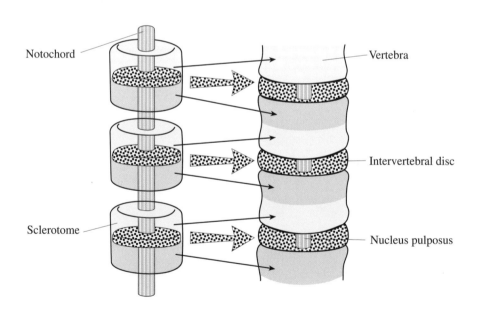

Notochord

Sclerotome

Vertebra

Intervertebral disc

Nucleus pulposus

5.3 The vertebrae form in relationship to the notochord

other natural fulcrums throughout the body. Stone noted that the disc between each vertebra acts as an orienting fulcrum for that local vertebral relationship. The intervertebral disc is literally a remnant of the notochord. The fulcrum within the disc can be thought of as a point of potency ideally located within its center (Fig. 5. 4). This is a suspended automatically shifting fulcrum that shifts within the phases of the Tide. It rises cephalad in inhalation and settles in exhalation. As seen in Chapter 2, the Breath of Life organizes form and shape by laying down fulcrums and axes in space. In this process, space is literally enfolded to generate the ordering matrix of form.

The vertebral column moves in relationship to the midline and to these automatically shifting fulcrums. Many practitioners consider the sphenobasilar junction (SBJ) to be the most cephalad fulcrum of the vertebral column and its major point of orientation. An awareness of the nature of these fulcrums can give the practitioner important information about the overall organization of the system. For instance, after an inertial fulcrum is processed, especially a vertebral or cranial base fulcrum, you may sense vertebral structures shifting back towards the midline and these automatically shifting fulcrums. No adjustment or force is necessary to achieve this. You may also sense the subtle rising of the vertebra cephalad in inhalation as the vertebral column as a whole subtly shortens towards the SBJ and Sutherland's fulcrum. An awareness of these dynamics can lead you directly to the fulcrums organizing eccentric and inertial patterns.

On Structural Balance

All structural dynamics relate to how vertebrae, and tissue structures generally, orient to the primal midline, suspended automatically shifting fulcrums, and to unresolved inertial forces. If a system is totally free of inertia, an ideal balance of structure, function, and motion ensues. If no inertial fulcrums are present within the body, the organization of structure around the midline is more likely to be symmetrical with an easy balance relative to the forces of gravity. Reciprocal tension motion would be completely oriented to the midline and to suspended automatically shifting fulcrums in an easy and balanced way (Fig. 5.5).[2]

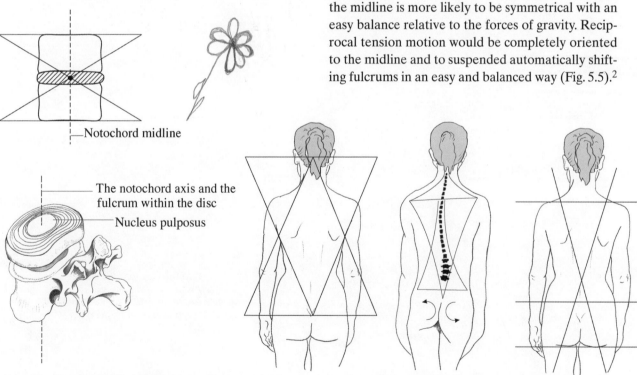

Notochord midline

The notochord axis and the fulcrum within the disc
Nucleus pulposus

5.4 The automatically shifting fulcrum within the disc

5.5 Images of structural balance

As we center life's conditions and inertial fulcrums are generated, our system must shift from this ideal balance to compensate for the conditions present, and structural compensations inevitably arise.

This does not mean that we become unbalanced or fragmented. Balance is always maintained, albeit in a compensated manner. Wholeness is never really lost; our system simply compensates for the nature of our unresolved experience, and these added forces must be centered within the whole in some way. The Breath of Life and its potency always maintain a balance of structure and function. But there is a price to pay for the need to contain and compensate for these unresolved forces. Tissues change in quality, form distorts, potency becomes bound in centering the conditions present, and vitality is reduced. The stage is set for the arising of pathology and pain. But even in the most pathologically desperate and painful conditions, balance is never really lost, the midline is ever-present, and a reorientation to the imperative of the Breath of Life is always possible (Fig. 5.6).

The issue is not about ideal structural balance, nor even about lesions, tissue and fluid effects and pathology. This approach is about resolving that which is unresolved within our system and reorienting to the Health that is never lost. It is about completing what we have not been able to complete and resolve, and sensing Health and Intelligence within all conditions. In the midst of a busy clinical practice, we must remember that this Health centers all of the conditions present, as a whole, all at once, within the totality of our body-mind-spirit experience.

Structure embodies the nature of our experience. The anatomical form of our body is a direct manifes-

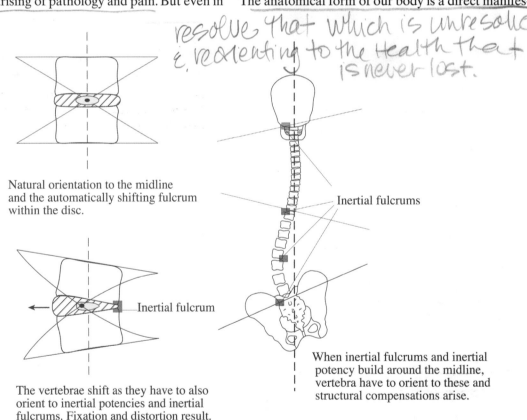

resolve that which is unresolved & reorienting to the Health that is never lost.

Natural orientation to the midline and the automatically shifting fulcrum within the disc.

Inertial fulcrums

Inertial fulcrum

The vertebrae shift as they have to also orient to inertial potencies and inertial fulcrums. Fixation and distortion result.

When inertial fulcrums and inertial potency build around the midline, vertebra have to orient to these and structural compensations arise.

5.6 Structural compensation

tation of the interchange between the ordering matrix laid down by the Breath of Life and the conditional forces of experience. Unresolved experience is centered as a whole within the body-mind. Structural balance is a direct manifestation of the centering function of the Breath of Life and directly expresses our life experience. The ability to relate to structural patterns and structural balance is a necessary clinical skill.

Anatomy does not lie; understanding structural positioning gives the practitioner an entry into the nature of that person's life experience and their healing processes. Structurally oriented healing forms, such as Osteopathy, Chiropractic, and Rolfing have evolved due to the importance of structural balance and midline inertial issues within the overall function of the body-mind. Structural readings are an essential part of the diagnostic process in these systems. Structural awareness is also seen within many forms of indigenous bodywork, such as Thai massage and manipulation, Chinese massage and acupressure, Ayurvedic massage, and many others evolving over many centuries. A working knowledge of structural issues is also essential for clinical efficiency in the biodynamic craniosacral approach.

I believe Osteopathy's orientation to Health is unique in Western medicine. Andrew T. Still, the founder of Osteopathy, consistently directed his students to listen for the Health as a starting point. Emphasizing Health challenges our prevailing modern medical culture that has such a combative and aggressive preoccupation with disease. Still's words inspire a deep examination of what Health is and how to hear its constant call. An orientation to Health deeply shifts the clinician's intentions and clinical work. It is something that must be developed and nurtured over time. It can be very hard to shift from our cultural conditioning. We tend to see disease as something to be conquered, and thus we polarize our experience of health and illness.

important perspective to healing & health & disease

VERTEBRAL FIXATION AND INERTIAL ISSUES

Vertebral fixation is a manifestation of tissue organization around inertial forces and their related fulcrums. Unless these inertial forces are resolved in some way, they will become organizing factors for vertebral motion and tissue quality. Their origins may be in falls, accidents, or birth processes. Postural issues and genetic overlays will also come into play. Some spinal issues will even have their origins in the prenatal experience. Due to the presence of inertial forces within the core of the system, vertebral motion and motility will become compromised, tissues will undergo changes in quality, and fluids will become static. As vertebrae orient to inertial fulcrums and the forces within them, orientation to the midline and primary respiration will be affected. Structural compensation will result. Mobility restrictions are thus compensatory to the action of inertial forces as they are centered by the potency within the system. When potency becomes inertial around the core of the system, vitality can be strongly affected.

Individual vertebral fixations commonly relate to inertial forces affecting a wide area within the spine and midline. Traumatic forces introduced into the longitudinal axis of the vertebral column can generate compressive issues within the vertebral column. These are called *axial forces.* Birth process is a common origin for this kind of wide ranging inertial force.

Patterns of vertebral fixation are called *lesions* or *somatic dysfunctions* in classical osteopathy. These terms denote an area of clinically significant tissue and fluid change and may include connective tissue contraction, bony fixation, local edema and fluid congestion, tissue changes such as thinning, dryness and/or densification, and tissue adhesion. These patterns may also include nerve involvement and facilitation. Loss of motility and mobility of tissues is the result.

As we have seen, the dural tube is a core link between cranium and pelvis, and specifically between occiput and sacrum. It should be able to glide relatively freely within the vertebral column between these two poles (see Fig. 4.3). The relationship between the dura and the vertebrae is most vulnerable within the intervertebral foramen. The layer of adipose tissue that lubricates the vertebral canal becomes thinner at these points. Any fixation or misalignment in vertebral dynamics will be directly transferred to dural dynamics at these vulnerable areas (see Fig. 4.4). If vertebral mobility and function are compromised, dural function, mobility, and motility will also be compromised, leading to inertial patterns. Furthermore, vertebral fixations can directly affect the central nervous system. Vertebral inertia can be directly transferred to nerves as they leave the vertebral canal, causing nerve facilitation.

As we enter an exploration into vertebral dynamics, it is important to reiterate that in biodynamic terms, inertial patterns are all expressions of biodynamic and biokinetic potencies. The art of this work is to facilitate a realignment to the embryological imperative and to the inherent ordering principle of the Breath of Life. As ones' appreciation of these factors deepens, the practitioner shifts from a lesion-based orientation to a focus on potencies and forces, and finally to the ordering matrix and the Breath of Life that centers it all.

ORIGINS OF VERTEBRAL FIXATIONS

Vertebral fixation and inertia can arise from many factors, including:

- Unresolved birth trauma.
- The forces of accidents and falls.
- The forces of traumatic experiences.
- Postural issues.
- Shock traumatization.
- Fluid congestion.
- Inflammatory processes and related tissue changes.
- Compensations for other inertial fulcrums and processes in the body.
- Pathogens and degenerative diseases.
- The forces of genetics.

SENSING VERTEBRAL INERTIA

In the clinical application above, you oriented to the primal midline in order to sense inertial issues within vertebral dynamics. You can also use the work learned in our previous chapter as a way into the dynamics of the vertebrae. This gives you another option for orienting to vertebral issues. From an *occipital cradle hold,* you can sense down the dural tube as in the last chapter. Very gently suggest/intend a superior tractioning of the dural tube as previously learned. Maintain a wide field of awareness when you do this. See if you can become aware of any inertia or boundary to this intention. If you do sense any inertia via either approach, see if you can locate the vertebral level that seems to organize the resistance. Working via dural traction or by an awareness of the primal midline, you will then practice some of your clinical skills in relationship to the inertial fulcrums perceived.

FLUID DIRECTION WITHIN THE SPINAL CANAL

In the process outlined below, you will be directing the potency within the cerebrospinal fluid to areas of vertebral inertia and fixation. The intention will be to begin a conversation about vertebral inertia and fixation via the potency within the fluids. Local issues may include vertebral fixations, fluid congestion, tissue contraction, tissue changes (such as densification or dryness of membrane), and nerve involvement. Dural tube and vertebral fixation will generate whole-body patterns and can also compensate for other inertial issues in the body.

Remember that the inertial fulcrums you discover are organized and maintained by inertial potencies and forces. Sensing the fulcrum that organizes an inertial issue is a skill that develops over many years. Keep the inquiry going and the information will come to you.

Once an inertial fulcrum is sensed, the intention is to access the potencies and forces at work and to initiate a process of reconnection and reorientation to natural fulcrums and to the groundswell of the Breath of Life. Starting with a mid-tide level of perception *the goal*

and widening your perceptual field from there, the deeper forces of the matrix and beyond may also be accessed. After a while this perceptual process becomes very organic and your perceptual field will naturally vary to match the level of action within and around the patient's system, shifting easily from mid-tide to CRI or Long Tide with a natural orientation to the Dynamic Stillness.

Clinical Application:
Directing Fluids along the Spinal Axis

In the clinical application below, you will sense areas of inertia and direct fluids and potency to them. As you direct fluid to the vertebra being palpated, you are also initiating a conversation with the tissues involved. While you monitor the response to your fluid direction, you may sense the vertebra moving. As it expresses motion, it is showing you its history. Remember to hold that with respect. A clear and present communication is being offered to you. Access the state of balance and orient to the Health that centers the conditions present. The only difference from previous work is that here you are using your skills in relationship to a specific vertebra instead of a wider area.

1. With the patient in the supine position (face up), hold the head in the occipital cradle position. Orient to the mid-tide. Monitor the quality of the fluid tide and its fluid drive. Initiate a conversation with the dural tissues by introducing a subtle cephalad traction via the occiput. Notice which vertebral level seems to be inertial.

2. Move the patient to a prone position and place one hand at the top of the head, superior to the foramen magnum. Place your other hand over the inertial area, with the center of your palm over the spinous processes. Tune into the cerebrospinal fluid and the fluid tide. Subtly direct fluids inferiorly from the foramen magnum through the spinal axis.

3. To initiate this conversation, intend a push against the fluids with a gentle sense of pressure from the hand on top of the head toward the receiving hand over the vertebral area. In essence, you are really directing the potency within the fluids to the inertial site. You suggest an intention and the potency takes over. As you direct fluids, you are engaging in a conversation. Listen for the response. You may perceive echoes from dense areas, lateral fluctuations of fluid, or spirals of fluid and potency around and within the inertial area.

4. Your lower hand monitors the response to the fluid direction. If there is strong fluid drive, the response will be almost immediate. You are listening for echoing of fluids from the resistant site, lateral fluctuations, vertebral and connective tissue motions and expressions of potency within the inertial area. First you may notice intensification of fluid drive and potency locally. You may sense a surge of potency within the fluids. You may sense potency and fluid being reflected back to your sending hand like an echoing against a rigid barrier. You may sense local patterns of lateral fluctuation near the receiving hand or expressions of potency within the vertebral and tissue patterns.

5. As you direct fluid to the area, the vertebrae being palpated may begin to express their patterns of inertia through motion. When motion is detected, listen for an inertial pattern to clarify. Help access the state of balance. Listen for a settling of the tissues into a state of balance and a deepening into stillness. The inertial tissue motions will seem to stop and settle. This is a state of dynamic equilibrium within all of the force factors and tensile patterns present. Within this, also listen for the initiation of inertial potencies and the welling up of potency within the inertial fulcrum. As the inertial potency centering the disturbance begins to be expressed, you may sense a deeper welling up of potency within the heart of the inertial pattern. You may also sense the biokinetic forces that maintain the disturbance being dissipated back to the environment as released heat and energy.

6. When the inertial forces have been processed, the tissue elements will begin to move again. The term unwinding has been used to describe what happens here, but I prefer other language. To me, this is not an "unwinding" process. This is an expression of reorientation and reorganization as discussed in Becker's three-phase process. When the inertial fulcrum that was organizing the resistance is resolved, the tissues will naturally reorient to the embryological fulcrums and midlines of the system. Give this realignment process the space and time it needs. Wait for a clear expression of the fluid tide and of tissue motility before you end contact.

Options

If you sense a specific vertebral fixation at a particular level of the spine, you may want to make a more specific and direct relationship to it. To do this, you can change the positioning of your lower hand by placing your index and middle fingers over the transverse processes of the specific vertebra being palpated. The fingertips are placed in the grooves on either side of the spinous process. This position gives more specific access to the individual vertebra (Fig. 5.7).

Another alternative is to first access a state of balance within the vertebral pattern, and then to direct fluid to the vertebral area. This reverses the sequence described above. Once you determine the vertebral level that is exhibiting inertia, place your hand over it and listen to its dynamics. As the vertebra shows you its patterns, help its tissues access their state of balance; then, within this state of balance, direct fluid from above. Continue to direct fluid until a reorganization of the vertebra is palpated.

BIOMECHANICS, BIODYNAMICS, AND SPECIFIC VERTEBRAL DYNAMICS

In order to have a clear physiological relationship to vertebra, it is useful to have an awareness of their mobility dynamics. The more specifically you can relate, anatomically and physiologically, to a particular inertial issue, the clearer will be your relationship to it. I would like to differentiate between the structural, biomechanical motions you might motion test for, and the inherent motions of motility generated within the phases of primary respiration. Biomechanics is about how we orient to gravity, how we use leverage, and how we move through life. Joints have mobility and allowable motions. We can flex and

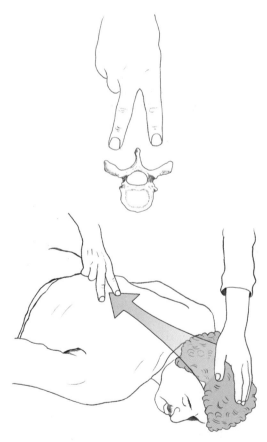

5.7   Direction of fluid through vertebral axis

extend our arms and legs and we can voluntarily move ourselves through the world.

However, a biomechanical orientation in clinical practice is not just about the natural biomechanics of joints and tissue structures. It is also about our clinical approach to the body's patterning and how we conceive of and relate to our human condition. In a purely biomechanical orientation, the human system might be conceived to be a mechanism with clockwork-like parts. This idea is derived from a vision of the universe which goes back to Descartes. A human being is likened to a clockwork mechanism, and perfect health is likened to the perfect functioning of all its parts. Within a classical biomechanical framework, the practitioner commonly orients to the allowable motion of joints and sutures and conceives of that motion in relationship to axes and direction of motion around those axes. Clinically, the practitioner may tend to orient to motion testing, resistance, and boundaries. The work then becomes based on releasing resistance and shifting lesions.

In the following sections, we will introduce the basic biomechanics of vertebral relationships and you will learn a specific clinical approach. This approach will allow you to explore the local tension dynamics and motion tendencies of a vertebra. The intention here is to acquaint students who may not have an understanding of biomechanics with some of these concepts and relationships. It will allow a more precise access to the inertial forces and issues within their dynamics. We are offering this in the context of a "conversation" with the tissues of the body. Motion testing will orient you to local mobility and resistance dynamics for learning purposes. We hope this will allow a clearer relationship to fixation and compensatory patterns. Once you have a sense of these motion dynamics, then a shift to a more biodynamic awareness is easier, and a sense of the precision of the motion generated within primary respiration becomes clearer.

Within a biodynamic context, the motions we listen for are those of motility, or inherent motion, within the inhalation and exhalation phases of the Tide. We orient to motility within the phases of primary respiration as we wait for the Inherent Treatment Plan to unfold. Motility will become conditioned relative to the forces at work within the system and will express motion relative to these forces. Mobility restrictions and voluntary axial motion are secondary to this deeper dynamic.

VERTEBRAL MOTILITY AND MOBILITY DYNAMICS

Vertebrae express their motility relative to the midline that they organize around. In inhalation, there is a subtle rising and shortening of the vertebral axis towards the SBJ. Each vertebra individually expresses a shortening top-to-bottom and a widening side-to-side. The shortening of the spinal axis is similar to the shortening of the neural axis in inhalation towards the lamina terminalis. This is the essence of their expression of primary respiration. All tissues within the body are following the action of the potency within the fluids as a unified field of action.

Each vertebra has four sets of articular surfaces called facets, two articulations with the vertebra above and two with the vertebra below, and a disc above and below also. Thus, each vertebra typically has six joint relationships, although there is no disc between C1 and C2. In the inhalation phase, space is generated within these joint relationships.

The mobility and voluntary motion of the vertebrae are largely governed by the facets of the articulations between them. In the lumbar area these facets are largely oriented vertically in an anterior to posterior plane. This allows for little individual rotation. The lumbar spine will generally rotate as a whole. It also gives some protection in lateral bending and allows the lumbar spine to express a good forward and backward bending. The motion of the thoracic spine is largely governed by the more transverse orientation of its facets, and by its relationship to the rib cage. The thoracics allow for more rotation and lateral bending than the lumbars. This helps compensate for the stability and containment offered by the ribs. The cervical area has the most allowable motion. Its facets are oriented more or less transversely, and this permits much rotation and lateral bending. Much

Much rotation is also allowed around the dens of the second cervical vertebra.

The ease of motion in the cervical area allows mammals to easily orient to their environment and to danger. In their orienting response, animals will momentarily freeze and then will calmly rotate the head via their cervical area to scan their surroundings. This high degree of cervical freedom has a cost. The cervical area is most vulnerable to whiplash injuries and to tension via the stress response. Proprioceptive and motion information goes directly from the cervical area to the locus ceruleus, an important pair of nuclei in the stress response. Thus, tension held within the neck area is commonly related to unresolved stress and autonomic cycling. The cervical area also bears the weight of the head and is thus vulnerable to postural stress.

where is this?

BASIC VERTEBRAL MOTION DYNAMICS

Vertebrae move in relationship to each other in very specific ways. Vertebral relationships, like any other joint dynamic, will have a natural range of motion. These dynamics are dictated by the relationships of the articular facets to each other, by the intervertebral discs between vertebrae, by adjacent structures such as ribs, and by the connective tissue and muscular relationships between and around them. The basic movements possible for the vertebrae are *forward and backward bending,* which occurs around a transverse axis, *rotation* or torsion, which occurs around a vertical axis, *side-bending,* which occurs around an anterior-posterior axis, *anterior-posterior glide,* and *lateral glide.* Finally, *compression* can occur between vertebrae, when one vertebra is compressed superiorly or posteriorly in relationship to another (Fig. 5.8).

In the following sections, you will learn to relate to vertebral fixations in specific ways. In this work, you will first palpate the *mobility* dynamics of the vertebrae. The vertebra can move in six basic directions and can become fixated in any of them. As you palpate these dynamics, you will sense the local tensions present and will help access the *point of balanced ligamentous tension.* This is similar to the point of balanced membranous tension previously discussed. Let's first list the important landmarks which allow you to know which vertebral level you are palpating. Once all of this is second nature, you will gain an intuitive knowing of which vertebra is involved.

Locating Vertebra via Spinal Landmarks

- Atlas: The atlas has no palpable spinous process. You can feel its transverse processes and articular masses slightly posterior to the mastoid process of the temporal bone (in the groove just posterior to the mastoid process).

- Axis: This is the first spinous process that you can palpate just below the foramen magnum. Laterally to this, you will be on its articular masses.

- C7: The next landmark is C7, the vertebra prominens. It is called this because it is usually the most prominent vertebra at the top of the shoulders, although sometimes T1 is actually more prominent. You can determine the vertebra prominence with the patient in a sitting position. Place one fingertip on the most prominent spinous process and another one on the spinous process above it. Then have the patient move their head forward and backward. When the head moves backward, if the upper vertebra is C6, it will move anterior and seem to disappear. If the upper vertebra disappears, it is C6 and the vertebra prominens is C7. If the upper vertebra does not "disappear" to your touch, it is C7, and in that case the vertebra prominens is T1.

- T7: In the prone position, T7 is commonly level with the bottom of the scapulae. In the sitting position, T8 is usually level with the bottom of the scapulae.

- T12: To find T12, follow the last floating rib up to the spine.

- L3: Usually located at the level of the waist.

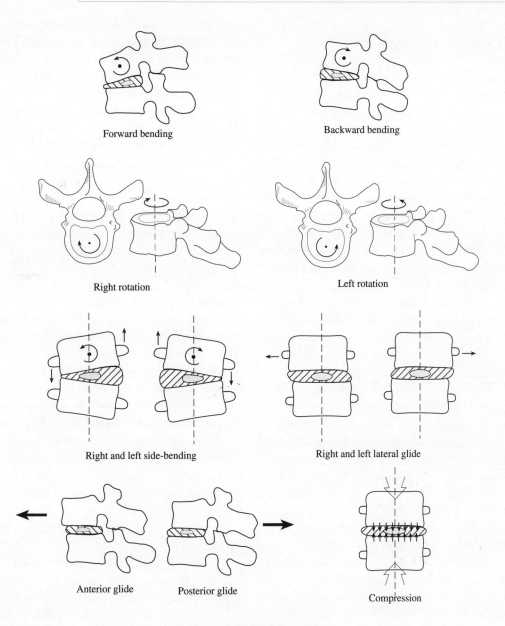

Forward bending

Backward bending

Right rotation

Left rotation

Right and left side-bending

Right and left lateral glide

Anterior glide

Posterior glide

Compression

5.8 Basic vertebral dynamics

- L4: Usually located level with the tops of the iliac crests.

- L5: The spinous process of L5 is often hard to feel. It is located in the hollow just above the sacrum.

THE POINT OF BALANCED LIGAMENTOUS TENSION

In the following sections I will introduce some basic clinical approaches to vertebrae and their motion tendencies. One classic approach is to motion test for the motions allowable within a vertebral relationship. There are different levels of motion testing within traditional manipulative practice and I will describe a few and then focus on balanced ligamentous tension.

One of the first kinds of motion testing I was taught was to literally move a vertebra around its axes of motion in order to discover the preferred directions of motion. This is traditionally called the *direction of ease* or *preferred motion*. For example, I might hold a vertebra and then physically move it around its axes in the different directions of potential motion, such as forward and backward bending, torsion, and sidebending. I would then choose the clearest motion preferences and take the vertebra in that direction until a barrier was perceived. Then a technique would be applied in an attempt to release the vertebra from the resistances holding it in that direction. This might have been a direct or indirect manipulation, an articular technique such as rocking the vertebra in certain ways, or a gentle functional approach that orients the tissues to physical respiration.

In a similar motion testing approach, I learned to inquire into the various motion tendencies of a particular vertebra around the classic axes and to *stack* the tendencies discovered. As each direction of ease was perceived, I would stack one tendency upon the next and very precisely reflect the mobility issues found at that vertebral level. At the culmination of the process, I would be holding the sum total of the conditioned tendencies of that specific vertebra. The next step was to access the point of balanced ligamentous tension within this stacked form. This was at first very tedious, but it did give me a good sense of the mobility dynamics of that vertebra.

In the work I will be asking you to explore, we will take another approach. This was taught to me in osteopathic apprenticeship, and I think it is a very gentle

way into the motion tendencies within a vertebral relationship. The heart of this process is to more openly explore the tension patterns perceived and to obtain a precise neutral within them: the point of balanced ligamentous tension. This is a local tension neutral within the relationships being palpated. I will describe this for the cervical area and then for the thoracic and lumbar areas.

WORKING WITH CERVICAL PATTERNS

In your previous session work you may have sensed cervical fulcrums, compressive issues, and related tissue effects. The cervical area has a relatively free range of motion compared to the rest of the spine. The dynamics of the atlas and axis are totally integrated with the occiput and cranial base. The mobility dynamics of the cervical spine are a unit of function with cranial base and occiput. The neck is a connecting link where the spinal cord, the throat, and many major nerves and vessels negotiate their way through a very narrow area. The cervical vertebrae also enable the orienting response, in which we turn the head to scan the environment and identify threat. Unresolved autonomic stress responses can generate tension in the cervical area. The neck often becomes tense as we constantly engage the orienting response in the everyday stresses of modern life. The cervical area is a common place for stress to be expressed as physical tension, vertebral fixation, and connective tissue restriction.

The dramatic and sometimes traumatic forces of the birth process can also leave an imprint in cervical dynamics. The cervical area often holds birth-related compressive forces and related effects such as compression, torsion, and cervical tension and pain. Tension headaches commonly have origins in cervical dynamics. Due to the continuity of connective tissue and membranous relationships, inertia in the cervical spine influences the cranial base and thus directly affects the dynamics of the sphenoid, occiput, and temporal bones. This obviously has important repercussions for the whole of the system. The fascia of the cervical area is also continuous with the fascia of the cranium, neck, thoracic, and abdominal areas. There are continuous fascial relationships from the base of the skull, through the cervical fascia, to the thoracic inlet, pericardium of the heart, the thorax, the respiratory diaphragm, the abdomen and pelvis (Fig. 5.9).[3]

Other considerations may also be important when relating to the cervical area. Tibetan Buddhists consider the neck to be the seat of ego. We "take it in the neck" when our ego processes are overwhelmed by our experience. The neck is also the traditional location of the throat chakra. This chakra is closely associated with issues revolving around space and boundaries. Thus, issues that especially relate to space seem to affect the neck and its tissue relationships. When the feeling of space in life closes down, the cervical area closes down. The cervical area tenses and contracts in response to stress and overwhelm. We contract to protect. It is a manifestation of an attempt to "hold things together." All of these stresses and lifestyle issues are part of the therapeutic journey.

The cervical area will also mirror other issues held elsewhere in the body. For instance, pelvic issues and patterns may be directly reflected, as will issues relating to the lower lumbar spine. The vertebral column functions as a single unit oriented to the primal midline and inertia in any part will be reflected in the whole.

Clinical Application: Cervical Patterns and the Point of Balanced Ligamentous Tension

This next exploration applies what we have learned to cervical patterns. Use Fig. 5.8 as a reference to refresh your image of motion possibilities generally. In the following application, you will begin your exploration of the cervical area in two ways. First, tune into the primal midline to sense any gaps in its expression. In the second process, you will engage the dural tube in a conversation about its ease of glide within the vertebral column. The former is a perceptual skill that commonly takes some time to

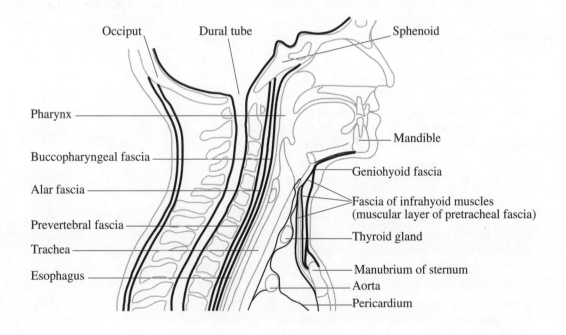

5.9   Continuity of fascial relationships

81

develop, but the primal midline will become clear the more you hold the intention to listen. The latter inquiry into dural glide is sometimes an easier way into the process for beginning students.

1. With the patient in the supine position, orient to the biosphere and mid-tide. With your hands in an occipital cradle hold, orient to the space around the person and slowly widen your perceptual field. As you do this, allow the primal midline to enter your perceptual field. Can you perceive this midline within the cervical area? Do you sense an uprising force within the vertebral and cranial base midline? Are there gaps in its expression? See if a specific area of the spine, with a specific vertebral relationship, comes to the forefront.

1. After this clarifies, very gently orient to the dural tube without narrowing your field of awareness. Then gently intend traction cephalad via the occiput. See if you can sense any boundary or resistance to this intention within the cervical area. Your traction is an intention placed into the tissue field via your hands, not a physical force. It is a conversation, not a demand. Try to sense the vertebral level within which inertia is located.

2. Once you sense an inertial issue, change your hand position to the specific vertebral level in the cervical area. Place the index and middle fingers of both hands on either side of the spinous process of that particular vertebra, over its articular masses. If you are working with the atlas, place your fingertips in the hollows under the occiput just posterior to the mastoid processes. You can also relate to the atlas by placing all of your fingertips under the occipital base pointing anteriorly toward the atlas (Fig. 5.10).

3. In this position, very gently begin to explore the tensions within and around the vertebral level being palpated. To do this, imagine that the vertebra you are holding has a fulcrum within the center of its body. This is an imaginary *neutral* within its dynamics. Randolph Stone would consider this the *neutral within its poles of expression*. Very gently explore the tensions present by moving the vertebra around this imaginary point. It is like holding a multidimensional children's teeter totter. First move it one way around the imaginary fulcrum and then another as you try to balance the tensions around it. As you initiate this exploration, the tensions present will come to the forefront, as will the preferred motions of that vertebra. There may be a tendency to narrow your attention in order to sense something. It is imperative not to do this as the potency may begin to react to your presence, and patterns will arise which are not inherent to the conditions present. Do not mentally or physically grab onto the tissues in any way as you explore this process.

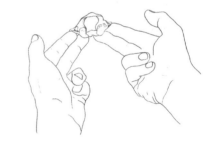

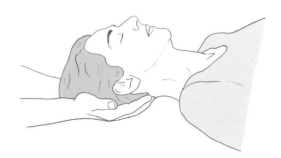

5.10   Cervical hold

4. Gently accommodate the tension patterns present until a settling into a point of balanced ligamentous tension occurs. At this point, all of the tensions present are reconciled around the fulcrum that generated them. When this precise neutral is obtained, the tissues will seem to settle into a stillness. From here, the inherent potencies may come into play and you may sense the inertia and fixation softening and the tissues expanding. You may sense a welling up of potency as the tensions settle into this local neutral.

Options

Fluid Direction

If the tissues being palpated seem very dense and inertial, and the potencies and inertial forces are deeply coiled, you may want to direct potency and fluid toward the vertebral area using the heels of your hands as you cradle the occiput. Direct fluids through the foramen magnum towards the vertebral fixation.

Lateral Fluctuation

In very inertial circumstances, you can also initiate a lateral fluctuation of potency and fluid between your palpating fingertips. Orient to fluids and potency and generate a lateral fluctuation by pushing potency from one set of finger tips to the other until a fluctuation is generated. Then let the fluctuation continue on its own and note the action of potency within the inertial condition.

GENERAL APPROACH TO THE CERVICAL COLUMN

The same principles applied to a single vertebra can also be applied to a group of vertebrae or a spinal region. The cervical vertebral column can become inertial and tense as a whole, making it difficult to work with specific fulcrums. Common origins of group involvement include whiplash and birth process. For example, the birth process may place the baby under continuous compressive forces affecting whole areas of the spine. The articular masses of the cervical column and their individual joint facets can become chronically compressed and fixed, losing independence and general flexibility.

It may be useful to approach the cervical area as a whole before doing the specific work described above. The next application will explore the tensions present within a larger area of the cervical column. This process may help resolve axially oriented traumatic forces and give you access to a wider area. After tuning into the system as above, and after assessing the ease of dural glide in the cervical area, you may want to work with a general process for the cervical area before the specific work described above.

Clinical Application: General Cervical Hold

In the following process, you will be placing your fingers in relationship to the cervical column as a whole. The intention will be to access a point of balanced ligamentous tension in relationship to the whole of the cervical spine.

1. With the patient still in the supine position, orient to the mid-tide. Place your fingertips longitudinally (vertically) along the articular masses of the cervical vertebral column. Your fingers should be together and should be pointing anteriorly in relationship to the patient's body (Fig. 5.11, next page).

2. Then very subtly and slowly suggest an anterior lift (toward the ceiling) on the articular masses. This is a very gentle intention that will initiate a conversation with these tissues. If you use too much pressure, the potency might respond defensively to your presence and you may simply lock things up. Once you gently initiate this intention, the tissues will begin to communicate their history to you. Listen to their story. It will be expressed as motion and tension patterns.

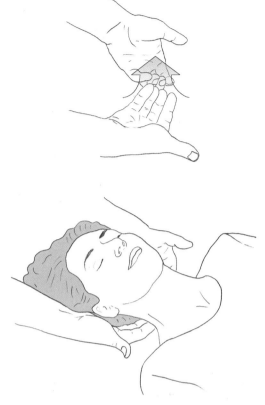

5.11 General cervical hold

Follow these motions and help access an point of balanced ligamentous tension. This is a local neutral within the overall tension patterns of the cervical area.

3. Within the balance point accessed, see if potency is expressed and wait for a sense of softening, expansion, lengthening and reorganization. How does the cervical area now relate to the primal midline and to suspended automatically shifting fulcrums?

Clinical Application: Thoracic and Lumbar Vertebral Relationships

The following exploration within the thoracic and lumbar vertebral areas is basically the same as for the cervical area. The intention will again be to explore the tension patterns present and to access the point

of balanced ligamentous tension. The main differences are the body positions of the patient and the hand positions of the practitioner.

1. With the patient in the supine position, again use the occipital cradle hold. Widen your perceptual field to see if the primal midline begins to clarify. Have patience with this. Notice where it is not obvious or where it is masked in its expression. Alternatively, you can observe these same phenomena from a sacral hold. See if you can sense the vertebral level within which this masking of the midline is present. You may sense a tissue pattern or tension from these vantage points. You may find that you can simply observe in stillness, during which an organization of tissue around an inertial fulcrum can be perceived, or a tensile pattern of some kind will come to the forefront. This may be observed as a distortion within the tissue field around a fulcrum, as a tension or pull within the connective tissues, or as fluctuant phenomena within the fluids. Fluids may be sensed to echo off inertial areas, or to move in some form of lateral fluctuation around the fulcrum.

2. Ask the patient to roll to a prone position. Standing at the side of the table, using your caudad hand, place your index and middle finger over the inertial vertebral area. An alternative hold is to use your thumb and index finger. See which hold is most comfortable and clear for you. Place your fingers over the transverse processes of the vertebra involved. This will be in the hollows on either side of the spinous process (Fig. 5.12). Again orient to the mid-tide. Hold a wide perceptual field that includes the inertial pattern. Do not narrow your perceptual field as you explore the tension patterns present.

3. Work as above to explore the tensions as though there is a fulcrum point within the heart of the vertebral body. Gently move the vertebra around this imaginary point. Let your fingers accommodate the tensions present and see if you can

access a local tension balance. A settling of the tissues will be sensed as the tensions are resolved around their fulcrum. Wait for expressions of

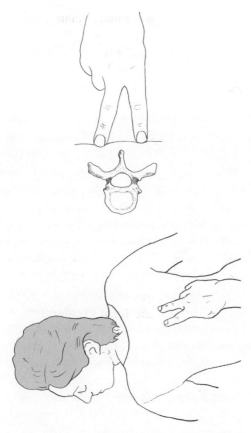

5.12 Thoracic and lumbar hand position

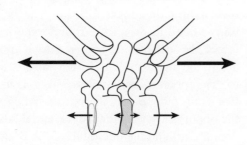

5.13 The vertebral disengagement

potency and for a softening and expansion of the tissues being palpated.

Options

Direction of Fluid

If a vertebra and its joint relationships seem very dense, you might direct potency and fluid to it. To do this, maintain your relationship to the vertebra within the point of balanced ligamentous tension as accessed above. Place your other hand on the top of the patient's head over the foramen magnum. Direct fluids from the cranium towards the vertebra involved.

Lateral Fluctuation

Alternatively, you can initiate a lateral fluctuation of potency and fluid within and around the vertebra being palpated. If you are holding the vertebra with your index and middle fingers, push fluid and potency from one finger to the other until a fluctuation is generated. This may activate the local potencies and initiate a healing process.

Axial Compression

You may sense two vertebrae compressed together towards the disc between them. The compressive forces involved may be very dense. If inertial potencies and forces cannot express themselves, a disengagement process may be helpful. Hold two vertebrae at the same time to determine if there is a clear sense of inertia and density between them. You can then use a conversation about space to help attain a point of balanced ligamentous tension. Hold the two vertebrae and gently traction them apart (Fig. 5.13). You are initiating a conversation about space within their relationship. When space is accessed, help access the point of balanced ligamentous tension.

Clinical Application:
Orienting to Primary Respiration

The above work gave you a chance to explore local motion and tension dynamics. Once you have a clear sense of these, then a shift to a biodynamic orientation is the next step. In this process, rather than working with local tension dynamics and allowable motion, you will orient to tissue motility within the phases of primary respiration. It is here that the work shifts to systemic neutrals, the state of balance, and to Becker's three-phase process. You will again relate to a specific vertebral level, but will work within the phases of primary respiration, rather than via motion testing and the point of balanced ligamentous tension.

1. With the patient in the supine position, hold either the occiput or sacrum and orient to the biosphere and mid-tide. Widen your perceptual field and see if the primal midline clarifies. Are there gaps in its expression? Is there density present anywhere along the vertebral axis? See if a specific vertebral relationship comes to the forefront.

2. When you become aware of a particular vertebral level, change your hand position. Use either the cervical hold or thoracic-lumbar hold described above. Orient to the actual motility and motion of the vertebra being palpated. In inhalation, you may sense a transverse widening within the vertebral tissue. Does the vertebra breathe within the cycles of primary respiration? What motions seem to be present within its phases?

3. Maintaining a wide perceptual field, listen for the deeper motility expressed within inhalation and exhalation. Have patience as you follow these motions. At some stage, a seeking may be sensed as tissues and fluids seek a state of balance in relationship to the forces which organize their dynamics. At most, without mentally or physically grabbing onto the potency, fluids, or tissues, simply slow things down. A state of dynamic equilibrium is attained not just within all of the forces and the tensions present, but systemically. It may seem that potency, fluids, and tissues are a unified field which settle into a stillness as a whole. This will have the sense of a settling into a depth where something begins to happen beyond the tensions and compensations held. It is the state of balance which allows something else to occur beyond the protective patterns and compensations held.

4. Listen, within the state of balance and its stillness, for expressions of Health. The state of balance is not a stillpoint; it is a state of dynamic equilibrium within all of the forces and tensions present. Orient to the underlying expression of primary respiration. Within the state of balance, you may still sense its inhalation and exhalation phases. See how deeply this state takes you into the ordering intentions of the Breath of Life. You may sense a shifting of potency within the fluids as the Inherent Treatment Plan unfolds. As the potency of the Breath of Life is expressed beyond the compensation present, the biokinetic forces which are maintaining the fixation may be dissipated back to the environment. You may sense this as heat and force vector resolution. As described in Volume One, you may even find that you go through the *mysterious gateway*. Here you may access the deeper potencies and forces within the Long Tide field of action as field phenomena and organizing matrix. You may sense a shifting of potency within the wider bioelectric field and space around the patient.

5. Once the inertial forces are resolved, the tissues of the vertebral area being explored will seek their natural organizing fulcrums. They will no longer need to organize around experiential forces. They will reorient to their natural fulcrums and to the primal midline. Listen and give space to this reorganization process. This is as important as any other part of this process. When given the opportunity, potency, tissues, and fluids will organize around the intentions of the Breath of Life. Give space for this reorganization process.

Does the vertebra move in a more balanced way in relationship to the primal midline? Does the vertebra express a more balanced motion and motility? What is its relationship to the primal midline? Can you perceive its expression as an organizing factor?

Vertebral Compression

Compression between vertebrae and within whole areas of the spine is very common. As always, compression patterns are generated by unresolved biokinetic forces introduced into the system as we experience the world. In addition, the vertebral column is always under gravity pressure when we are in the upright position. This compressive gravity force is energetically balanced by the uprising force within the primal midline. The vertebral column ideally functions as though each vertebra is hung from above. The joint relationship between each vertebra is then allowed space, and the disc and nucleus between each vertebra acts as a hydraulic piston that spreads the compressive gravity force through the disc and maintains the joint space and flexibility (Fig. 5.14).[4] Adding to this fluidic sense is the fact that each vertebral artic-

ular joint is a synovial joint. In essence, vertebrae should be floating within their relationships.

As we experience life, unresolved inertial forces may build up around the vertebral axis. This can begin with the womb experience and continue through birth process and onward. As inertial forces and potencies build within and around the vertebral axis, the joint space and the hydraulic action of the disc may become compromised. As inertial forces build up around the vertebral core, potency can become bound in centering the unresolved biokinetic forces. This can lead to lowered vitality and lowered fluid drive. The action of the fluid tide may be sensed to be depressed and sluggish. Vertebral relationships within the spinal column may become inertial and compressed, and a loss of mobility is inevitable.

Vertebral Disengagement

In the next section, we will use the conversation of disengagement to help access space between two vertebrae. Disengagement is a natural process. In the inhalation phase of primary respiration space is generated within every suture and joint. Compressive forces will compromise this natural process. In this case, the space within vertebral joints will close down, and the natural disengagement within the inhalation phase will be affected. The intention here is to help access space within the relationship and to re-establish the natural disengagement process. As you will see, it is the action of the potency within the phases of primary respiration that processes the inertial forces present and re-establishes space.

Clinical Application:
Vertebral Disengagement

1. Identify which vertebral relationship to work with using one of the approaches described above. You may sense for the gap in the expression of the primal midline, use dural traction to sense vertebral issues, or direct fluid through the vertebral axis to sense the response.

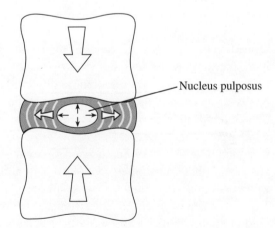

Nucleus pulposus

5.14   The intervertebral disc and its nucleus as a hydraulic piston

2. With the patient in the prone position, place the index and middle fingers of one hand over the transverse processes of one vertebra, and then place the index and middle fingers of the other hand over the other vertebra. Alternatively, you can use the thumb and index finger of each hand. Maintain a wide perceptual field and orient to the biosphere and the mid-tide. Maintain an awareness of the unity of potency, fluids, and tissues. Orient to the inhalation and exhalation phases of primary respiration.

3. Within the phases of primary respiration, sense the motility of the vertebrae you are holding. Can you sense the vertebrae breathing? In the inhalation phase is there space generated between the vertebrae? Is there a sense of a subtle widening, shortening and rising during inhalation?

4. Very gently and subtly intend the two vertebrae apart. Intend this as a conversation about space. Simply help access the available space. When space is accessed, a number of processes may come into play. Orient to the phases of primary respiration. You may sense an intensification of potency over a number of cycles within the space accessed. As this builds, the inertial forces present may be processed. You may sense a drive of potency into the inertial area and disengagement is then perceived to occur from within. Alternatively, you may sense that the potency-fluid-tissue field settles into a state of balance. When this occurs, listen for expressions of Health to arise within the neutral accessed. You may sense the processing of various kinds of biokinetic forces, force vectors, etc. Listen for the reorganization of the vertebrae to the midline and for a clearer expression of motility and motion (see Fig. 5.13).

Axial Forces and Disengagement

It is not unusual to encounter unresolved longitudinal or axial forces affecting a whole area of the spine and leading to a wide area of vertebral compression. There may be specific vertebral fulcrums involved, but the biokinetic forces generating them affect more than one vertebral segment. Axial compressive forces originate from unresolved birth trauma or other traumatic or shocking experiences. They are almost always traumatic in origin. They generate a core condensation of potency and related tissue contraction and compression. This need to protect must be appreciated and respected. Here our work is not about fixing anything; it is about the resolution of traumatic forces and unresolved experience. One way to approach inertial issues within the midline is to relate to the axial force present as a whole. Here you can engage in a conversation with these forces via the intention of disengagement through the whole vertebral core of the body.

The idea is to bring the intention of space to the vertebral midline as a whole, and to shift your view in such a way as to perceptually open to the deeper ordering forces at work. Within the mid-tide level of perception, you are in relationship with the action of the potency as an ordering principle within the fluids of the body. Here you are in the realm of embodied forces. You will meet the embodiment of inertial potencies and unresolved biokinetic forces that are active in the system. As you help access the state of balance, these potencies and forces come into play. In this application, you will also practice widening your perceptual field toward the horizon to see if deeper potencies are engaged. These potencies are more directly a factor of the ordering matrix and midline generated by the action of the Long Tide.

As you widen your perceptual field towards the horizon, you open to the Long Tide and its field phenomena. Listening within this wider perceptual field is like a call to these deeper potencies. It starts a conversation with the wider and deeper forces at work. Here field phenomena may come into play, and the wider ordering forces may be appreciated. The Long Tide may seem to enter the space from a much wider field of action. Perceptually, it may seem like meeting a wider matrix that orders the form of that particular human being. Ordering winds may be sensed. You may perceive motions around and within the body that seem to permeate and radiate everywhere. The midline may clarify as its phenomena come to the forefront. The wider forces perceptible within the Long Tide may be appreciated.

Clinical Application: Disengagement and the Vertebral Axis

Next we will use an intention of disengagement and space to relate to whole areas of the spine, a wider area of biokinetic force. The axial forces present may generate specific inertial fulcrums within vertebral dynamics, but the force must be engaged as a whole through the midline for efficient clinical results.

1. Find a comfortable position for both you and the patient and place your hands in an occipital cradle hold. Establish elbow fulcrums and avoid backpressure within the fluid system via the heels of your hands. Let your hands float on the tissues as well as you can and orient to the biosphere and the mid-tide level of perception. Let your hands be immersed within fluid, and widen your perceptual field to the biosphere. Hold the whole body and the energy field around it within your field of awareness.

2. Listen to the system from the occiput and allow an awareness of the primal midline to enter your perceptual field. Within this wider field, simply orient to the primal midline. Now with a subtle intention of inquiry, intend a cephalad traction via the occiput. Orient to the vertebrae rather than to the dural tube. You are tractioning the vertebral column, not the dural tube within it. The intention is to bring a conversation about space to the whole vertebral axis and to the forces at work within it. This is not a demand. Very subtly intend space through the vertebral axis until you sense a boundary to this intention. The intention is to engage the forces at work, not just their tissue effects (Fig. 5.15).

3. As space is accessed, orient to the phases of primary respiration. Listen especially to the inhalation phase. As you listen to the action of potency within the inhalation phase, you may sense a drive of potency within the space accessed. As this drive builds over a number of cycles, a natural disengagement of the forces and tissues may occur. You may sense a drive of potency into the inertial area, and disengagement is then perceived to occur from within.

4. Alternatively, you may sense the tissues and fluids settling into a state of balance. Once the state of balance is obtained, widen your perceptual field toward the horizon. Let your hands float

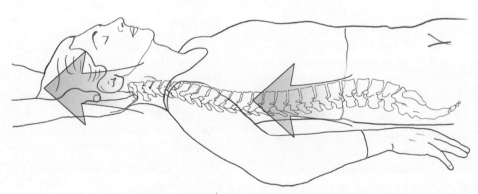

5.15 Axis disengagement via occipital cradle

within potency and gently widen your perceptual field to the boundary where it still feels safe and contained. Let yourself settle into this wider field of listening. In time, you may sense the deeper, slower tidal phenomenon of the Long Tide. The primal midline may become even more obvious here. Allow your listening to include a much larger field of action. Maintain your intention of disengagement through the midline as you do this.

5. Listen with an awareness of the intention of disengagement within the state of balance. The inherent biodynamic forces may begin to express their healing intentions. You may have an experience of potency moving from the midline, through the tensile fields of the body. You may have a perception of the shifting of potency from the field into the body, to specific inertial issues. You may have a direct perception of the biodynamic forces processing biokinetic forces and disengaging the compressive issues. The biokinetic forces resolve and disengagement is perceived to truly occur from outside-in and inside-out.

Like a mysterious gateway, the shift in your perceptual field can bring you to formative organizing forces. The intention of disengagement and the state of balance can bring you to the ordering matrix itself. The motion of the potency of the Breath of Life through the inertial fulcrums, like a fountain spray of life, is most clearly experienced here as the force which disengages and resolves the inertial issue.

OTHER CONSIDERATIONS

Tuning into the midline brings up a whole cluster of topics. Katherine Ukleja, D.O., a senior tutor at the Karuna Institute, shared some interesting thoughts with the staff team. Katherine said that she had the sense that Breath of Life is a divine carrier wave that the soul is riding into incarnation. Along with the blueprint comes the consciousness of a unique being. She

has noticed in session work that reorienting to the midline function of the Breath of Life seems to help the "rider on the Tide" process deep karmic imprints that may have little to do with this particular life, but may express lifetimes of experience. Furthermore, that being is also taking on the karma and the genetics of a generational family line. When the possibility arises to reconnect all of this to the source and its ordering matrix, a deep healing of personal and generational karma, or *miasmas,* as these are called in homeopathy, may occur.

In my own clinical practice, I have also noted how midline structures seem to reflect the energy of wider issues. The midline is protected from these core issues via a direct condensation of potency and contraction of tissue. The midline is protected from difficult conditions. Potencies condense around the midline and vertebrae literally become denser around the notochord and primal midline. Their dynamics seem to reflect the whole of our history, including past life and generational issues. I know that these thoughts may stretch the belief systems of some readers, but I would suggest that you really keep an open, non-judgmental listening and see what is valid in your practice. Taking all of this into consideration, it is no wonder that classical spinal adjustments can yield powerful results. I would, however, advise a subtle and sensitive approach to these issues. With a deep, responsive listening, something happens beyond the forces being centered, and the healing process will proceed from the "without to the within and within to the without"[5] with depth and stability.

1. This is after William Larsen, *Human Embryology* (Churchill Livingstone Inc., 1997).

2. This is after Kapandji, *The Physiology of the Joints* (Churchill Livingston Inc., 1974), and Randolph Stone, *Polarity Therapy Volume One* (CRCS Publications, 1986).

3. This diagram is after Netter, *Atlas of Human Anatomy* (Ciba-Geigy, 1989).

4. This is after Kapandji, *The Physiology of the Joints* (Churchill Livingston Inc., 1974).

5. A favorite saying of Randolph Stone.

6

Pelvic Dynamics

· ·

The inferior pole of the structural midline, the pelvis and sacrum, is highly interdependent with the structures above. The involuntary motion of the sacrum between the ilia is one of the definitive aspects of the classic Primary Respiratory Mechanism. Ease of motility and mobility within pelvic tissues and relationships is crucial in the dynamics of the midline and the system as a whole.

In this chapter we will:

- *Review the anatomy of the pelvis.*
- *Note how inertial issues within sacral relationships are transferred directly to dural dynamics.*
- *Palpate sacrum, innominate, and general pelvic motion dynamics.*
- *Explore the specific patterns of the sacrum and innominate bones.*
- *Relate to compressive forces in lumbosacral and sacroiliac joints.*
- *Explore intraosseous distortions of the sacrum.*

OVERVIEW

The pelvis is the foundation of midline structural dynamics and a common site for inertial issues. Iner-

tial issues here will directly affect the reciprocal tension membranes via the firm attachment of the dural tube at S2. Compressive issues here will also directly affect the motility of the central nervous system via the connection of the filum terminalis to the coccyx which can tether the spinal cord. Sacral compression can even lead to facilitation issues in the brain stem and cerebellum due to constant drag on the central nervous system.

Inertial forces in the pelvis and sacrum will also strongly affect the expression of the fluid tide throughout the system. The fluid systems of the body convey the potency of the Breath of Life to cells and tissues as potency. The inhalation surge of the fluid tide arises from the pelvis. The lumbosacral cistern is a key site for fluid potentization. Inertial potencies held within the inferior pole will affect the drive and vitality of the whole system.

In classic traditions such as the yogic system of India, the sacrum and lumbosacral waterbed are considered to be sites of powerful potential energies. This energetic quality is represented as a coiled serpent, the kundalini energy of the sacral area. The sacrum is also considered to be a site of crystallized energy and of life force held in reserve. The pelvic chakra (water chakra) is traditionally located at the base of the sacrum in the lumbosacral junction. The root chakra (earth chakra) is located between the apex of the sacrum and the coccyx. Chakras are organizing centers along the midline that order specific orbs of structure and function. The pelvic chakra relates to grounding energies, nurturing feelings and intentions, and sexuality and self-view. The root chakra relates to foundation, support, and a sense of stability and centeredness in life. When inertial issues are held within pelvic dynamics, these qualities can become distorted, withheld and contracted. Traditional cultures looked at the human system as a conscious energy system, and the pelvis was considered to be a root, or foundation of that system.

These dimensions may come into play when working with the pelvis, and the pelvis can reflect these in its patterns and shapes. I have had many patients with issues relating to self-worth, sexual confidence, an ability to nurture and be nurtured, and a loss of ground and contact, who have benefited greatly from biodynamic approaches with pelvic issues.

The chakras can be palpated by orienting your perceptual field to these phenomena. One way to do this is to hold your hand a few inches above the patient's spine. Let your awareness encompass the whole biosphere with the entire ordering matrix. Starting from the coccyx, slowly move your hand superiorly. Do not narrow your field of awareness as you do this. Move from the coccyx to the occiput a number of times. After a number of passes, you may begin to sense localized vortices and/or pulsations within the midline. These will have different qualities expressing their distinct locations and functions.

ANATOMICAL RELATIONSHIPS

The whole pelvic bowl, including bones, joints, muscles and connective tissue, operates as one unit of function. Unifying all the components is a strong ligamentous stocking of connective tissue that supports the lumbar vertebrae, surrounds the sacrum (Fig. 6.1), anchors the muscles, and stabilizes all the relationships. The sacrum can be visualized as hanging from the lower lumbar area within this stocking. As it hangs, ideally it is floating within the fluids of its joint relationships.[1] It is important to understand the ligamentous relationships of this stocking and to be able to sense its integrated dynamics. Ligaments that

stabilize the relationship between the fifth lumbar vertebra and the pelvis and those stabilizing the relationships between the bony structures of the pelvis are of particular interest.

The ligamentous relationships of L5 and the pelvis include:

- Caudad continuations of the anterior and posterior longitudinal ligaments that connect the body of L5 to the first sacral segment.

- The ligamentum flava that connects their laminae.

- The inter- and supraspinous ligaments of the spinous processes.

- The iliolumbar ligament stabilizes the relationships of L5 to the pelvis. It radiates laterally from the transverse processes of L5 via two main bands. The cephalad band attaches to the crest of the ilium and the caudad band connects to the base of the sacrum where it blends with the anterior sacroiliac ligament.

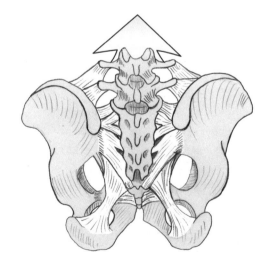

6.1 The sacrum hangs in the ligamentous stocking from the lumbar vertebra

Lumbosacral Junction

The primary joint between the pelvis and the lumbar vertebrae is the lumbosacral junction, including all joint and connective tissue relationships between L5 and the sacrum. The two articular facets and the intervertebral disc between L5 and the sacrum are often found to be in compression. Biokinetic forces of trauma and stress are commonly expressed as inertia within these pelvic tissues (Fig. 6.2).

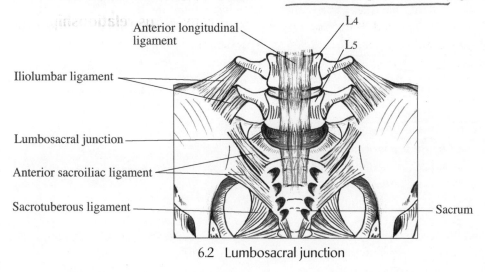

Anterior longitudinal ligament

L4

L5

Iliolumbar ligament

Lumbosacral junction

Anterior sacroiliac ligament

Sacrotuberous ligament

Sacrum

6.2   Lumbosacral junction

The Sacroiliac Joint

The sacroiliac joints form another major joint relationship of the pelvis. The joint has L-shaped articular surfaces that allow for the variety of pelvic motions required for walking, running, sitting and stretching. The joint allows both rotational and gliding motions. It commonly has a lower and upper compartment. These compartments are generally formed by concavities in the articular surfaces of the sacrum and convexities in the articular surfaces of the ileum. Many variations in the internal topography of the joint surfaces are possible. Many people have one large compartment rather than two. Some have a small third compartment at the level of S2, and some have one type of articular surface on one side of the pelvis and another on the other side. It is also possible to find that the sacral surface is convex rather than concave and that each joint surface of the same sacrum is different (Fig. 6.3).

The articular surface of each bone is covered with a cartilaginous plate. The cartilage covering the sacrum

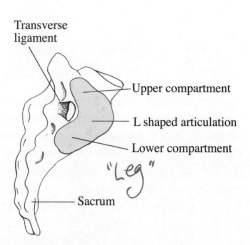

Transverse ligament

Upper compartment

L shaped articulation

Lower compartment

"Leg"

Sacrum

6.3   The sacrum, its articular surfaces, and the transverse ligament

93

is thicker than that found on the ileum. The cartilaginous plates are in close association and are connected by softer fibrocartilage. At the anterior and posterior ends the joint surfaces are connected by fine interosseous fibers. Posteriorly, at the level of S2, these interosseous fibers thicken to form what is sometimes called the axial or transverse ligament of the sacroiliac joint. The transverse ligament helps to create the sacrum's transverse axis of rotation at S2 (see Fig. 6.3).

The sacroiliac joints are synovial joints. There are joint capsules (fluid filled sacs) around each sacroiliac joint. Fluidic potency and circulation are thus essential in their functioning. The synovial fluids enable ease of motion and the mobility necessary within the dynamics of the joint. These fluids carry the potency of the Breath of Life, and the quality of fluids is a major factor in the maintenance of joint mobility.

The sacrum and its sacroiliac joint surfaces form a wedge-shaped, upside-down pyramid that is wedged into the innominate bones at the sacrum's articular surfaces and secured by its connective tissues. A series of coronal sections through the sacroiliac joints shows this wedging mechanism. At the first section, at the level of S1, the distance between posterior sacroiliac joint margins is slightly greater than the anterior margins. This is the start of the anterior-posterior wedge shape (Fig. 6.4a). At this level the articular surfaces of the sacroiliac joints also taper closer together as they move inferiorly. The joint's apex is truncated caudally, so there is also an upside-down pyramidal wedging of the sacrum into the innominate bones.

In another section through S2, the posterior width is distinctly greater than its anterior width and the two joint surfaces again narrow together medially (Fig. 6.4b). The sacrum's apex is again truncated caudally. So at the level of S2, there is a clear wedging of the joint surfaces. A third section, through S3, shows an interesting change. At this level, the anterior width is greater than the posterior (Fig. 6.4c). There is generally also a wider dimension transversely across the two joint surfaces. Hence, its apex is truncated cephalad.[2] This change in the wedging at S3 within the joint surfaces helps to stabilize the joint in its motion. The

wedge shape of the sacrum's joint surfaces, and their interlocking concave-convex form, resist downward pressures of weight, and the second sacral segment (S2) thereby becomes the natural axis for the motion of the sacrum. This is reinforced by the interosseous axial ligament at the level of S2.

Although this is a general description of typical joint surfaces, variations in joint structure are extremely common. The wedging can be opposite to that described above. I have even seen different directions

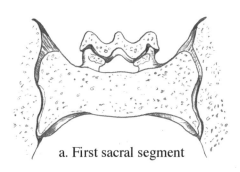

a. First sacral segment

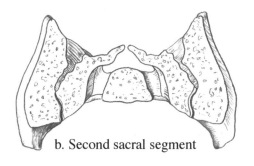

b. Second sacral segment

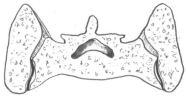

c. Third sacral segment

6.4 Coronal sections through the sacroiliac joints

of wedging from one side of the same sacrum to the other. Variations of the topography of the articular surfaces have been mentioned above. The sacral surfaces are generally concave, commonly with two joint concavities, many times with one long L-shaped concavity and sometime with three concavities. I have seen many variations of these surfaces and have seen specimens with convex rather than concave surfaces.

There are commonly two "legs" of the L-shaped sacroiliac joint: an upper, relatively horizontal leg, and a lower, relatively vertical leg. Each leg can have a compartment or depression corresponding to the shape of the iliac articular surface.

The legs can hold compression independently of each other. Compressions of the upper leg of the L tend to be transferred to the upper aspects of the ligamentous stocking that maintains stability in the lumbosacral relationships. The iliolumbar and lumbar vertebral ligaments can become involved, and lower- to mid-lumbar pain, tissue, and fluid congestion and nerve facilitation may result.

Compression in the lower leg of the L will tend to be transferred to the sacroiliac ligaments such as the sacrospinous and sacrotuberous, and sciatic pain radiating in the buttocks and legs may result. Bilateral compression of both legs of the L is also common and can result in pain distribution in any direction. The interosseous ligaments around the joint may also become involved, with resulting restriction in mobility. Pain is often transferred to the opposite side of the pelvis, away from the compressed sacroiliac joint. The compression can also be transferred diagonally across the ligamentous stocking to the opposite side.

Ligaments Connecting
the Sacrum to the Ilia

Understanding and accurately visualizing the relationships of the ligamentous stocking that connects the lower lumbar area, the sacrum, and the innominate bones together, is a key to effective clinical work. The ligamentous stocking, as a unit of function, is a self-locking mechanism and helps to stabilize the pelvis and its joint dynamics. The transfer of the downward force of weight through the lumbar area to the pelvis is buffered and resisted by the connective tissue structure. This helps to stabilize the sacrum and its sacroiliac joints. We are first going to look at the ligaments that connect the sacrum to the ilia around the sacroiliac joints themselves. These are the anterior sacroiliac, posterior sacroiliac, and interosseous ligaments. Although we describe them individually, all these ligaments function as one ligamentous unit (Fig. 6.5, next page).

Anterior Sacroiliac Ligament

The anterior sacroiliac ligament consists of numerous bands that form a sheet-like ligament. It connects the anterior surface of the lateral aspect of the sacrum to the margin of the auricular surface of the ileum and its preauricular sulcus.

Posterior Sacroiliac Ligament

The posterior sacroiliac ligament consists of numerous fibers that are oriented in a number of directions. Its superior part is sometimes called the short posterior sacroiliac ligament. It is nearly horizontal in orientation and connects the first and second transverse tubercles of the posterior surface of the sacrum to the tuberosity of the ileum. Its inferior part is sometimes called the long posterior sacroiliac ligament and it is oblique in orientation. It connects the third transverse tubercle of the sacrum to the posterior superior spine of the ileum and merges with the superior part of the sacrotuberous ligament. It is a strong ligament, creating one of the chief bonds of the joint.

Interosseous Sacroiliac Ligament

This ligament consists of a series of short, strong fibers that connect the tuberosities of the sacrum and ileum. It lies deeper than the posterior ligament and connects the borders of the joint. It creates a strong band posterior to the articular surface at the level of S2 and defines the classic osteopathic axis of rotation for the motion of the sacrum.

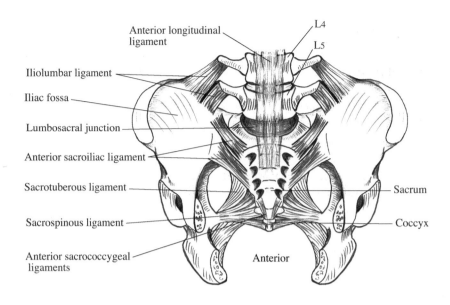

Anterior longitudinal ligament

L4

L5

Iliolumbar ligament

Iliac fossa

Lumbosacral junction

Anterior sacroiliac ligament

Sacrotuberous ligament

Sacrum

Sacrospinous ligament

Coccyx

Anterior sacrococcygeal ligaments

Anterior

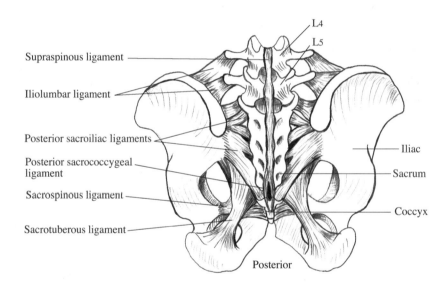

L4

L5

Supraspinous ligament

Iliolumbar ligament

Posterior sacroiliac ligaments

Iliac

Posterior sacrococcygeal ligament

Sacrum

Sacrospinous ligament

Coccyx

Sacrotuberous ligament

Posterior

6.5 The major ligaments that stabilize the sacroiliac joints

Ligaments Connecting the Sacrum to the Ischium

The ligaments connecting the sacrum to the ischium help to stabilize the joint. They are an integral part of the ligamentous sock that holds and stabilizes the lumbosacral area. These include the sacrotuberous and sacrospinous ligaments.

Sacrotuberous Ligament

The sacrotuberous ligament is a broad fan-shaped complex of fibers that connects the posterior inferior spine of the ileum, the fourth and fifth transverse tubercles of the sacrum and the caudad part of its lateral margin and the lateral margin of the coccyx, all to the inner margin of the tuberosity of the ischium. Its caudal border is continuous with the tendon of origin of the biceps femoris muscle and many of its proximal fibers are continuous with the posterior sacroiliac ligament and sacrospinous ligament. It is also continuous with the interosseous ligament and joint capsule.

Sacrospinous Ligament

The sacrospinous ligament is a triangular sheet that is attached at its base to the lateral margins of the sacrum and coccyx and at its apex to the spine of the ischium. Its fibers are continuous with the sacrotuberous ligament and also blend with the sacroiliac joint capsule.

These ligaments form a unified ligamentous stocking that holds and stabilizes the sacrum and lower lumbar vertebrae and also affords attachment for various pelvic muscles. The ligamentous stocking is an important aspect of the self-bracing mechanisms of the pelvis and its integrity is essential for ease of lumbosacral and craniosacral functioning.

Neuroendocrine–Immune Implications

The sacrum should be perceived to be floating within its joint relationships. If it is not, the dural tube and CNS can become tethered in their expression of motility and mobility. This can become a major inertial factor in the system, leading to facilitation within the brain stem and initiation of hyperarousal states via the hypothalamus-pituitary-adrenal axis.

Chronic lumbar muscle contraction will be transferred directly to the ligamentous stocking and can cause related contractions in ligamentous fibers. The contractions can then be transferred on to the sacroiliac joints. Chronic tissue contraction can cause nerve facilitation and inflammatory responses. These will cause chronic nociceptive input (pain input) to be sent to the dorsal horn cells of the spinal cord. These cells may then become sensitized, and chronic pain and a vicious cycle of facilitation may result. Similarly, vertebral fixations can generate nerve facilitation, hyper- or hypotonic nerve response, tissue contraction, and chronic inflammatory responses.

Frank Willard, Ph.D., points out that the ligamentous structures of the lumbosacral area contain many nociceptive nerve fibers (pain receptors) and efferent sympathetic fibers. These are capable of secreting proinflammatory neuropeptides that interact with immune cells in the surrounding tissues. Chronic stimulation through nerve facilitation and tissue contraction can result in chronic low-grade inflammatory responses that are thought to play a major role in chronic pain and degeneration in the lumbosacral area.[3]

Furthermore, chronic nociceptive input into the dorsal horn neurons of the spinal cord can generate wider effects within the system. Cycles of central nervous system facilitation can be set up and the hypothalamus-pituitary-adrenal axis can become sensitized. The neuroendocrine-immune system will become adversely affected, and the system may become overwhelmed.

To resolve these inflammatory responses, we use our understanding of states of balanced tension, fluid dynamics, and expressions of the potency of the Breath of Life within disoriented and sensitized cells and tissues.

THE INVOLUNTARY MOTION
OF THE SACRUM BETWEEN THE ILIA

The sacrum is a roof more than it is a back wall for the pelvis. It is situated in a relatively oblique position in the pelvis with its base much more anterior than its apex. As a midline structure, the sacrum's motion is traditionally described as flexion and extension. In the inhalation phase, the sacrum subtly rises cephalad and expresses an intraosseous widening as its segments uncoil. The subtle cephalad rising of the sacrum is an important motion. If the cephalad lift of the sacrum in the inhalation phase is restricted by inertial issues, the motility of the central nervous system will be affected. The central nervous system is connected to the coccyx via a continuity of pia mater called the filum terminalis. In inhalation, the sacrum also expresses rotation around a transverse axis located at S2 (the second sacral segment). Its base rotates in a superior and posterior direction, while its apex rotates in an inferior and anterior direction around S2. This is its classic flexion motion. In our description of the anatomy of the sacrum and its ligamentous relationships above, you may remember that its wedge-shaped articular surfaces, and the transverse ligament located at the level of S2, help to generate this axis of rotation.

Movement of the sacrum is accompanied by movement in the surrounding tissues. The innominate bones express external and internal rotation. As the sacrum expresses inhalation, the innominate bones widen and externally rotate. As the sacrum expresses exhalation, the innominate bones narrow and internally rotate (Fig. 6.6).

As the fluid tide ascends in inhalation, the sacrum, dural tube, and central nervous system also ascend as they shorten and widen. These movements are happening as part of the body's unified motility. All fluid and tissue motion is a single unit of function, and as we describe separate structural motion, we are artificially breaking down this unit of function. This is useful for clinical purposes, but it must be remembered that all tissue motility and motion is expressed as a whole within the body physiology. All of these interrelationships were originally orchestrated during embryological development via the action of potency both within the bioelectric field as a whole, and within the fluids more directly. The organization of all inherent motions within the body is generated by, and orients to, the potency of the Breath of Life. All these parts ideally orient to the primal midline within the bioelectric field. This midline is a function of the whole field and is an expression of the action of the Long Tide as a field phenomenon. These were originally laid down during embryological formation and continue to be laid down in every moment. Thus, the motility and motion of the sacrum ideally orients to the midline and to automatically shifting fulcrums such as Sutherland's fulcrum and the SBJ.

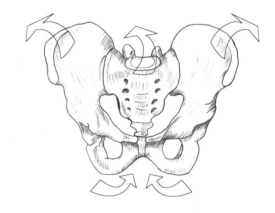

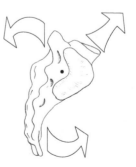

6.6   Inhalation of the sacrum
within the innominate bones

INHERENT MOTILITY OF THE SACRUM

As we have seen, all cells and tissues in the body, including the sacrum, express an inner breath or motility. This is most easily sensed within the mid-tide. In the inhalation phase, you may sense a welling up of potency and fluid within sacral tissue and a widening and uncurling of the sacral segments. This sense of widening and uncurling is a manifestation of the sacrum's motility, or inner expression of the Breath of Life. In the exhalation phase, the opposite may be sensed; the sacrum will narrow and curl up. This inner motion is within the cells and tissues of the sacrum and is most important. I have palpated many patients whose sacrum expressed interosseous motion between the ilia in some way, yet could not express this internal motility. Instead of curling and uncurling, the sacrum seemed inwardly inertial.

When the sacrum expresses some external motion, without expressing internal motility, it is commonly a consequence of intraosseous birth forces, or other traumatic forces of some kind that are present within the tissue of the sacrum. These intraosseous forces can generate many clinical issues within the system. The classic osteopathic phrase for these kinds of patterns is "intraosseous lesion." I prefer to use the word, "distortion," as this gives a better sense of its nature. Intraosseous distortions of the sacrum will strongly affect the expression of potency within the fluid tide. The inertial potencies centering the intraosseous forces commonly dampen down the inhalation surge of the Tide. On a tissue level, spinal nerve roots leaving the sacral canal can also be affected. This may be expressed as nerve facilitation, local inflammation, sacroiliac and low back pain, and various kinds of pelvic visceral symptoms. The intraosseous pattern can also be transferred superiorly and be expressed within the dynamics of the occiput, cranial base, and brain. Furthermore, the intraosseous issue may contribute to a tethering of the central nervous system via the filum terminalis. Thus, the motility of the CNS may be compromised.

SACRAL MOBILITY DYNAMICS

Before exploring the craniosacral dynamics of the pelvis, it is also useful to have a general understanding of its basic mobility. As we have seen, the sacroiliac joint is L-shaped and allows both gliding within its articular surfaces and rotation around its axis of rotation at S2. If you are sitting down and your ischial tuberosities (sitz bones) are fixed, as you bend forward and backward, the sacrum moves around the fixed ilia. The sacrum simply forward-bends and backward-bends on the ilia (flexion and extension) with both rotation and gliding around S2. But as you walk, or move freely without fixing the ilia, the two bones move in relationship to each other with both rotation and gliding at their L-shaped joint surfaces. Due to the L-shaped joint structure, and to the combined rotation and gliding dynamic of the joint, the sacrum both rotates and side-bends at the same time as it expresses movement in relationship to the ilia. Fixations of the sacrum are thus commonly expressed as flexion or extension patterns combined with torsion where there is both a side-bending and a rotation component (Fig. 6.7).

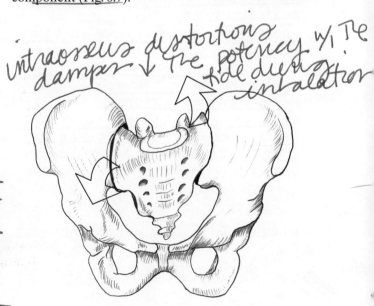

*intraosseus distortions dampen ↓ the potency w/ the
tide during inhalation.*

6.7   Torsion in sacral dynamics

Approaching Clinical Applications

The pelvis can be a sensitive or emotionally charged area. When approaching the pelvis, the practitioner must keep this in mind. The sacrum may hold issues relating to sexuality, self-worth, and nurturing. Negotiating safe contact is critically important here. The pelvis can hold a history of trauma that may involve physical and sexual abuse, falls, and accidents. It is important to explain your intention to your patients, and why you are contacting this area. It is also important to give them some power in the relationship by giving them easy ways to signal any discomfort, such as lifting a hand, or simply saying "no." At every step, explain what and why you are about to engage in a particular contact, and negotiate that gently and gradually. Do not attempt to override protective patterns because you might overwhelm the patient. Patients may not verbally communicate feeling overwhelmed to you, but the system will. The goal is to access the Health within, not to activate symptoms or emotional processes. If emotional processes arise, know what you are in relationship to. There is a huge difference between a true emotional completion and a traumatic recycling of emotional energies. In a true emotional completion it is clear that the patient is grounded in the present. There is a sense of something moving through their system and completing as space is accessed. In a traumatic recycling of emotional energies, things may speed up dramatically and the patient may seem to be caught up in their emotions with little space. It may seem as though they are re-experiencing the trauma rather than processing it and letting it go. For review, see the chapters in Volume One on trauma skills.

Clinical Application: Sensing the Motility and Motion of the Sacrum

The sacrum is ideally sensed to be hanging freely within its ligamentous stocking and floating within its synovial joint relationships. Listen for this sense of floating as the sacrum expresses its motility and motion. If it cannot float, as is often the case, then the fluidic nature of the joint relationship is compromised. Also listen for a subtle rising of the sacrum at the beginning of the inhalation phase. If the sacrum cannot express this, the central nervous system may be tethered and its motility will be affected.

1. With the patient in the supine position, make contact with the sacral hold. Sit at the lower caudad corner of the treatment table with your chair pointing toward the diagonally opposite shoulder. Ask the patient to lift the pelvis off the table so you can place your hand under the sacrum as previously described. Your fingertips should be pointing cephalad and the patient's sacrum should be comfortably nestled in your hand. The heel of your hand should not be pressing against the sacrum. Your elbow should be near or under the knee so that your wrist is not at a sharp angle. Your hand should be comfortable. After establishing your practitioner neutral and wide perceptual field, imagine that your hand is sinking under the table and is giving the patient's sacrum space to talk to you. Even though the patient's weight is on your hand, you should still have the sense that your hands are floating within fluids.

2. Orient to the biosphere and mid-tide. Within this widened field, listen to the motion of the sacrum within the phases of primary respiration. As you perceive sacral motion, it may be perceived to be part of a unified tensile tissue field. An awareness of the whole body is not lost. See if you can sense both its outer motion and its inner motility as it widens and uncurls in inhalation and narrows and curls up in exhalation. Stay with this awareness for some time. Do you sense a subtle rising at the beginning of its inhalation motion? Spend as much time as necessary for clarification of the motility and motion of the sacrum. Do not chase or rush after patterns.

3. Wait for a deepening into primary respiration and a clarification of a pattern. As you listen, allow yourself to sense any inertial fulcrums and

bone is a connective tissue

related tensile patterns present. These may include rotations, torsions, and compressive issues. You may sense related connective pulls and strains placed upon the sacrum. For instance, there may be a contraction in the ligamentous sack within which the sacrum is supported. This contraction may orient to a fulcrum within the lumbar area or elsewhere. Alternatively, there may be a connective tissue strain through the body relating to a major joint such as a shoulder or knee, or even to an organ, such as the liver or stomach. Remember that bone is a connective tissue, and bony dynamics are a unit of function with all connective tissue patterns within the body. As you sense a pattern clarifying, orient to the fulcrum that organizes its motion. Follow the perceived pattern around its organizing fulcrum. This inertial fulcrum may be a local one, within the sacroiliac or hip joint for instance, or may be related to a more distant fulcrum somewhere else in the body.

4. Listen for the state of balance. Wait for a settling into this systemic neutral. Notice how the system attempts to express its healing processes within the state of balance. Open your perceptual field to the unity and one-thing-ness of potency, fluid, and tissue. Remember Becker's three-phase healing awareness. Listen for something to happen within the stillness of the state of balance. Listen for a change in the potencies. This may be perceived as pulsation, permeation, fluid drive, fluctuation, heat, expansion, or other expressions. Listen for the inertial potencies to be expressed and for biokinetic forces to be processed. As usual, you are listening for expressions of Health, such as pulsation of potency and fluid fluctuation.

5. You are waiting for a permeation and expansion of potency and a softening and expansion of the tissue elements. As this occurs, allow the tissues to reorganize and listen for a sense of greater ease in sacral motion. You may also become aware of an increased sense of potency as the sacrum expresses its motility. You may also have a greater sense that the sacrum is floating in its joint relationships. A literal rehydration of the joint relationship may have occurred. Fluids are now free to express themselves as the inertial potencies are processed. You may notice that the inertial fulcrum organizing the pattern has shifted or dissipated and that the inertial pattern has resolved. Simply accessing the state of balance may allow the system to express its potency and resolve the issue. Sometimes further conversations are required due to the density and chronic nature of the inertia.

Clinical Highlight: Kundalini Forces

The sacrum literally means "sacred bone." It is the traditional seat of vitality in the human body. It is also the traditional location of kundalini energy. Kundalini energy is basically the storehouse of potency within the sacral waterbed. Mystical and tantric traditions have practices to rapidly open this storehouse of vitality. These practices are not to be taken lightly and must be learned under the guidance of a master of those traditions. Energy can be unloosed too quickly and disturbances can arise within the body-mind process. I have had a number of "Kundalini refugees" whose systems became very disturbed with the use of extreme breathing practices geared to "raise the Kundalini." They presented a very unintegrated and dissociated state; the clinical focus revolved around EV4s, working with resources, and establishing neutrals within their systems.

INNOMINATE BONE MOTILITY AND MOTION

The innominate bones have a number of important articulations: the two sacroiliac joints, the pubic symphysis, and the hip joints. The sacroiliac joint was described above. The pubic symphysis is the articulation between the two pubic bones. It has an inter-pubic fibrocartilaginous disk that connects the two bones and allows slight movement. The hip joint is a ball and socket joint. The acetabulum is a cup-shaped cavity on each innominate bone that receives the head of the femur. The acetabulum is anteriorly located on the innominate bone and is also located anterior-inferior to the axis of rotation of the innominate bone as a whole (Fig. 6.8).

Motility

In inhalation, the innominate bones widen transversely, seem to move apart at the ilia, and express external rotation; in exhalation, the innominate bones narrow at the ilia and rotate inwardly (see Fig. 6.6).

Mobility and Inertial Issues

The possible motions of the innominate bone joints include anterior and posterior rotation and gliding motions around the sacroiliac joints, lateral shifts or shears, and superior and inferior shifts or shears (vertical shifts). The innominate bones can become fixed in any of these directions. Vertical shifts always originate in external trauma, usually occurring due to falls or accidents (Fig. 6.9). Any fixation within the sacroiliac joints will be transferred to the pubic symphysis and the hip joints, and can generate compensatory fulcrums in these areas. Furthermore, these issues can generate compensatory patterns in cervical, occipital and cranial base dynamics. Any of these patterns may be encountered in a general exploration of the motions of the pelvis.

It is common for one innominate bone to prefer, or be fixed in, posterior rotation while the other prefers, or is fixed in, anterior rotation. This generates

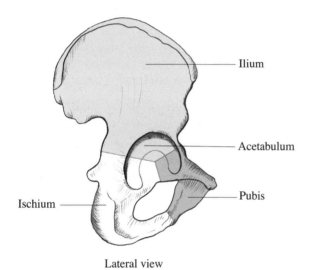

Lateral view

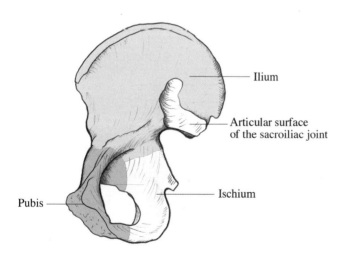

6.8 Anatomy of an innominate bone

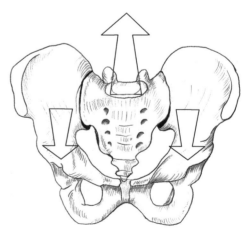

6.9 Superior vertical shift of the sacrum within the ilia

torsion across the relationships of the pelvis. It is also common for both innominate bones to prefer posterior rotation, with one more posterior than the other. This also generates torsional forces across the pelvis.

When torsion occurs, the sacral base is usually forced into a posterior and inferior position on the most posterior innominate bone side. This is because as the innominate bone rotates, its posterior superior iliac spine rotates posteriorly and inferiorly, and the sacroiliac joint follows. As the sacrum is forced inferiorly and posteriorly by the innominate bone, it must rotate and side-bend at the same time. It is then forced into a torsioned position (Fig. 6.10).

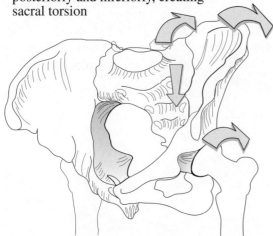

Posterior rotation of the innominate bone forces the sacrum to rotate posteriorly and inferiorly, creating sacral torsion

6.10 Mechanics of Sacral Torsion

The leg on the side of the posteriorly rotated innominate bone is usually found to be physiologically short (as opposed to anatomically short). That is because the acetabulum follows the posterior rotation of the innominate superiorly, and the head of the femur is rotated relatively superior, generally yielding a short leg on that side.

Thus, a common structural picture on the side of a posteriorly rotated innominate bone is:

* A physiological short leg on that side
* An inferior and posterior sacral base on that side
* A torsioned relationship between the sacrum and innominate bones.

Clinical Application: Sensing Motility and Motion of the Innominate Bones

In this next section we will explore the motility and motion of the innominate bones at the ilia.

ASIS

1. With the patient in the supine position, place your hands over the anterior aspects of the pelvis at the anterior superior iliac spines (Fig. 6.11). See if you can let your hands float on the tissues with the sense that they are immersed in fluid. Orient to the biosphere and mid-tide. As you do this, see if you can sense the motility and motion of the pelvis. You may notice some interesting tissue motions. First there is the basic inherent motion of the ilia. Within the phases of primary respiration, you may sense them transversely widening apart in inhalation and narrowing together in exhalation. You may also become aware of various shapes and patterns of motion.

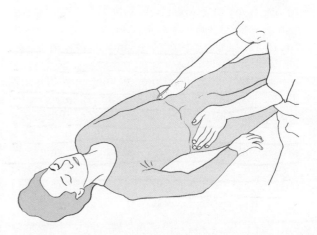

6.11 Hand position for the innominate bones

103

For instance, you may sense that one ilium prefers inhalation and the other prefers exhalation. You may also sense torsioned, sheared, and compressed tissue patterns. Simply listen to the motility of the innominate bones within the phases of primary respiration.

2. Some of the issues described above may be noticed. One ilium may be more posteriorly rotated than the other. The pelvis as a whole may be side-shifted either left or right, or one or both innominate bones may be vertically shunted. Notice all of this. Listen, remain oriented to the whole body and the expression of inhalation and exhalation and wait for a pattern to clarify. See if you can sense the organizing fulcrums for these motions.

3. Help access the state of balance. Listen for expressions of Health. Note any fluctuations, pulsation, permeation, fluid drive, etc. Notice how the system expresses its Health within the stillness and wait for a sense of resolution and reorganization.

Clinical Application: Sacropelvic Patterns

In our initial exploration, we will be tracking both sacral motility and motion and the related motility and motion of the pelvis as a whole. You will be holding the transverse structures of the pelvic diaphragm and its related fascia as well as the bony structures of the pelvis. In this position, the intention is to start a conversation with the tissues, fluids, and potency of the area and to see what their healing priorities are. The simple act of being present and holding a wider perceptual field initiates this conversation. When you bring a wide awareness to a person's system with a neutral yet active listening, and when you maintain respectful boundaries as you do this, that system will communicate to you. It will tell you its life history and give you perceptual access to the Health within.

1. With one hand under the sacrum as explained above, place your other hand over the pubic symphysis (sacro-pelvic hold). Slowly work the heel of your hand caudad from the abdomen until the edge of the heel of your hand is over the pubic symphysis. Your fingers are generally pointing cephalad (Fig. 6.12). In this position, allow your hands to float within fluids. Orient to the midtide. Notice how the pelvis expresses its motions within the inhalation and exhalation phases of primary respiration. See if you can sense the potencies and the drive underlying the tissue motions. Notice how all of this is organized in relationship to the midline function. How do the tissues organize themselves around their history?

2. As you tune into this, notice the quality and patterning of the sacro-pelvic motion. What organizes this? We are always interested in origins because they are about present conditions and present organizing factors. From what does this pattern originate? Where is the fulcrum that organizes this? The pelvis may express almost

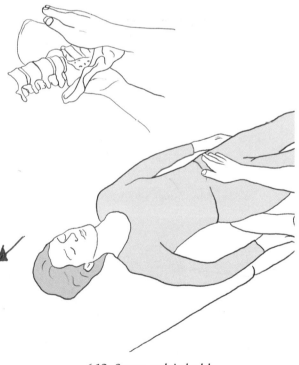

6.12 Sacro-pelvic hold

any kind of motion, and this may be organized around an inertial fulcrum located almost anywhere. It may be helpful to review the anatomy of the fascial and connective tissue relationships in the male and female pelvis.

3. How do the tissues move you as your hands float within fluid? What story is told? Notice any inertial fulcrums that seem to organize the motions and motility of what is being communicated. On a tissue level you may note compressive forces at work within the sacroiliac joints, hip joints and lumbosacral junction. Follow these dynamics as usual, wait for something to engage from within, and for a pattern to clarify. Help access the state of balance around the organizing fulcrums. Listen for the initiation of potencies and for self-healing processes. Listen for expansion of potencies and tissues, softening of boundaries, and reorientation of tissues to the midline as the inertial forces are resolved.

There are many possibilities for patterning in this area. You may have perceived tissue compression and related patterns involving any of these locations. For instance, on a tissue level, you may have sensed the sacrum pulling up into the lumbar area, or moving around the lumbosacral junction. You may have also sensed the sacrum pulling into, or moving around, one of its sacroiliac joints. Alternatively, you may have sensed a general lack of motility and motion of any kind. You may have also noticed these issues via the fluids as fluid fluctuations, spiraling of fluid, and fluid rebound. These are common phenomena within the pelvis.

RELATING TO SPECIFIC INERTIAL FULCRUMS

In the following exploration, we take two approaches to meeting and having a conversation with the related tissues, fluids, and inertial potencies. In the first approach, simply listen and follow the priorities of the system as the dynamics are shown to you. As the conversation unfolds, follow the patterns being expressed and help the tissue elements access the state of balance. This will initiate a conversation with the inertial potencies that maintain and center the compressive pattern.

In the second approach, use the principle of disengagement to access space and to initiate a further conversation with the inertial forces. Suggesting space begins a conversation about the potential space within a relationship and invites inertial potencies to be expressed. It becomes a conversation about space and the Health centering the conditions present. The intention will be to access space within the joint relationships and allow inertial potencies to be expressed within the compressive situation.

RELATING TO LUMBOSACRAL COMPRESSION

Compressive forces are often found within the relationships of the lumbosacral junction, leading to tissue compression and fluid congestion. The lumbosacral junction is the transition point between the lumbar vertebrae and the sacrum. At this point the weight that is carried through the bodies of the vertebrae is transferred to the sacrum and pelvic arch (Fig. 6.13).[4]

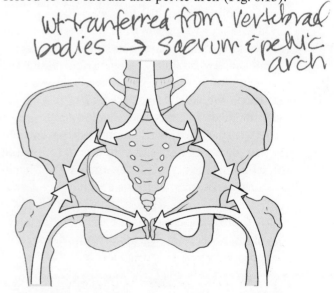

6.13 Weight transfer via the lumbosacral junction

Membranous and ligamentous strain patterns from other areas of the body are often transferred to the lumbosacral connective tissues. Postural issues and trauma of various sorts, including falls and accidents, can be reflected here. Birth trauma and birthing forces are another potential source of stress here. These various experiences introduce biokinetic forces into the tissue field that may affect the dynamics of the lumbosacral junction in many ways. Remember the discussion above about the ligamentous sock that surrounds the sacrum and lower lumbar area. Also remember that many nociceptive fibers are found within these connective tissues (see Fig. 6.1).

While monitoring the motion at the sacrum above, you may have sensed a pull superiorly into the lumbosacral junction, or a sense of motion expressed in some way around the lumbosacral junction. Initially, the important thing will be to access the inertial forces organizing the compressive pattern. There will be local forces within the joint dynamic and there may be remote fulcrums that are also maintaining the disturbance. Hold the whole of the person in your awareness. Maintain a wide perceptual field and notice the dynamics that arise within it. Within a state of balance, the system may naturally initiate the potencies that are maintaining all of this.

In the following explorations, we will be creating a relationship with the lumbosacral junction to follow its patterns and relate to its compressive issues. Initially, we will be simply listening and helping the tissues, fluids, and potencies involved access a state of balance. We will then use the skill of disengagement to initiate a further conversation about space.

In the first step of the exploration, simply listen to the system via a lumbosacral hold and follow the dynamics that are revealed. The intention will again be to access the state of balance within the inertial relationship. The second phase of the exploration will be to initiate a conversation about space via an intention of disengagement. The inquiry is, "what space is available and accessible given these forces at work?"

There is always potential space available for the expression of inertial potencies.

Clinical Application: Lumbosacral Junction

1. The patient is in the supine position. With one hand under the sacrum as above, place your other hand in a partial fist under the lower lumbar vertebrae. Your fingers should be against the spinous processes from L5-L3. If the lumbar curve is too flat to achieve this, let the spinous processes fall in the indentation between your fingers and the heel of your hand, or just use your fingers to make contact with the lumbar spine. The inferior aspect of your hand should be just touching or very close to your lower hand at the sacrum (Fig. 6.14).

2. In this position, widen your perceptual field to the biosphere and the mid-tide. Follow the dynamic of the relationship between the sacrum and lumbar spine. The sacrum will organize its motion around compressive forces within the lumbosacral junction. For instance, you may sense a cephalad pull at the sacrum towards the lumbosacral junction. If the compressive forces are dense, you may not be able to sense much motion at all. The motility and mobility of the sacrum may seem to be compromised.

3. With this awareness, follow any pattern that emerges and help access the state of balance. Simply listen and help slow things down until a state of balance is attained. The state of balance is inherent within the inertial forces centering and maintaining the compressive pattern. Your role is simply to help access it. Listen for expressions of Health, reorganization and realignment to the primal midline.

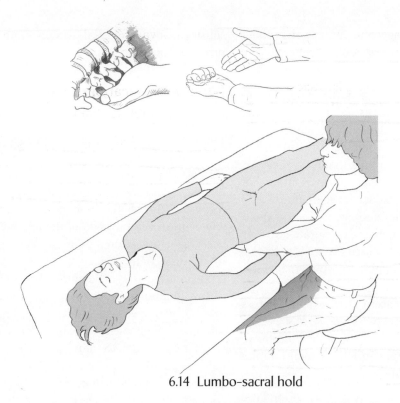

6.14 Lumbo–sacral hold

DISENGAGEMENT AND THE LUMBOSACRAL JUNCTION

Accessing a neutral within the dynamics present is often all that is needed to resolve the biokinetic forces within an inertial fulcrum. Inertial potencies will be expressed, and you may sense a welling up and permeation of potency within the relationship. This may include your awareness of the Long Tide and the deeper forces at work within the system. You may sense the biokinetic forces that were maintaining the compression being dissipated back to the environment. The compressive forces will resolve and the lumbosacral junction may be sensed to expand. The biokinetic energies of force vectors from birth and accidents are often processed. They may be perceived to literally leave the body.

Sometimes, however, the compressive forces are so dense, and the tissue and fluid effects so chronic, that a further conversation is useful. In this next exploration you will be engaging in a conversation about the potential space within the joint relationship and using the conversation skill of disengagement. You will be inquiring into how much space is available within the relationship and will then help the tissues access their state of balance. This is not a demand, but a conversation with the tissues and forces at work within the compressive fulcrum.

1. Maintain your lumbosacral hold as above. With your cephalad hand under the lumbar vertebrae, subtly intend a stabilization of the lumbar area. Using this hand, gently engage the tissues in an intention to wait. After stabilizing the lumbar area, subtly intend a caudad traction via the sacrum. This is offered as an inquiry, not as a demand. Within the mid-tide this can be perceived to be a more direct conversation with tensile forces. As you intend traction, a conversation begins and the tissues can show the potential space available within the relationship. It is not

just about a disengagement of tissues; it is about disengagement of the very forces maintaining the compression.

2. As you intend traction, a limiting boundary to the traction may be accessed, representing the amount of space available. The boundary feels as if further traction would be stressful for the system. Do not lock up the tissues against this boundary which could create stasis instead of the desired state of balance. The intention is to traction enough to initiate a conversation about space, but not so much as to generate stress or more tension. Once a sense of space is accessed, listen for the action of potency within that space. How does potency manifest here? Does it well up or drive into the area? Do the fluids express this? Do the tissues express a sense of seeking a neutral, a state of balance? Slow the fluid-tissue motions down, if appropriate, to facilitate the accessing of this state.

[margin note: respect boundaries]

3. Listen for expressions of Health, permeation of potency, and for a softening and expansion of the tissues. The biokinetic forces that have maintained the tissue compression will be processed as this occurs. The sacrum may be sensed to literally float toward the feet.

4. Wait for the sacrum to express its motility with greater potency and drive. This will be sensed as a stronger fluid drive in the system and a fuller motility (widening-uncurling, narrowing-curling) within the sacrum itself.

You may engage in several cycles of expansion, processing of compressive forces, reorganization of tissues and states of balanced tension. There may be a number of biokinetic issues maintaining the compressive pattern. These may resolve in a gradual and staged manner. For instance, the forces of a fall may resolve, then the tissues may reorganize and a different inertial issue may emerge. A new state of balance may then be accessed, allowing these forces to be processed, and then another inertial issue may come to your attention. It may seem as though potency is shifting from one inertial issue to another as each is processed in turn.

PRIMARY AND SECONDARY COUPLING OF COMPRESSIVE ISSUES

Lumbosacral compression is often coupled or associated with other compressive issues in the body such as occipito-atlanto-axial compression, intraosseous occipital issues, and compression at the SBJ. Compressive forces held anywhere within the midline of the system will be mirrored throughout the midline. If the lumbosacral compression is primary, then the others tend to express a compensatory compression. Clinically, we relate to these as a single unit of function.

It is common for secondary compressive fulcrums to arise in compensation for a primary issue as a factor of inertial potencies at work. Potency acts as a unified field in order to maintain order and the best balance possible. As the system holds inertia, more of this unified field will become inertial in order to compensate for the forces present within the system as a whole. As the greater field of potency becomes inertial in various ways, compressive forces will be transmitted through the tensile tissue field to other relationships.

Lumbosacral compression may strongly affect dural function and ease of dural glide. Fluid dynamics will also be affected. The patient may be more prone to lower back issues. Chronic low-grade inflammation is often associated with lumbosacral inertia. The connective tissues go into protective contraction, muscles go into spasm, and joint compression results. Nerve facilitation and pelvic visceral issues may also arise, generated by lumbosacral compression.

DISENGAGEMENT AND THE SACROILIAC JOINTS

Next we will begin to explore inertial forces found within the sacroiliac joints using an approach similar to the above process, first listening and helping access the state of balance and then exploring disengagement and space. Compressive fulcrums are common here. Review the anatomy of the sacroiliac joints and the pelvis generally. Know the male and female anatomy. In previous explorations, you may have sensed a specific inertial fulcrum located within a sacroiliac joint. You may have noticed that the sacrum moves around a specific S/I joint, or that it seems to be hinging in its motion around the joint. You may have noticed connective tissue strains or pulls originating from a sacroiliac area. Alternatively, you may have sensed fluid dynamics, such as fluctuations and rebounds, organized around an S/I joint.

Remember that the sacroiliac joint is L-shaped and quite variable in its structure and surface topography. Follow what is presented without excessive preconceptions of ideal joint motion, in order to be able to perceive the unique characteristics of the individual patient. Facilitate the ideal for that particular person.

Clinical Application: Sacroiliac Joints

As you palpated and listened to the system, you may have sensed a compressive pull through connective tissues towards a sacroiliac joint or you may have perceived the sacrum moving around a compressive fulcrum within an S/I joint. A sense of torsion within sacral dynamics may have been perceived, or perhaps a hinge-like motion between the ilia or around a sacroiliac joint. You may even have sensed a compressive wedging of the sacrum between the ilia. Very little pelvic motion at all will then be perceived. These various compressive patterns are all organized by inertial forces. These forces are expressions of unresolved experience. They may resolve by following the dynamics expressed and helping to access a neutral, the state of balance. However, the compressive forces present may be very dense and deeply coupled, and the tissue structures involved may have undergone real qualitative changes and be chronically compressed and inertial. The space within the joint literally closes down, and the fluids within and around the joint become static. There may not be enough space available for potency to initiate a healing process and resolve the compressive issue. You may need to make a more specific relationship to the joint. As above,

you may want to assist the resolution of the compression by engaging in a conversation about space via an intention of disengagement. Remember this work is as much about space as about form. Inertial forces resolve in space.

The first step is to simply listen. In the *sacral hold,* follow the dynamics expressed and sense the organizing fulcrum. Help the tissues access a state of balance if necessary, and listen for potency to come into play and biokinetic forces to be processed. You have worked with this intention at the sacrum before. This may be all that is needed to resolve the inertial issue. If the compressive forces are dense and chronic, a further conversation with the tissues may be required.

1. The *sacroiliac hold* is a new hand position for exploring S/I patterns. First hold the patient's sacrum as previously learned (Volume One), then place the forearm (near the elbow) of your other arm on the lateral aspect of one iliac crest and the fingertips of the same arm on the lateral aspect of the other iliac crest. Your arm is arched over the pelvis and bridging the space between the two ilia. You now have a clear relationship with the two iliac crests as you maintain the original sacral hold (Fig. 6.15).

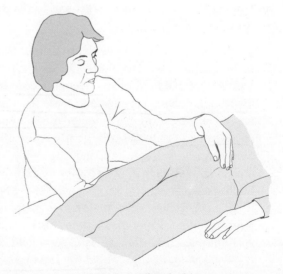

6.15 Sacroiliac hold

2. Synchronize your perceptual field to the mid-tide. Orient to the phases of primary respiration. Follow the expression of tissue motility within these phases. Include the innominate bones in this exploration. Access the state of balance and be open to reciprocal states of balance within potency, fluids, and tissues. Remember that you are always working with the unit of function of potency, fluids, and tissues. Hold the whole of this within your perceptual field as you assist in accessing a neutral within the dynamics perceived.

3. Listen for expressions of Health within the stillness of the state of balance. Listen for the initiation, permeation, and expansion of potencies. Listen for responses within the fluids and tissues. Wait for reorganization and reorientation of the tissues to their natural fulcrums and the midline function.

Clinical Application: Disengagement and the Sacroiliac Joints

In this next section we use the same hand position to explore potential space within the S/I joint relationship via the intention of disengagement. In this process you will be stabilizing the innominate bones as you bring the conversation of disengagement to the S/I joint area.

1. Again, maintain a wide perceptual field that includes the whole biosphere. Do not narrow your perceptual field as you begin the conversation about disengagement and space. To initiate this conversation, gently intend the two iliac crests together. To do this, gently bring the elbow/upper forearm and fingertips of your arched arm together. This narrowing of the front implies a widening effect in the back at the S/I joints, as if the iliac crests are levers to open the joints on either side of the sacrum. This is a suggestion of traction, not a forceful command, as if you are gently asking, "Would you like to move this way?" Intend the iliac crests together until

space is generated within both S/I joints. When space is accessed, you may sense that the sacrum begins to express motion of some kind, or settles into your hand.

2. When this occurs, subtly add a caudad traction at the sacrum. Both of these intentions, one at the iliac crests and the other at the sacrum, initiate conversations about space and potential within the two sacroiliac joints. Do this subtly, as a conversation with the tissues. "How much space can you allow here?" "Can you express your potential space here?" This is not a demand; it is an inquiry.

3. Once space is accessed, listen for the action of potency. If a neutral is sought, listen to the seeking phase of Becker's three-phase process. Help access the state of balance within the relationships. Here another conversation is added. "Can you access the state of balance?" "Can you access stillness here?" "Can you express your potency here?" Listen for expressions of Health within the neutral accessed. Listen for fluid fluctuations and pulsations of potency around and within the inertial fulcrum.

4. As inertial potencies are expressed within the state of balance, the biokinetic inertial forces will begin to resolve. You may sense that the sacrum begins to float footward. The sacrum may resolve its inertia in stages, in a ratchet-like manner. An inertial issue will resolve, the tissues will reorganize, and then another layer of experience may be accessed. Each time, access the state of balance in order to help resolve the inertial forces encountered.

5. After you perceive the resolution of the sacroiliac compression, monitor the sense of sacral motion and potency. Is the Breath of Life expressing itself more fully and in a more balanced manner? Is potency more available? Is there better drive within the fluid tide? Does the sacrum lift cephalad in inhalation? Is there easier motion and motility?

6. At the end of these sessions, check the sacrum for both mobility and motility. Have these improved? Is there a greater sense of fluid drive within its expression of motility?

Be patient because the process may take a number of sessions. Respect the timing of the patient's system. In an ongoing clinical practice, first orient to primary respiration and wait for the Inherent Treatment Plan to unfold. Listen to the fluids and potency of the system with a wide perceptual field and wait for the treatment plan to engage. Sense where the healing forces need to work first. You may be surprised to realize that something else must occur before the compressive forces within the sacroiliac joints resolve. This "something else" may be located anywhere else in the body. You may sense potency shifting to other areas that need attention, before the sacroiliac issue can be addressed.

Fluid Approaches and Options

We have several clinical options for working with sacroiliac issues, all based on the use of conversations with potency and fluids. Let's use a few examples of clinical applications to discuss these approaches. In the work above, you may have met a situation that seemed chronic and intransigent. The sacroiliac tissues may have become very condensed, and the fluids may be very inertial. Again these are all results of inertial forces and potencies. Although the sacrum should ideally be floating within the sacroiliac joints, the joint relationships may have been perceived to be dry or dense, and to lack fluidity. Directing fluids to inertial fulcrums within the state of balance may assist in processing the inertial forces present.

Clinical Application: Direction of Fluids

1. Maintaining the sacral hold, place your other hand on the front of the body with the palm over the inguinal ligament area anterior to the sacroiliac joint being addressed. From this position tune into fluids and direct fluid from the anterior hand to the sacroiliac joint (Fig. 6.16).

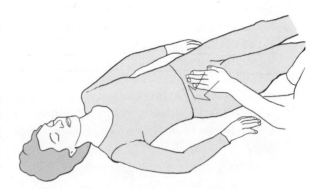

6.16   Direction of fluid to a sacroiliac joint

2. Sense the response of the fluids to this intention. Notice any echoing of fluid and potency from the compressed area. Notice how the fluids and potencies around and within the area respond. Wait for the inertial potencies within the fulcrum to express themselves in some way and for an expansion and welling up of potency to emerge within the relationship. Directing fluids begins a conversation with the whole field of potency and fluid, and the inertial potencies within the fulcrum may then respond.

3. An alternative to the above process is to make a more direct relationship to the joint. To do this, move your hand from the sacral hold. Place your cephalad hand under the sacroiliac joint being addressed. Using this hand, place a "V" under the joint, using your index and middle fingers to span the joint with the posterior inferior iliac spine between the fingers.

4. Place your caudad hand over the anterior inguinal area. The palm of that hand should be centered over the inguinal ligament. With the hand under the joint, use your V-spread to access the state of balance across the sacroiliac joint.

Then, with your anterior hand, direct fluids from the inguinal area to the V-spread. Sense the response of potencies and fluids to this intention. Wait for a sense of expansion and welling up of potency within the V-spread area.

5. If the potencies still seem very inertial, add an intention of disengagement to begin a conversation about space. You have the posterior superior iliac spine (PSIS) between your V-spread fingers. The intention is to subtly traction the PSIS laterally in order to access potential space within the sacroiliac joint. Continue to direct fluid to the area. Listen to the response of fluids and potency. See if you can sense inertial potencies being expressed within the joint and biokinetic forces being dissipated. Then return to the original sacral hold, listen for changes, and follow patterns that are shown to you.

LATERAL FLUCTUATION

Lateral fluctuation conversation skills can also be helpful with sacral and pelvic issues. You may sense various forms of fluid or potency fluctuations around an inertial fulcrum. These may take almost any form. They may be pendulum-like, swinging back and forth, or they may be expressed as figure eights or spirals. These fluctuations are the expression of potencies and fluids in direct relationship to the inertial fulcrum being addressed. They are compensatory motions generated by the presence of the inertial fulcrum. Please remember that enhancing lateral fluctuations can be activating, and this method should be avoided in acute or painful situations. This process is most appropriate for very inertial and dense areas.

If the compressive forces are so dense that little or no reorganization seems to occur, you can artificially start a lateral fluctuation. As you are listening to the system via the sacral hold, start a lateral fluctuation of fluid and potency across the sacroiliac joints. Use the thumb and little finger of your palpating hand to do this. The intention is to subtly push against the swings of the pendulum and to create a stronger flux

of fluid and potency. This generally encourages a greater expression of potency within the area. Any time the fluid fluctuation becomes stronger in an area, more potency becomes available. This may encourage expression of potencies within the inertial fulcrum. At first, the uptake of your suggestion may be sluggish. Gently persevere. The fluids and potency within the area will begin to respond. As this occurs, you may have a sense of potency welling up in the area.

Clinical Highlight

While I was working in a clinic in London, a thirty-five-year-old man was referred to me. He had been suffering from ongoing sacroiliac pain for over a two year period. He remembered a fall off of a horse four years before and a past sense of tightening in the area. When his pain was most intense, it was disabling, and he was in a depressed state. He entered my office space bent over with contraction and pain and needed to be helped onto the treatment table. He was literally crying with pain and despair. The current intense bout had been going on for almost a month.

Upon palpation I found that his system was literally shut down; there was both local inflammation and tissue shock in the lumbosacral area and a general sense of autonomic activation throughout his body. The first thing I tried to do was create some kind of sense of resource for him. I tried to help him access a relatively comfortable position and then tried to orient him to some sense of felt resource and space. We worked verbally and with CV4s and stillpoints over a number of sessions in order to help downregulate his activation and help him access a sense of space and stillness within himself. I also showed him a parasympathetic recovery position from the work of Randolph Stone. This involved him lying on his left side with a pillow between his knees, placing his left hand over the rear of his neck and his right hand over his butocks with his fingers in the crease between his buttocks. He found this a very comforting position to use at home.

He found that the sessions gave him some additional resources, and his S/I pain gradually lessened. By the tenth session his autonomic activation had greatly reduced, and his system was better able to orient to primary respiration and the Inherent Treatment Plan. For the first time, I really was able to perceive the wholeness of his system, and his fluid-tissue field felt unified. Then a powerful sequence of events took place. His potency began to shift within the fluids and an issue within his thoracic area was attended to. I supported this process as mid-thoracic compression softened and his structural midline lengthened. The tissue field then distorted around the right O/A area, and an old compressive issue was attended to. Once this completed, the potency shifted to the occipital bone and an intraosseous compression. As the intraosseous forces resolved, his central nervous system came to the forefront along with a related cranial base pattern. The occipital, cranial base, and CNS issues were all related to very early experience and birthing forces. As these resolved, another level of autonomic clearing occurred with an electric-like release down the sympathetic chain.

It was only then that the treatment plan could shift to the pelvic area. It took many sessions for his system to do what it needed to begin to relate more directly to the S/I issue and the pain that it generated. Over a number of subsequent sessions I was able to support work in the pelvic area with some of the processes described in this chapter. An intraosseous birth pattern within the sacrum came to the forefront. As this occurred, he remembered an early childhood image of a fall off a bicycle. It appeared that a coupling of these forces with his horse accident had occurred. When these uncoupled, a general reorientation of his tissue field around the midline occurred, along with a real lightening of his sense of pressure and fragility. When the biokinetic forces within and around the sacrum fully resolved, a major shift within the tissues of his pelvis occurred, and the motility of the whole pelvic area realigned to the midline. By the twentieth session, his pain had completely subsided and his depression had lifted. Basically, he felt hopeful and had relief from pain for the first time years. Over the course of the later sessions, I also taught him some stretching and chi kung exercises that empowered him to relate to his sacroiliac area with much less fear.

The main points here are that the technique described above is used within the context of the Inherent Treatment Plan, and that it is also helpful to give patients methods that empower them to take their healing process into their own hands.

INTRAOSSEOUS SACRAL ISSUES

If you cannot sense the presence of primary respiration and midline orientation after the above work, you may be encountering an intraosseous distortion of the sacrum. An intraosseous distortion is a pattern of compression or inertia within the bone itself. The segments of the sacrum have mobility at birth, but intraosseous issues can occur due to biokinetic forces placed on the young sacrum. Issues may also be generated during the toddler period when infants learn to walk and have many falls on the bottom. Trauma to the pelvis may also generate intraosseous distortions within the sacrum.

Clinical Application:
Intraosseous Inertia within the Sacrum

With intraosseous inertia the segments of the sacrum may seem compressed together, and the sacrum as a whole may not express a fullness of motility. This is a common issue. The sacrum may feel lifeless and dull, or dense and compressed, even if it is expressing some kind of outer motion. This is commonly missed. Do not fixate on the structural expression of motion. Look deeper than the basic flexion-extension motion. Listen to the inner story of the tissues. Is the bone itself breathing the Breath of Life? Look to its motility.

1. If you sense compressive forces at work within the sacrum, bring this awareness into your palpating hand. Follow the sense and quality of these forces and facilitate space within the sacrum. Remember that the sacrum is a living, flexible, fluid tissue. Potencies, fluids, and tissues are one unified function. Engage the sacral tissues and encourage space by spreading the hand holding the sacrum in all directions. Bring the intention of spread to the fingers and palm of your hand as an intention, not a command. The intention is to access the potential space available within the tissues of the sacrum.

2. When space is accessed, listen for the expression of potency. See if there is a manifestation of potency and a processing of inertial forces. If it seems that the tissues are seeking a neutral, help the tissues access the state of balance. Within the state of balance, maintain your awareness of the inner sense of the sacrum. You are waiting to perceive an expression of the potency of the Breath of Life within the bony tissue. You may sense pulsation, the welling up of potency and fluid, and lateral fluctuations within and around the sacrum.

3. You can also use the skill of lateral fluctuation discussed above as you relate to the intraosseous inertia. After intending spread, if things seem

very dense, you can initiate an expression of lateral fluctuation. These fluctuations may even be perceived within the intraosseous tissues of the sacrum.

4. To do this, use your thumb and index finger on one side and the little finger and lateral aspects of your hand on the other. Enhance, or start, a lateral fluctuation from side-to-side across the sacrum as though you are amplifying the swings of a pendulum. Listen for the action of potency and fluids within the tissues of the sacrum. You are waiting to sense a literal rehydration of the bony tissue of the sacrum and a greater expression of potency and motility. The sacrum may be sensed to soften, spread, and open like flower petals.

Intraosseous inertia within the sacrum can have important consequences for the vitality of the system. Inertia in sacrum/coccyx relationships will strongly affect the expression of the fluid tide and of tissue motility throughout the body. If the sacrum is holding intraosseous inertia, the ability of the whole system to express primary respiration may also be compromised. A long time ago an osteopathic old timer said to me, "If the system doesn't respond to your work, look to the sacrum!"

1. F. H. Willard, "The Anatomy of the Lumbosacral Connection," in *Spine: State of the Art Reviews* 9(2), May 1995 (Hanley & Belfus, Inc.).

2. Description of joint surface topography based on *Gray's Anatomy,* twenty-ninth American Edition (Lea and Febiger).

3. Ibid., Willard.

4. This is after Kapanji, *The Physiology of the Joints* (Churchill Livingston Inc., 1974).

7

The Occipital Triad

···

Now we turn our attention to the other end of the core link of the Primary Respiratory Mechanism. At the superior pole of the spine is the occipital triad of the occiput, atlas (C1), and axis (C2). As we found with the inferior pole, these three structures are intimately linked together due to the continuity of ligamentous relationships. In addition continuity here is derived from their common embryological origins. The occiput originates from sclerotomes and can be considered to be a modified vertebra. Thus, the occiput, atlas, and axis form a functioning embryological unit. Inertial issues within the triad will be directly transferred to the cranial base, the dural membrane system, and below to pelvic systems. The old maxim "as above, so below" certainly holds true for midline structures.

In this chapter we will:

- *Introduce the dynamics of the occipital triad and its relationship to the dural tube.*

- *Discuss the intraosseous possibilities of the occiput.*

- *Learn clinical approaches to occipital-atlas-axis issues.*

The Occipital Triad

The junction between the cranium and cervical vertebrae is commonly called the O/A (occiput/atlas) junction. This highlights the close relationship of the occiput and its condyles with the articular surfaces of the atlas. However, it is of utmost importance also to understand the continuity of their relationship with the axis. These three bones and their associated connective tissues form a clear local unit of function (Fig. 7.1).

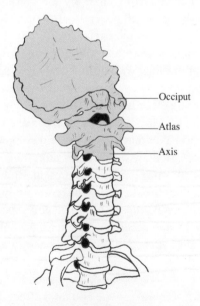

Occiput

Atlas

Axis

7.1 The occipital triad

A fluidic model is necessary to accurately understand the functioning of the occipital triad. Ideally, the atlas should be floating within the synovial fluids of its joints, and the axis should be hanging fluidly from the occiput via the ligaments supporting the dens. The atlas ideally floats between the occiput and axis as the axis fluidly hangs from the occiput on tension fibers. As we will discuss thoroughly in Chapter 13, connective tissues are basically fluidic in nature. Their fibers float within a semiliquid field. Connective tissue relationships are also fluid relationships, and together they all form a unified liquid crystalline matrix. All connective tissues, including bone, are fluidic and energetic in nature. The whole triad system should function with space between its components. Both atlas and axis should be floating within their synovial fluids. Tissues rest on fluids and the whole hierarchy is organized by the Breath of Life.

ANATOMY AND THE BIGGER PICTURE

Understanding and accurately visualizing the anatomical relationships of the occipital triad is an important starting point, so we want to take time to really understand the specifics of this area. The clearer you can be about the living anatomy, the more efficient and effective you will be as practitioner. However, it is possible to become overly focused on details here.

In a biodynamic understanding, resistance and symptomology within the body-mind are factors of the interplay between inherent biodynamic potencies and unresolved biokinetic forces. Always remember: when tissue inertia is present, these deeper forces are at work. You may perceive fluid congestion, tissue compressions, tissue changes, adhesions, etc., but the focus must be on the forces present. Biokinetic forces that affect the occipital triad commonly originate in trauma, including birth trauma and experiences such as shock and accidents. Potencies become inertial to contain overwhelming experiences and will act to center the disturbance. An inertial fulcrum is generated by the conjoining of these dynamic forces. These, in turn, generate tissue and fluid effects both locally and throughout the body. As you deepen into the slower tidal phenomena, these forces are perceived ever more clearly. These can be directly appreciated by the practitioner and patient, and the work becomes much more efficient and effective. When you work with the inherent potencies and forces involved, the work naturally takes on a deeper meaning.

It is important to remember that inertial processes are always centered within the wider ordering matrix generated by the action of the Long Tide. Tissues organize in relation to the ever-present expression of this matrix from the time of conception to the moment of death. Tissue inertia is a reflection of deviations from this principle. When we recognize these deeper processes, sessions are not just about the release of resistance or changes in symptoms, but center on the resolution of inertial forces and realignment to origin or source. As we get into anatomical and clinical specifics, let's not lose sight of this big picture.

LIGAMENTS THAT SUPPORT AND PROTECT THE OCCIPITAL TRIAD

Before approaching clinical issues, let's review some basic anatomy. We will look at the following ligamentous relationships from the most superficial to the deeper relationships. Inertial issues can be found in any one ligament or in a combination of ligaments (Fig. 7.2).

Superficial Relationships of the Occiput, Atlas, and Axis

The main ligaments that lie superficially in relationship to the deeper ligaments are the anterior atlanto-occipital membrane, the anterior atlanto-axial ligament, the posterior atlanto-occipital membrane, and the posterior atlanto-axial ligament.

- *The anterior atlanto-occipital membrane* is broad and dense and connects the anterior margin of the foramen magnum with the superior border of the anterior arch of the atlas. It is strengthened in the midline by a cord-like thickening that connects the basi-occiput with the tubercle of the

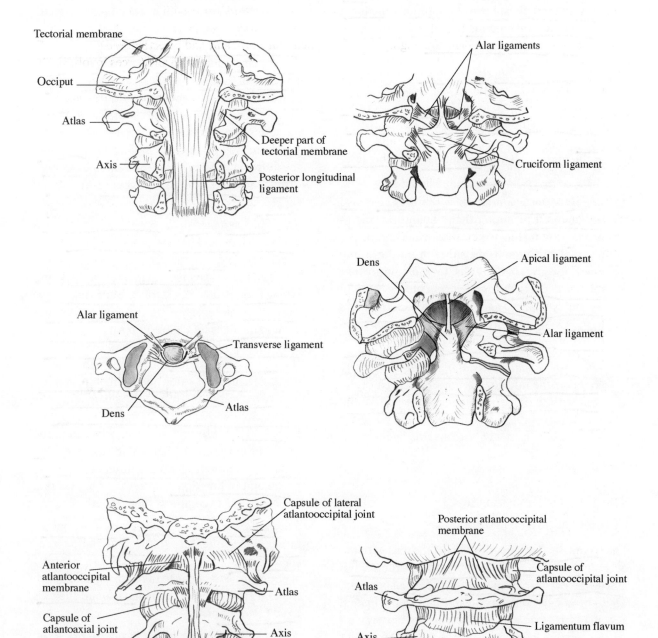

7.2 The layering of the membranes of the occipital triad

anterior arch of the atlas. This thickening is continuous with the anterior longitudinal ligament of the vertebral column. It is closely associated with the alar and apical ligaments.

- *The anterior atlantoaxial ligament* serves a purpose similar to that of the anterior atlantooccipital ligament in that it connects the inferior border of the atlas to the superior border of the axis anteriorly. It is also strengthened by a rounded cord in the midline that is continuous with the anterior longitudinal ligament.

- *The posterior atlantooccipital membrane* is also broad, but it is thinner than the anterior membrane. It connects the posterior margin of the foramen magnum to the superior border of the posterior arch of the atlas. Its most important relationship is to the dural membrane itself, where it is firmly attached anteriorly. Compressive forces in the O/A junction can be directly transferred to the membrane system via this relationship.

- *The posterior atlantoaxial ligament* posteriorly connects the inferior border of the arch of the atlas with the superior aspect of the arch of the axis. It serves the same purpose as the posterior atlantoaxial ligament above and the ligamentum flavum below.

The Deeper Relationships of the Occiput, Atlas, and Axis

The ligaments that directly connect the axis with the occiput are the tectorial membrane, the cruciate ligament, the two alar ligaments, and the apical ligament. These ligaments create a critically important, unified system of triad relationship. These tissues closely connect the occiput, atlas, and axis. The tectorial ligament is superficial to the cruciate ligament, which is in turn superficial to the alar and apical ligaments

- *The tectorial membrane* can be thought of as a cephalad extension of the posterior longitudinal ligament of the vertebral column. A strong, broad band, it covers the ligaments of the dens and is in close relationship with its transverse ligament. The tectorial membrane connects the posterior surface of the axis to the occiput just anterior to the foramen magnum on the basi-occiput. It blends with the cranial dura mater where the dura mater attaches to the basilar portion of the occiput. Compressive forces in the cervical area and the spine generally can be directly fed into the dural system via this relationship. If the tectorial membrane is in contraction, the occiput, atlas, and axis will all become compressed together.

- *The cruciate ligament* is composed of the transverse ligament and its extensions superiorly (crus superious) and inferiorly (crus inferius). Its center part, the transverse ligament, is a thick and strong band that arches across the atlas and straps the dens in place. There are synovial membranes around the dens that allow it to rotate within the space made by the anterior arch of the atlas and the transverse ligament, like a peg and socket joint. The superior extension of the cruciate ligament goes from the transverse ligament to the basi-occiput above, where its upper fibers merge with dura. Its inferior extension attaches to the posterior border of the body of the axis. The cruciate ligament helps bind the three bones into a single unit of function. Contractions held within it will obviously compress them together.

- *The alar ligaments* are strong cords that connect either side of the dens to the condylar parts of the occiput. They pass obliquely and laterally superior from the dens to the occiput. Along with the apical ligament, they help suspend the axis from the occiput.

- *The apical ligament* extends from the tip of the dens and connects it to the anterior aspect of the foramen magnum, suspending the dens from the occiput. The apical ligament can be considered to be a rudimentary intervertebral disc, and it contains traces of the notochord. It is thus closely related to both the early embryology of the system and to the midline expression of the Breath of Life within the system. Its fibers also merge with cranial dura.

INERTIAL ISSUES

Inertial forces and related strains can be held in any or all of the above ligamentous relationships. The joint capsules themselves can and will organize around compressive forces. Contraction of the posterior atlanto-occipital membrane, and adhesion between it and the dural membrane, will strongly compromise the mobility of the dural tube. It is also common for the alar and apical ligaments to be in contraction and thus to hold the whole triad system in compression. The cruciate and tectorial ligaments may also tense and contract due to the presence of inertial forces, and these contractions will often be coupled with bony compressions. Because their upper fibers merge with the dura mater and dural tube, compressive issues in the occipital triad can be transferred directly to the cranium (including reciprocal tension membrane and sutures), spine, and sacrum.

Bony structures and their related ligaments are a unit of function. They are a continuity of form. Because of this, inertial patterns outside the Primary Respiratory Mechanism are traditionally called "ligamentous articular strains." Resistances found within bony relationships are always associated with membranous or ligamentous strains. Joint compression and patterns of fixation will always involve the local ligaments that maintain the joint's stability. We will explore these local dynamics in the clinical sections below.

Inertial issues within the occipital triad can have far-reaching consequences for structure, fluid circulation, and nerve function. This area serves as a concentrated gateway for the entire body. Some inertial issues include:

Structure

When exploring dural tube and spinal relationships, you may notice a sense of compression or congestion at the top of the spine. This area is very prone to compressive and torsional patterns due to birth trauma, traumatic experiences, and postural issues. If the occipital triad becomes inertial, the cranial base and dural motion may be strongly affected. The whole vertebral column will also be affected, and reflections will be found within all its other relationships. Compressive patterns at this superior pole of the spine will also be reflected in the lower lumbar area, especially at the lumbosacral junction. All sorts of symptoms can be generated by these conditions.

Fluid Circulation

Occipital triad inertia can also greatly impact fluid movement, affecting arteries, veins, and cerebrospinal fluid. The vertebral artery threads its way through the transverse processes of the cervical vertebra and makes a nearly right-angle turn between the atlas and occiput, while the carotid artery is located at either side of the triad structure, and the basilar artery and Circle of Willis are just superior to the occiput. Compression within the occipital triad can compromise the blood supply to the brain stem (Fig. 7.3). The veins

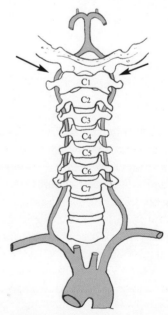

7.3 The vertebral artery and its ninety-degree turn

119

draining the head are similarly affected. The internal and external jugular veins and the vertebral veins can be compromised by occipital triad compressions. This can generate a backpressure in venous sinus drainage and a general sense of fluid congestion, producing a marked effect on the quality of fluid drive and potency in the system as a whole. Inertia within the occipital triad can also create backpressure into the cranium that restricts cerebrospinal fluid circulation, negatively affecting the essential transmutation interchange between potency and fluids.

Nervous system

Nerve function is similarly vulnerable to compression and congestion within the occipital triad area. The jugular foramina, passageways for the glossopharyngeal, vagus, and spinal accessory nerves, are particularly important. Intraosseous compressions in the occiput and compressions between the occiput, atlas, and axis will affect the jugular foramina and may cause impingement of the vagus nerve, with potentially severe repercussions throughout the body including disorders of the heart, lungs, digestive organs, and neuro-endocrine-immune system.

CLINICAL APPROACHES

There are three basic areas of clinical exploration in this chapter. Our first approach focuses on the forces that may be held within the bony dynamics of the occiput itself. The dynamics of the atlas and axis will be strongly influenced by these unresolved forces and their related tissue effects. This chapter contains a simple clinical approach to compression across the occipital condyles generated by intraosseous forces. Later (Chapter 16) we will explore more detailed intraosseous issues. Our second exploration focuses on potential inertial issues between the atlas and the occiput (O/A junction). The third focuses on the unified function of occiput, atlas, and axis and the essential relationship between the axis and occiput.

INTRAOSSEOUS OCCIPITAL DISTORTIONS

Inertial fulcrums can be located anywhere within the body. If they are located within the cells and tissues of an individual bone, then inertial issues are generated within the dynamics of that bone. The tissue of the bone will be affected by these forces in some way, and its form and motion will distort to comply with them. Basically, an intraosseous distortion is an inertial issue located within the tissue of that particular bone. It is very common to find these kinds of inertial issues within the tissue of the occiput. For example, the atlas may actually become wedged between the condylar parts of the occiput due to intraosseous inertial patterns.

Palpating an intraosseous distortion feels like a movement pattern or tendency toward a particular shape within specific area of a single bone, as compared to articular distortions that feel as if they involve two or more structures in relationship to each other. A particular bone may be sensed to be dense or inertial, and tissue motility throughout the cranium may be organized around it. Because intraosseous distortions commonly originate in prenatal and birth experiences, you can sometimes feel that you are holding an infant's head in your hands as you palpate an adult skull. You must respect the infant's experience as you hold the adult skull. Respectful contact and patience are especially important in working with intraosseous distortions because these patterns generally arise from trauma. Discharge of shock affect and similar phenomena can be common as these patterns resolve. We will look at intraosseous issues in much more detail in Chapter 16.

The occiput is in four parts at birth: the squamous portion, the two condylar parts and the basi-occiput (Fig. 7.4). These parts can be forced into compressive and/or torsioned relationships during the birthing process. Common inertial patterns include rotations of the squama of the occiput relative to the rest of the parts, torsioning across the condylar parts and the foramen magnum and compressive telescoping of the occipital structure towards the SBJ. The form of the occiput can distort based on the forces at work

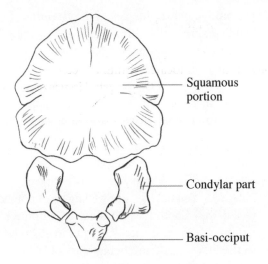

Squamous portion

Condylar part

Basi-occiput

7.4 The occiput at birth

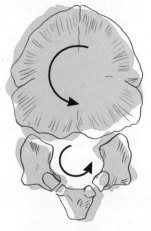

Rotation with torsion
across condylar parts

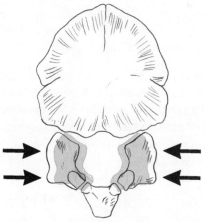

7.5 Common intraosseous distortions
of the occiput

because bone is living tissue, not like the dry and hard examples of dead bone used for anatomical study.

During birth process, forces can be introduced into the occiput that cause its parts to compress, or telescope, together. As the parts of the occiput are forced to compress together, the tectorial membrane and the alar and apical ligaments will be pulled superiorly. This typically compresses the axis and atlas as a unit superiorly into the condyles of the occiput. You can thus end up with a common compressive picture in which the condyles of the occiput, atlas, and axis are all compressed together. These same forces can also generate medial compression within the condylar parts of the occiput. This will, in turn, wedge the atlas between its articulations and compromise both its motility and mobility.

Intraosseous distortions of the occiput will always affect the dynamics of the atlas and axis. The atlas and axis will be pulled superiorly by compressive forces and will also be affected by intraosseous torsions within the occiput. The atlas can become wedged in its articulation with the occipital condyles if there is medial compression generated by the telescoping or compression of structure. On a very basic level, learn to listen to the dynamic forces involved, and the inertial forces that organize the tissue patterns will become clear (Fig. 7.5).

Clinical Application: The Condylar Spread

If you sense a medial compression of the condyles and a wedging of the atlas into the condylar parts, you can suggest a lateral spreading across the foramen magnum. In essence, you are engaging in a conversation with the tissues via the intention of space across the foramen magnum. This, in turn, initiates a conversation about disengagement between the condyles of the occiput and the articular surfaces of the atlas.

1. Place your hands under the occiput in an occipital cradle. Orient to the mid-tide. Listen to the fluid tide and then include the tissues being palpated. Do not narrow your perceptual field as you orient to the tissues of the occiput. See if a sense of compression and narrowing across the foramen magnum comes into your awareness. If you have a sense of restricted motion, block-like motion or inertia between the condyles and atlas, you may want to focus more directly on the condyles.

2. To do this, change your hand position from the occipital cradle to a condylar spread position. Spread the heels of your hands apart so that your fingertips point towards the occipital condyles. Make contact with the condyles by imagining that you are extending your fingers towards them. Again orient to the mid-tide and the motility of the tissues within the phases of inhalation and exhalation (Fig. 7.6).

3. In this position, intend/suggest a spread across the foramen magnum. This is a very subtle intention brought to the tissues as an inquiry. In this, you are engaging in a conversation with the tissues. "What is possible here? Can you give yourself space? What is this really like?" Once again the intention is to access enough space so that the biodynamic potencies of the Breath of Life can be expressed within the state of balance. A traditional way to intend a lateral spread across the condyles is to gently bring your elbows together. This will encourage a lateral spreading of your fingertips and this intention will be transferred to the condyles and foramen magnum.

4. As space is accessed, listen for the action of potency. Sometimes when space is accessed, there is a build-up of potency and processing of inertial forces. You may sense a welling up of potency or a drive of potency into the area. Commonly a state of balance is accessed that directly relates to the inertial fulcrum being palpated. You can assist this if necessary. Subtly slow any motions down and listen for a settling into the state of balance. Be open to the expressions of fluids and potency within this stillness. Listen for Becker's *something happens*. Listen for expressions of Health.

5. When the biokinetic forces resolve, you will sense a lateral spreading of the condylar parts and an expansion across the foramen magnum. You may also sense a de-wedging of the atlas from the condylar parts.

Option: Lateral Fluctuation and Condylar Dynamics

If the forces and their tissue effects are very dense, you can initiate lateral fluctuations of potency and fluid in order to stimulate the inertial potency within the tissue. If you do note an expression of potency arising, you can start lateral fluctuations within the tissues of the occiput. You can do this, as previously learned, by intentionally pushing against the fluids and potencies within the inertial tissues, first in one direction, then the other between your palpating fingers. In the condylar hold, initiate a lateral fluctuation from the index and middle fingers of one hand to the index and middle fingers of the other. See if you can sense fluctuations arising within the occiput

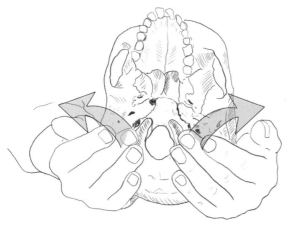

7.6 Condylar spread hold

itself. Remember that bone is a connective tissue and connective tissue is a fluidic matrix. This will often initiate an expression of potencies within the inertial fulcrum.

TUNING INTO THE OCCIPITAL TRIAD

In this next section, we will explore the occiput-atlas-axis triad and tune into its dynamics. We will first explore the occipito-atlanteal junction (O/A junction) and then widen our view to include the axis. If needed, review the anatomy of the occipital triad area before undertaking the applications below so that your conversation will be precise and accurate.

The first step will be to tune into the area and to see if any inertial patterns clarify. Three approaches are suggested here. The first is using an O/A hand position to listen for the expression of the primal midline. A second approach is via awareness of the fluid dynamics of the area. A third approach is to use skills of traction to engage the dural tube membranes in a conversation about ease of glide. These approaches all involve the skills and conversations learned previously; the only new aspect of the lesson is the anatomical detail of this area.

The questions are the same. Do you sense a clear expression of potency, fluids, and motility through the area? How have the structures organized themselves? Is there balance in their expression of motility and motion? Do they orient to the midline? If not, how have they organized themselves? Are there inertial patterns expressed as shapes of motion and mobility dynamics? How does the fluid tide express itself within these dynamics? Is there fluid backpressure or lateral fluctuation present?

At the end of each process, sense for tissue reorganization, expressions of motility and mobility, ease of dural mobility, and for the expression of the fluid tide. Compare the new expression with the initial presentation. It is always important to establish baselines so that you can judge how the system is responding to treatment. Three possible baselines are the quality of potency and fluid drive of the system, how tissue motility and motion orients to the midline and to suspended automatically shifting fulcrums, and ease of dural mobility and glide.

The following exercises employ the same skills developed in working with vertebral patterns, applied to the superior pole of the vertebral column. Tissue patterns perceived may include any of the allowable motion dynamics that we described previously in vertebral relationships. These include forward- and backward-bending, rotation, side-bending, anterior-posterior shifts, lateral shifts and superior and/or inferior compression.

Clinical Application: O/A Junction and the State of Balance

1. In this first exploration, we will learn a new hold, the *occipito-atlanteal hold* (*O/A hold*). With the patient in the supine position, cradle the occiput so that your hands curl around the squama with the pads of your fingers against the occipital ridge and the tips of your fingers pointing anteriorly, toward the atlas. Your hands should be held together supporting the occiput (Fig. 7.7). Imagine/intend that you are extending your fingertips anteriorly until you sense that you are in contact with the atlas. Do not use a heavy pressure to do this. Use your intention. It should feel as if the atlas is floating on your fingertips. Again orient to the biosphere and mid-tide.

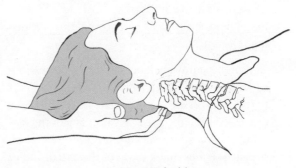

7.7 O/A hold

2. As you come into relationship with the atlas, it will begin to show you its movement tendencies. How does the atlas express its motility? How does it express motion? Notice how the atlas moves within the phases of primary respiration.

3. You may perceive the atlas expressing particular motion tendencies. While you sense this, include the motion of the occiput. See if you can hold the whole occiput-atlas experience within your perceptual field. Do not narrow your field down as you do this. You are orienting to a particular field within a much wider one.

4. You may sense compressive forces at work within the relationship of the atlas and occiput. These will give rise to tissue compression and fixation. Do not initially try to follow or engage these. Wait for a sense of unity to arise and a clarification of inhalation and exhalation. Wait until a pattern clarifies. It may seem like *something engages from within,* there is a shift in the potency and a particular tissue distortion comes to the forefront.

5. Listen for the state of balance. This is a subtle process; the most active role for the practitioner is to have a gentle intention about slowing down any motions or patterns being expressed. Wait for a settling of the tissues into a state of balance. You cannot make the system access this state, but you can assist it in finding its own inherent balance. On a tissue level, you are waiting for a state where all the tensions in O/A relationships access a state of equilibrium. It will feel like the tissue field settles and stills around the organizing fulcrum.

6. Within the state of balance, listen for expressions of Health. See if you sense inertial potencies being expressed. As these potencies are expressed, you may sense a processing of the biokinetic forces that had maintained the compressive tissues, and a sense of the expansion of potencies within the area. On a tissue level, you are waiting for a sense of softening of the resistance, expansion, and a floating free of the atlas in its relationship with the condyles of the occiput.

7. Listen for reorganization of the relationships of the occipital triad and realignment to the primal midline. You may also sense that the atlas reorients itself between the axis and occiput.

In many situations simply accessing the state of balance may be all that is needed. However, if the inertial potencies are chronic and the compressive forces at the O/A junction are very deep, more specific conversations may become necessary.

Clinical Application: Disengagement and the O/A

Compression of the atlas into the condyles of the occiput is common. Compression of the O/A is commonly combined with rotation and torsional forces. The following disengagement process for O/A compression has been called an *O/A spread.* Here you will be bringing an inquiry into space to the relationship between the atlas and occiput.

1. In the *O/A hold,* sense the atlas on the tips of your fingers. Again, this is an intention rather than heavy pressure. You may have become aware of compressive forces that fix the atlas within the condyles of the occiput and keep the tissues from freely floating within fluids.

2. In this position, you will be intending space, or disengagement, within the relationship between the atlas and occiput. To initiate this, spread the heels of your hands and tips of your fingers apart. You must have the sense that you have engaged the atlas with your fingertips. The intention is to initiate a conversation about superior-inferior space within the relationship. This intention is transferred to the tissues. Your fingertips traction the atlas inferiorly, while the heels of your hands place a subtle superior intention at the occipital squama. Do not narrow your field of awareness down as you do this. Maintain a wide

perceptual field that senses the whole body as a tensile field of action (Fig. 7.8).

3. Wait for a sense that space has been accessed. You may sense a softening and spreading of tissues. The atlas may feel freer. Help access the state of balance. Wait within the state of balance and notice how the system expresses its potencies. Listen for expressions of Health and a permeation of potency into the tissues.

4. When the inertial forces are resolved, you may then sense an expansion of potency within and around the fulcrum. As this occurs, note that the tissue elements also express expansion. You are waiting for the atlas to disengage from the condyles and reorient to the midline. Remember that when tissues orient to an inertial fulcrum, they must orient to the midline in an eccentric way. Wait for a sense that the atlas and occipital condyles are floating away from each other. Wait for the completion of the reorganization and realignment stage of Becker's three-phase awareness process.

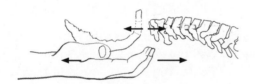

THE UNIT OF FUNCTION

After exploring the specific patterns of the O/A relationship, we next take a wider approach. The occipital triad is really one single unit of function, operating as a complete system that can be approached as a whole including bones, ligaments, and the fluids of the joint capsules.

Clinical Application: Occipito-Axial Relationships

In this next section, we will widen our inquiry to include the whole of the triad relationship by contacting the occiput and axis and spanning the atlas. In this position, you will listen to the motility and motion of the whole triad area, wait for a pattern to clarify and help access the state of balanced tension.

1. From the *O/A hold,* slide your fingertips inferiorly until they contact the axis. We call this the *occiput-axis hold.* The first palpable spinous process inferior to the foramen magnum is the axis. Spread your fingers transversely along the posterior arch of the axis. You are still supporting the occipital squama in the palms of your hands. You will now be cradling the occiput with your fingers posterior to the axis (Fig. 7.9).

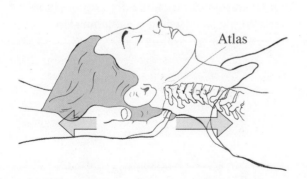

7.8 O/A hold with an O/A spread

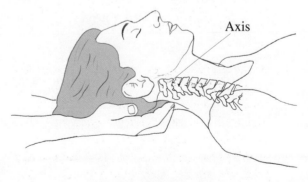

7.9 Occiput–axis hold

2. In this position, sense the motility and motion within the phases of primary respiration. Allow the potency-fluid-tissue field to communicate its priorities to you. Allow the work to unfold within your palpation contact. Follow the dynamics present and help access the state of balance. Wait for the resolution of the forces involved, expressed as an expanding and softening tissue reorganization.

Clinical Application: Disengagement and the Ligamentous Field

If there are compressive issues within the triad as a whole, you may sense that the ligaments between the occiput and axis are contracted, and the occiput, atlas, and axis do not have independent motion. There will be a sense of compression and congestion and a lack of mobility in the area. In this next approach, we start a conversation with the inertial ligaments and encourage space and the state of balance within the whole unit of function.

1. In the occiput-axis hold as learned above, initiate a conversation about space with all of the ligamentous and joint relationships of the occipital triad. This is similar to the approach above in the occiput-atlas hold. To initiate this conversation, spread the heels of your hands and tips of your fingers apart. Sense how you have engaged the axis with your fingertips. This is a suggestion, an intention, not a heavy pressure or force.

2. Intend this spreading of the tissues until you perceive that space is accessed. You may sense more motion as this occurs and/or an intensification of the action of potency within the relationship. Help access the state of balance.

3. You are now directly engaging the ligamentous relationships between occiput and axis in a conversation about history and Health. See if you can specifically sense which ligaments or joint capsules are most inertial and contracted.

4. Orient to fluids and potency. Listen for expressions of Health. Wait within the stillness of the state of balance for expressions of inertial potencies, expansion, softening of the resistance barrier, and reorganization of the triad relationships. You may sense the ligaments involved softening and lengthening. Note how the occiput, atlas, and axis have reorganized their motility and motion after these forces have resolved.

FLUID APPROACHES

In all of the above approaches and relationships, pay attention to the expression of the fluid drive and potency within the state of balance. You can use fluid skills (directing fluid, lateral fluctuation) if the inertial forces within the relationships of the occipital triad are very deep. In the occipital triad hand positions, you can direct fluids with the heels of your hands from the cisterna magna to the fulcrums and relationships below. You can also use your fingertips to subtly initiate lateral fluctuations. If the area seems congested, intentionally push against the fluids within the relationships, first in one direction then in the other, to draw potency into the relationship.

8

Patterns of the Cranial Base

The motion dynamics of the cranial base are a central theme in the classic cranial understanding of the whole human system. Sutherland considered the cranial base, and more specifically its sphenobasilar junction (SBJ), to be a key fulcrum within the system, allowing access to the entire history of the patient. When cranial base issues arise and resolve in session work, the entire system responds. We will introduce cranial base dynamics in this chapter and suggest some clinical approaches to its inertial issues.

In this chapter we will:

- *Learn ways to inquire into cranial base patterns as holistic distortion patterns of the whole cranial tissue field.*
- *Discuss implications of these patterns.*
- *Learn to relate to these patterns therapeutically.*

THE CRANIAL BASE AND THE SPHENOBASILAR JUNCTION

The cranial base and the SBJ is traditionally considered to be the functional heart of the cranium and a natural fulcrum for midline vertebral relationships. Sutherland considered the sphenobasilar junction to have functions similar to those of a joint with a disc.

Hence, it is sometimes also called the sphenobasilar symphysis (SBS). Sutherland reported seeing a number of fetal skulls with actual discs between the sphenoid and occiput, showing that embryologically the sphenoid and occiput can be considered to be modified vertebrae. The SBJ is located at the most superior pole of the embryological notochord. At birth, the joint is a synchondrosis—a cartilaginous bridge—making it more stable than a disc joint. It retains the function of a synchondrosis throughout life (Fig. 8.1).

In the traditional biomechanical concept, the sphenoid bone is considered to be the keystone, or the major gear, of the cranium. As the sphenoid bone rotates and expresses its motion, the other midline bones are said to rotate in the opposite direction. This is like a child's game of gears in which there is one master gear that drives all other gears (Fig. 8.2). As we shall discover, bones are not really gears, nor are their motions mechanical, but the traditional concepts may help you orient to their motions and interrelationships.

Beyond the cranium, all tissue patterns organized around the midline will be expressed within and around the SBJ in some way. If there were no inertial patterns held in the system, then motility and motion around the SBJ would be expressed with balance and ease.

Major cranial nerves pass through or near the cranial base via foramina in and between its bones. Impingement or stress along these nerves can generate nerve facilitation issues with effects throughout

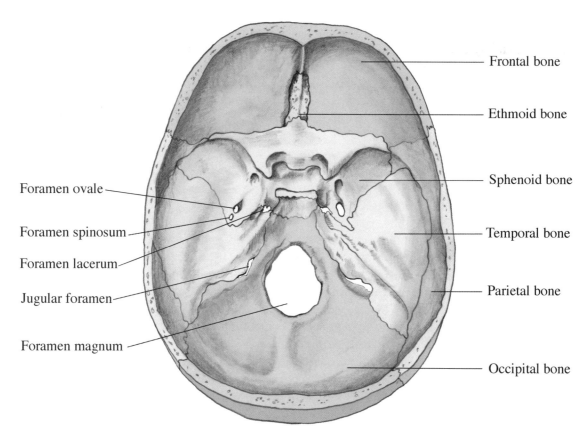

Frontal bone

Ethmoid bone

Sphenoid bone

Foramen ovale

Temporal bone

Foramen spinosum

Foramen lacerum

Parietal bone

Jugular foramen

Foramen magnum

Occipital bone

8.1 The cranial base

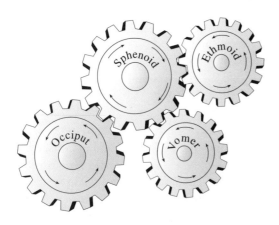

8.2 The "gears" of the cranium

the whole body. Major arteries and veins are near the SBJ and also pass through these foramina. Patterns of inertia and compression within the relationships of the cranial base can affect the functioning of all these blood vessels. The brain stem rests directly on the basilar portion of the occiput just below the SBJ, so distortions here can also affect autonomic nervous system processes and the whole neuroendocrine-immune system.

Another important cranial base participant is the pituitary gland, the master gland controlling many metabolic and stress response functions. The pituitary gland rests in the saddle of the sphenoid bone within the sella turcica. It is strapped into this saddle by dural membrane called the diaphragma sella. Patterns of dysfunction within the bones and membranes of the cranium will be directly fed into the pituitary via these relationships, thereby affecting the entire neuro-endocrine-immune system.

As we investigate the dynamics of the cranial base, we may sense how all structures within the cranium are a unit of function. They are totally interrelated in their dynamics. Cranial base patterns are really patterns of distortion throughout the cranium. Birth issues are often manifest within these dynamics. Many of the deepest inertial patterns originate in very early life experience. Prenatal and birth experiences significantly shape the membranous-articular relationships of the cranium, and these patterns can be important gateways into this material.

Reciprocal Tensions and Sutherland's Fulcrum

Since we are looking at a membranous-articular system, we must appreciate the suspended automatically shifting fulcrum located within the straight sinus: Sutherland's fulcrum. Sutherland's fulcrum is ideally located within the anterior aspect of the straight sinus where the falx and tentorium meet the great vein of Galen. This fulcrum is the natural fulcrum for all of the membranous-articular motion within the cranium. In its organizing function, Sutherland's fulcrum is a concentrated point of potency that naturally expresses the respiratory cycles generated by the Breath of Life. It is the reference point for the reciprocal tension motion of the whole cranium. It is around this fulcrum that all forces are ideally resolved and balanced, and through which ease of motion is maintained. Bone is a connective tissue. The motions of the cranial bones are totally integrated with those of the reciprocal tension membrane. Sutherland's fulcrum is the natural point of resolution for the reciprocal tensions and tension patterns within the cranium. Both the falx and the tentorium can be considered to be suspended from this fulcrum point. If there were no inertial patterns within the system, then the membranous-articular motion of the cranium would be in lovely fluid balance around this automatic shifting fulcrum. This

includes the motion of cranial bones and of the cranial base.

If the system is centering inertial patterns, then this point of resolution will shift away from its ideal location. This makes an awareness of its dynamics essential for practitioners. If this point of balance shifts closer to its ideal location within the straight sinus, then you know that something has really been resolved (Fig. 8.3).

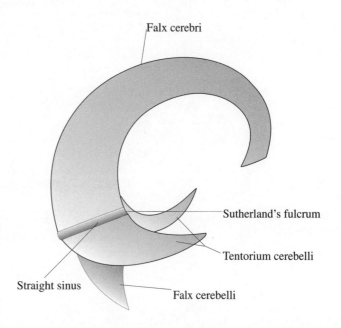

Falx cerebri

Sutherland's fulcrum

Tentorium cerebelli

Straight sinus

Falx cerebelli

8.3 The reciprocal tension membrane and Sutherland's fulcrum

Classic Motion Dynamics of the SBJ

In inhalation, the sphenobasilar junction rises and the tissues of the sphenoid and occiput expand and widen. This is an intraosseous inner breath. As this occurs, the occipital squama and greater wings of the sphenoid dive caudad (footward). This diving is traditionally described as a rotation around transverse axes in opposite directions (i.e., the occiput rotates in the

129

direction opposite to the sphenoid). Within the inhalation phase these motions are classically called *flexion*. The opposite motions, in exhalation, are called *extension* (Fig. 8.4). All midline bones (vomer, ethmoid, and sacrum) are said to rotate in a direction opposite to the sphenoid (Fig. 8.5).

Within the slower tides, the motion around the SBJ is sensed to be fluidic and integrated. The SBJ is at the heart of the arrangement of the bones in the cranium. As the tide ascends, the SBJ ascends like the center of a flower and all of the other bones widen and open like the petals of the flower, opening to the sun. The SBJ is the fulcrum around which this occurs. This is not a mechanical motion, it is fluid and organic. Bones are fluidic forms, and their motility is expressed as an inner organic filling and widening and a reciprocal settling and narrowing. As the SBJ shifts, the whole membranous-articular flower-like dynamic organized around it will also shift. This, in turn, all orients to Sutherland's fulcrum as a unified connective tissue dynamic.

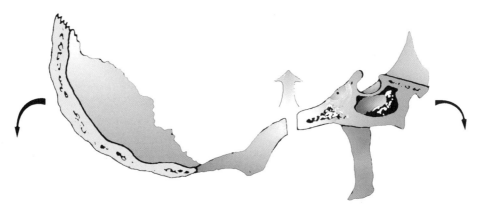

Inhalation around the SBJ

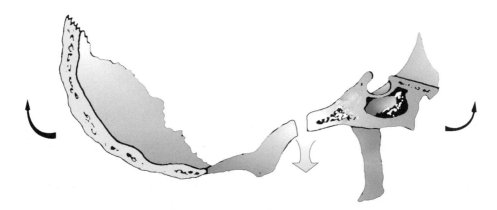

Exhalation around the SBJ

8.4 Inhalation/Exhalation of sphenoid and occiput

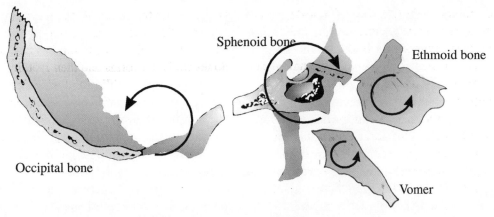

8.5 Midline structures in inhalation phase

THE CRANIAL BASE AND INERTIAL ISSUES

In the following applications, we will be exploring patterns of fixation. In these patterns, the tissues of the cranium become conditioned to express certain motions, or fixed in certain patterns, due to the inertial forces affecting them. These may be local forces within the SBJ itself or forces remote to its immediate dynamic. A fixation within the cranial base may be generated as a result of direct traumatic forces, or in compensation for inertial fulcrums found almost anywhere within the body.

The unresolved issues held within the body-mind will be expressed around the SBJ in particular ways. Sutherland discovered that inertial patterns expressed at the SBJ can be broken down into particular components, and that these can be named, tested for, and eventually perceived intuitively. He outlined six particular patterns that may be expressed around and within the SBJ. In the following sections you will begin to explore these patterns and learn to perceive them. You will basically learn to ask the tissues some specific questions. Learning to ask the right questions will help you appreciate the form of the various patterns and will allow you to be in a clearer relationship to them.

Motion testing gives an entry into the motion allowed within the joint relationship. It is the first step in learning about these patterns. Later we will realize that motion testing, especially within the deeper and slower tidal rhythms, is not really necessary. Indeed, it may get in the way of the inherent intentions of the Breath of Life as it orchestrates the healing process. Simply listening to the system within the phases of primary respiration will emerge as a more effective approach.

PATTERNS OF THE WHOLE

The cranial base should be approached cautiously and respectfully. All of the compensations expressed around the SBJ are patterns of experience and must be met with respect and inquiry. In relating to cranial base patterns, we are relating to our patient's whole mind-body process and the whole of their history. The SBJ pattern is just the tip of the iceberg. The SBJ shows the embodiment of that history and how experience is being centered by the potency of the Breath of Life. These patterns are symbols of a much greater dynamic, a much wider and deeper orb of experience. It is not a matter of needing or wanting specific changes, nor of fixing anything, but of opening up to possibility and potential. It is up to that person and the depths of his or her system to make the choices and sense the possibilities. The Breath of Life does the healing. It is not up to the practitioner to impose solutions onto the patient's system.

Patterns here result from forces and pressures applied to the system. For instance, due to a trauma, strong forces may enter the cranium and become entrapped and inertial. If the experience cannot be resolved at the time of the trauma, the forces involved will be centered by the potency of the Breath of Life in some way. The potency of the Breath of Life will also become inertial to center the disturbance.[1] Inertial fulcrums result that generate tensile distortion patterns. These tissue distortions are also manifestations of Health. They are an expression of Intelligence at work. They are patterns of containment and compensation. They are the best possible expression of health that the system can maintain, given all of the inertial forces it is centering.

A common origin of SBJ patterning is the birth process and birth trauma. Other origins can include falls, accidents, or emotional shock. Patterns originating in other parts of the body can also be expressed in some way at the SBJ.

Along with the motion dynamics perceived, there may be a whole psycho-emotional history to hear. The patterns you perceive are life patterns. You are in relationship to the embodiment of that person's life history. The inertial patterns can tell a larger story than the simple motion dynamics being expressed. In this psycho-emotional wholeness, life statements become the organizing fulcrums of personality and self. Life statements are deeply ingrained beliefs about self and the world it inhabits. These can be held just as rigidly as any physical fulcrum. These psycho-emotional structural patterns will be part of the larger trauma schema of a person's experience and must be approached with clarity and respect. Employ verbal skills for dealing with overwhelm and activation of traumatic cycling if these processes arise during session work.

BIOMECHANICS AND BIODYNAMICS OF THE CRANIAL BASE

Sutherland based his model of motion and his terminology on the biomechanical concepts that prevailed at that time in the osteopathic profession. Thus, the traditional description of cranial base motion is biomechanical in theory and language. The biomechanical approach states that bones move around axes of rotation, motion transfers mechanistically from structure to structure, and the whole system operates like a clockwork apparatus. This viewpoint is why terms like flexion/extension and internal/external rotation were used to describe bony motion and all tissue motion in the body.

These concepts are transformed in a craniosacral biodynamic approach. Inherent motion is seen to be much more organic and fluidic. Motility is directly perceived as an inner breath that arises all at once within the whole person. Potency, or life force, is sensed to be the organizing and driving factor. "Axes of rotation" and similar biomechanical phrases are at best just approximations of reality. The deeper sense of motility and motion is that of an intraosseous inner motion, a welling up within each structure during the inhalation phase yielding an expansion and widening of that structure. The subsiding of this surge is the exhalation phase, palpable as a settling in the tissues. Interosseous motion between structures is really an expression of this deeper inner motility. It is the drive of the potency within the fluids that naturally generates both intra- and interosseous motion. The quality of these motions is organic and fluid when perceived through the slower tidal rhythms. Bones are part of a unified tensile tissue field, a liquid crystalline matrix.

This chapter uses conventional terminology, but this usage is mainly for the purpose of learning. Traditional language may help a newcomer orient to the basic patterns and probabilities for individual bones and for groups. But the intention is to go far beyond the mechanistic viewpoint as learning gives way to actual clinical practice. A craniosacral biodynamic approach is much more effective in the long run.

PERCEPTION AND THE SPHENOBASILAR INQUIRY

In the following sections we will learn to perceive the basic patterns potentially found around the SBJ. In all of the processes described below, we will be welcoming the SBJ into our perceptual field without losing a sense of the form and dynamics of the whole cranium.

The intention will be to maintain a wide perceptual field and gently become aware of the particular motions and forms around and within the SBJ. Let them come to you. Listen, don't look. Be soft and wide in your focus. Because the SBJ reflects the experience of the whole system, sensitivity and fine-tuning of perceptual skills is needed. Specifically, all the instructions about maintaining a wide view and avoiding crowding the system are especially relevant. This work entails an essential retraining of our perceptual processes. Cranial base dynamics will be much clearer, and the relationship to the whole much more obvious, if you maintain this wide field. The information you receive will be more accurate, and the Inherent Treatment Plan more obvious, with a soft, wide perspective. Motion testing tends to draw us closer and make us focus on specifics, but this tendency must be resisted in the exercises below. After a while the need to motion test drops away as your relationship to the system deepens and the treatment plan speaks to you. In essence, you will find that you form a deeper and deeper relationship to the Breath of Life and to the forces it generates in the human system. As this occurs, the work orients more and more towards stillness and space.

The mid-tide, the 2.5 cycles per minute rhythm, is the preferred starting point for all these exercises. Work here is oriented towards the forces at work within the human system, be they biodynamic or biokinetic. As you palpate within the mid-tide, the motility of individual structures will be perceived to be part of a greater tensile field of action. The motions of the sphenoid bone and of the occiput will be sensed to be part of a unified dynamic. The felt-sense is that you are not just palpating individual structures, but are sensing a unified fluid-tissue field. Within this greater whole, you can still perceive the motion of the individual bones. Listening from a mid-tide level helps transform motion testing into a more intuitive process of inquiry.

SPHENOBASILAR INQUIRY AND MOTION TESTING

Cranial base patterns are traditionally learned via motion testing. In the following sections I will introduce these palpation intentions with a particular mindset. We will be initiating an inquiry, rather than testing for position or fixation. Asking the right questions will help you appreciate the form of the various patterns and will allow you to be in a clearer relationship to them. Questions are posed by your direct hand contact via subtle suggestions of motion introduced into the fluid-tissue field. The answers come as patterns of distortion throughout the whole field, not just as motions around the SBJ. The goal is to be able to hear the story of the system as this Inherent Treatment Plan unfolds and to perceive how these patterns are reflected within the whole person.

KNOW YOUR ANATOMY

Familiarity with the relevant anatomy is an essential prerequisite. With a solid knowledge of the anatomy, all of these dynamics can be sensed as you listen to the motions of the SBJ and cranial bowl with your gentle attention. See if you can visualize their form in your mind's eye as you sense them in your hands. The more accurately you can identify the fulcrum and visualize the surrounding anatomy, the more the patient's system will express itself and respond to your questions. Somehow the patient's inner intelligence can judge your knowledge of anatomy, and will adapt its expression to match. An analogy is the degree of meaningful contact that is possible when traveling in a foreign country; the more we know the language, the deeper will be our capacity for meaningful relationships. The language of the body is anatomy, so really understanding the tissues and how they work greatly enriches your practice.

Practicing the movements with skull models and disarticulated bones is one of the best ways to develop thorough and accurate capacity to visualize anatomy. Having a set of disarticulated bones to play with can be invaluable. Hold them and rotate the bones into the patterns. Use them to practice the treatment processes. Initially it is important to be able to picture these patterns. Once you are familiar with them, they become more of a felt-sense through your palpating hands. Another training aid is using modeling clay to mold the bones of the cranial base and reciprocal tension membrane. Play around with the shapes with these clay models, moving the whole clay form into the patterns. You may gain a better sense of these patterns as distortions, rather than as patterns of rotation of individual bones.

CLASSIC CRANIAL BASE PATTERNS

There are two categories of inertial patterns found within the dynamics of the SBJ. These are called *physiological patterns* and *non-physiological patterns*. Physiological patterns are those that are naturally allowable within the biomechanics of the SBJ; these include flexion-extension, side-bending rotation and torsion. Non-physiological patterns are those that are not normally allowable within SBJ biomechanics. These include lateral and vertical shears and compression. For each of these patterns, we will use a two-step learning process. First we will learn how to ask the right questions, and second, we will explore ways of resolving the patterns revealed in response to our questions.

We will be using a way of motion testing that acknowledges that these patterns are distortions throughout the entire cranium. These are not the traditional ways of posing these questions. Classic approaches are covered in many other books and courses. I teach these alternative methods in foundation courses as they acknowledge the unified nature of the fluid-tissue field.[2]

In the following clinical applications, you will be using one of the vault holds learned in previous chapters. In all of the work outlined below, the patient is in the supine position. From the vault hold, you will intend a deepening into a specific direction of motion, a very subtle momentary intention in that direction. It is a suggestion, "Do you like to move in this way?" This has the quality of asking a question, rather than directing or making a demand on the system. Once you ask the question, wait and listen to the answer. The question is an impulse, a momentary suggestion. Do not guide or push the system in that direction. After your suggestion in a particular direction, let the fluids take the tissues. Sense how far the tissues float in that direction. This process makes the pattern clearer both for yourself as practitioner and for the patient's system. It is a reflective process (Fig. 8.6).

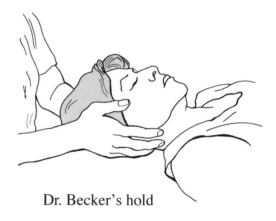

Dr. Becker's hold

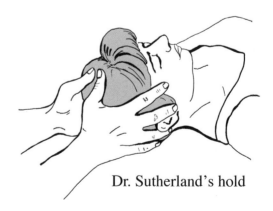

Dr. Sutherland's hold

8.6 Two traditional vault holds

PHYSIOLOGICAL PATTERNS

Clinical Application: Inhalation and Exhalation

First we will simply listen to the now familiar motions of inhalation-flexion and exhalation-extension using either or both of two hand positions. *Sutherland's hold* is a vault contact with the index finger at the greater wing of the sphenoid and the little finger on the occiput. *Becker's hold* is similar but uses the thumb to palpate the sphenoid. Try both of these to get a feeling for which works better for you. In inhalation, as the SBJ rises, the sphenoid and occiput are said to move into flexion, and as it descends, they are said to move into extension. In reality, a flower is a better analogy than a clock for visualizing this basic movement.

1. In either of the two vault holds, negotiate your contact with the patient's system and orient to the mid-tide. First tune into the fluid tide, then include the tissues. Once you are generally aware of tissue motility and motion, then orient to the SBJ. Do not narrow your perceptual field; simply include an awareness of the sphenoid bone and the occiput via your hand contact.

2. First ask the patient's system, "Do you like inhalation?" As the SBJ rises in inhalation, can you sense the "flower petals" of the cranium (the cranial bones arranged around the SBJ) opening and widening? Include the fluid field in this sense. At the beginning of an inhalation phase, as you sense the SBJ rising, simply amplify this sense of the flower petals opening. Your fingers follow that sense of welling up and filling as though they are spreading in all directions. This is a momentary intention of spreading. Let the fluids take the tissues and see how far the tissues move in inhalation.

3. Then ask the question, "Do you like exhalation?" In the exhalation phase, see if you can sense the SBJ settling and the flower petals closing and narrowing. The intention in your fingers is the

opposite of the above. At the beginning of exhalation, amplify this sense of closing and narrowing by subtly narrowing your contact to the cranial tissue field. Your fingers gently close and narrow the flower petals. It is just a momentary intention; you are not guiding the tissues that way. Sense which direction the fluid-tissue field prefers (Fig. 8.7).

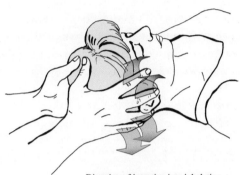

Direction of intention into inhalation
Fingers spread as "flower petals" spread

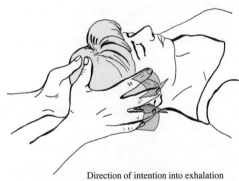

Direction of intention into exhalation
Fingers close as "flower petals" close

8.7 Palpation intentions
in inhalation and exhalation

4. Ask yourself which direction the system seems to prefer. If the system prefers the inhalation direction, it is called an *inhalation pattern*. If it prefers the exhalation direction, it is called an

exhalation pattern. Listen to the pattern via the motion of the fluids and tissues. Can you sense the location of the fulcrum that organizes that pattern? Being able to sense the organizing fulcrum is a key to effective work with any pattern.

Clinical Application: Facilitation of Sphenobasilar Reorganization

With each exercise, we will follow our initial identification of the pattern with approaches to resolve the forces at work using skills taught previously. We are not using new techniques or processes, but rather applying what we already know to new areas.

1. In the *vault hold* and listening via the mid-tide, let the tissues come to you as you hold a relatively wide perceptual field. Again ask the fluid-tissue field the appropriate question about the preferred direction. This time, help access the state of balance. Follow the motion in that direction until the pattern clarifies. Help access the state of balance and subtly suggest a slowing down of the motions perceived. Do not physically or mentally grab on to the tissues as you intend this. Listen for expressions of Health within the state of balance. These may include fluid fluctuations, expressions of potency within the inertial fulcrum, and a welling up of potency from the wider field through the fulcrum. Listen for a change in the potency within the state of balance.

2. Wait for a processing of inertial forces. You may sense a welling up of potency, the generation of heat, and even the resolution of a force vector in the form of streaming of heat or energy along a particular pathway. This generally indicates that a traumatic force vector of some kind is being dissipated back to the environment.

3. When a resolution of the inertial forces occurs, you may sense an expansion of potency, fluids, and tissues in your hands. Once inertial forces

are resolved, the inertial potencies that were centering their action can reorient to the midline and express their natural motion. This in turn allows the fluid and tissue world to do the same. Allow the tissues to express their inherent motion and listen to how they reorganize and realign to midline phenomena such as automatically shifting fulcrums.

If the inertial forces are very dense, you can initiate other therapeutic conversations such as lateral fluctuation or the direction of fluids towards the inertial fulcrum.

Cranial Patterns in Inhalation

In a classic inhalation-flexion pattern, the SBJ is fixed or held in a superior position. In essence, the flower petals of the cranial bones, and all cranial structures, are then fixed in inhalation. In an extreme fixation, the person's head may look widened and feel block-like. The cranium may have a rounded look with wide, prominent cheekbones and wide orbits. The eyeballs may seem to be protruding, and the hard palate could be flattened. Viewed from the side, the head will look shorter front-to-back. From a front view, the head will seem wide side-to-side. The person's body may appear externally rotated (feet and hips in an open position) and wide.

Cranial Patterns in Exhalation

In a classic exhalation-extension pattern, the SBJ is fixed or held inferiorly. All cranial structures will then also be held in exhalation. The resulting patterns are basically the reverse of the above. In the front view, the cranium may appear narrow side-to-side and the face will seem narrow. The eye orbits will appear narrowed and sunken and the hard palate will be arched. You may also see a narrow forehead, sunken eyes, hollow cheeks and a prominent sagittal suture. In a side view, the head will seem longer front-to-back; in the front view it will look narrowed side-to-side. The person's body may seem internally rotated and narrow.

SPHENOBASILAR SIDE–BENDING ROTATION

The next physiological pattern is called side-bending rotation. In this pattern, the greater wing of the sphenoid and the squamous portion of the occiput have been forced together on one side. Structures on one side are crunched together and structures on the other side are widened apart. This widening can be perceived as a bulge, called the side of the convexity. The side of the narrowing is called the side of the concavity. In biomechanical terms, side-bending rotation is said to occur around two vertical axes located within each bone. The sphenoid and occiput have been forced to rotate in opposite directions around these axes and may become fixed in a side-bent position. In the classic description, on the narrowed concave side, the structures are relatively internally rotated and on the bulged convex side, they are relatively externally rotated. Remember that this is actually a pattern of distortion sensed throughout the cranium, not just a simple rotation around axes.

On the side of the bulge, there is also a tendency for the structures to rotate inferiorly. This may create a perception that the structures on the convex side, such as the occipital squama and the sphenoid's greater wings, are lower than the structures on the concave side. All cranial bones on the bulged side, such as the temporal bone and parietal bone, will express external rotation relative to those on the opposite side. They are held in an inhalation-flexion position relative to the opposite side that is in an exhalation-extension position. The rotational component is sometimes masked or overridden by other membranous pulls and patterns so it may not be obvious until these other patterns have been resolved. For instance, a strong inferior fascial pull on the concave or narrowed side may cause an inferior rotation on that side, overriding the tendency to rotate inferiorly on the convex side (Fig. 8.8).

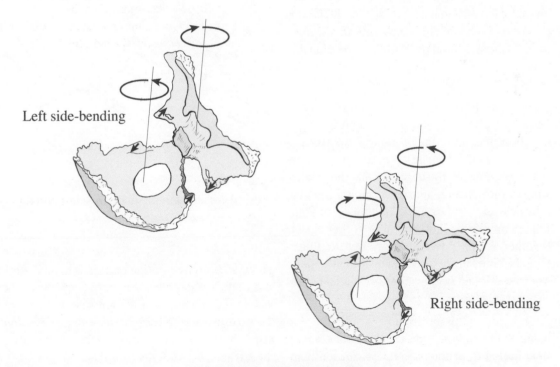

Left side-bending

Right side-bending

8.8 Sphenobasilar side-bending

Clinical Application:
Side-Bending Rotation

The side-bending process is the same as explored above for inhalation-flexion and exhalation-extension. Just as flexion-extension are allowable motions within the dynamics of the SBJ, so is side-bending. If no side-bending fixation is present, then when you test for these patterns, either side may gently bulge and recede to a small degree. You may sense some side-bending motion on both sides with a balanced and easy feel. If there is a side-bending fixation present, one side of the cranium may seem to be more convex, and the system will prefer this direction more definitely. Within the mid-tide, this will be sensed as a distortion within the entire cranial articular-membranous system, rather than a rotation around axes.

1. In the *vault hold,* orient to the mid-tide. Tune into the fluid tide and then include the tissues. Orient to the wider sense of inhalation and exhalation through the fluid-tissue field of the cranium. Again see if you have a sense of the flower petals opening and closing. Within this whole, listen to the shape and quality of the basic inhalation-exhalation motions of the sphenoid and occiput.

2. Then begin the inquiry into the nature of side-bending rotation. This is more about asking a question than directing or guiding the tissues. Very subtly intend/suggest a narrowing on one side of the cranium by suggesting that the greater wing of the sphenoid and the occipital squama move closer together. Imagine that all of your fingers on one side momentarily gather closer together as they ride the tissues. Let the fluids take the bones in the direction of your intention. Your other hand simply monitors the response to your suggestion.

3. As you intend this, notice any expression of a bulge on the opposite side. Do the tissues like to float in that direction? See if you can sense an overall distortion throughout the cranium as you

monitor for the bulge on the other side. It is like you are holding a fluid-tissue ball in your hands and you are sensing for a distortional shape in its whole form. You may also sense the rotational component coming into your hands, as the bulged side may rotate inferior.

4. Repeat this on the opposite side. You are waiting to sense which side has the larger (or narrower) convexity or bulge (Fig. 8.9).

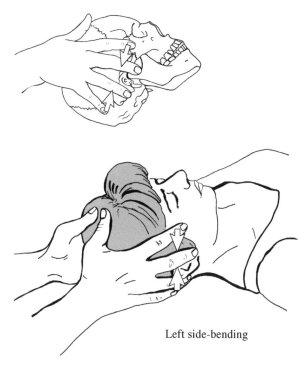

Left side-bending

8.9 Palpation intention in side-bending

The side-bending rotation pattern is named after the side of the greater convexity or bulge. So, if you sense a greater convexity on the right side of the cranium, the pattern is termed a *right side-bending rotation* (or just right side-bending). If the greater convexity is on the left side, it is called a *left side-bending rotation*. If there is no prominent side-bending pattern, the system will allow an equal amount of side-bending motion on both sides. There will be a sense of ease in this, and the inhalation-exhalation motion will not be held in a side-bent position.

Facilitation of Sphenobasilar Reorganization of Side-Bending Patterns

After the inquiry above, we will work to facilitate resolution of inertial forces just as we did before.

1. If you sense a greater convexity, or bulge, on one side, then again intend/suggest side-bending rotation to that side. Follow the tissues in their preferred direction and help access the state of balance. Subtly suggesting a slowing down of the motions may be all that is needed. This is a subtle negotiation with the potency, fluid, and tissue elements where your palpating hands accommodate the motions sensed and gently slow things down to help access the state of balance.

2. Within the stillness of this state, listen for expressions of Health. You may sense expressions of potency, fluctuations of fluid, and deepening stillness within and around the inertial fulcrum. Wait for a general sense of expansion within the tissues, a reorientation to the midline, and a greater fullness and clarity in tissue motility. Use other skills of conversation if the inertial forces seem particularly dense.

CRANIAL PATTERNS IN SIDE-BENDING ROTATION

In side-bending rotation, the structures on one side of the cranium are closer together than the structures on the other side. There is a narrowing on one side and a bulging out on the other. On the side of the concavity, the greater wing of the sphenoid may be fixed posteriorly towards the temporal bone, and the squama of the occiput may be fixed in an anterior position towards the temporal bone. This may generate a number of overall cranial patterns.

The sphenoid will be rotated posteriorly around a vertical axis on the concave side, while the occipital squama on that side will be rotated anteriorly. As the temporal bone follows the occiput in its motion, the occipital squama will hold the temporal bone in internal rotation. The frontal bone will follow the greater wing of the sphenoid posterior and may have a flattened, internally rotated look, and the eye orbit on that side may be narrowed. On the convex side the opposite will be seen. The greater wing and occipital squama will be forced apart, and the temporal bone will be held in external rotation. The frontal bone on this side may also have a widened, externally rotated look to it, and the eye orbit may be widened.

SPHENOBASILAR TORSION

Torsion is a third physiologically allowable SBJ motion. Classically, torsion is said to occur around an anterior-posterior axis from glabella to inion running through the center of the body of the sphenoid and SBJ. The sphenoid and occiput rotate in opposite directions around this axis, and a torsion occurs within their tissues especially at the SBJ where the synchondrosis distorts in a twisting fashion. Play with disarticulated bone models to become familiar with this. Connect the sphenoid and occiput with play dough or any pliable clay-like medium. Notice how the clay twists as you rotate the bones.

A torsion fixation occurs when the sphenoid and occiput have become fixed in one direction or the other, yielding a torsion pattern in cranial relationships. Within the slower and deeper rhythms, this is perceived as a distortion within the tissue field as a whole rather than as a mechanical rotation around a set axis. The axes may initially help you become familiar with these patterns, but don't take them too literally. We are really talking about a distortion within the whole cranium and tissue field, not just a simple rotation between two isolated bones. When the cranium is forced to distort into a torsion pattern, the sphenoid and occiput express inhalation-exhalation accordingly. Within the phases of primary respiration, one greater wing will be perceived to be superior to the other while the occipital squama on the opposite side will also be superior (Fig. 8.10).

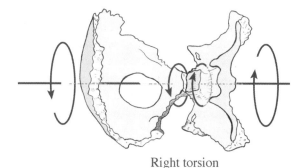

Right torsion

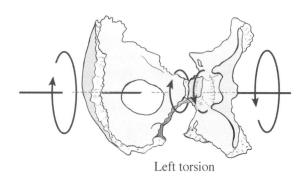

Left torsion

8.10 Sphenobasilar torsion

Clinical Application: Torsion

We will begin with an inquiry into the presence of torsion around the SBJ. As above, the intention is to sense if there is a preference for a torsion fixation in one particular direction.

1. Using either vault hold, orient to the mid-tide. First tune into the fluid tide and then include the tissues. Again sense that you are holding a unified fluid-tissue field. Sense the flower petals opening in inhalation as the SBJ rises. Sense the motion of the occiput and sphenoid as part of this whole.

2. To inquire into torsion, imagine that you have a transverse axis or axle through the palms of your hands. Subtly rotate your hands in opposite directions around this axis. Gently transfer this rotation to the greater wings of the sphenoid bone and to the occipital squama. Your hands are subtly intending a torsion throughout the fluid-tissue field of the cranium. This intention asks, "Do you like to distort this way or that way?" It honors the fact that we are really relating to patterns of distortion in the tissue field rather than a simple rotation of bones around axes. First ask the question one way and then the other. See which direction the fluid-tissue field prefers to express this torsional distortion.

3. See how far the tissues like to float in the preferred direction. If there is a torsion fixation present, the system will float into torsion easier and further on one side than the other. If there is no torsion fixation, then a slight torsion motion will be found with balance and ease in both directions (Fig. 8.11).

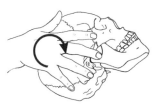 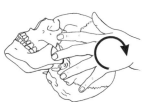

Right side   Left side

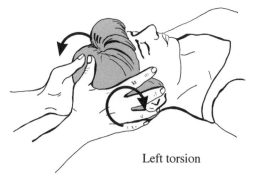

Left torsion

8.11 Palpation intentions in torsion

Torsion is named after the side of the superior sphenoid wing. If the greater wing is high on the right side, it is called *a right torsion pattern.* If it is high on the left, it is called a *left torsion pattern.*

Facilitation of Sphenobasilar Reorganization of Torsion Patterns

The following treatment process is the same as those described for the other patterns above, just applied to a different pattern.

1. Maintain your orientation to the mid-tide. Intend/suggest the torsion discovered above. As you intend/suggest a rotation of your hands in the preferred direction, follow the motion and help the tissues access a state of balance. This is a negotiation not just with the tensions but also with the forces that generate the tension. The state of balance is a systemic neutral, a dynamic equilibrium within the whole system. You will sense a settling, not just in the local tissues, but in the system as a whole. When this neutral is attained, listen for expressions of Health.

2. Within the state of balance listen for fluid fluctuations and expressions of potency. You may sense pulsations of potency, vector-like motions of potency, a drive of potency within the fluids, or a more holistic permeation of potency throughout the field through the fulcrum. This has a quality of softness to it, yet is powerful and clear in its healing intentions. You are waiting to sense a softening and expansion of the relationship. Listen for the realignment of potencies, fluids, and tissues to midline phenomena.

CRANIAL PATTERNS IN TORSION

In torsion, the superior greater wing is in a relative extension position while the inferior greater wing is in a relative flexion position. The facial bones follow the motion and position of the sphenoid bone. On the superior greater wing side, you may see an extension-like pattern in facial structures. The structures on the high side may have an internally rotated, narrowed look with a narrowed eye orbit and internally rotated facial structures relative to the low wing side. On the inferior greater wing side, you may see a widened eye orbit and externally rotated structures.

The occipital squama on the superior greater wing side will express a relative flexion pattern. It will be in an inferior position relative to the high greater wing because it is rotated in the opposite direction to the sphenoid bone. Since the temporal bone follows the occiput, the temporal bone will express external rotation on the side of the low occipital squama. In torsion, the anterior structures (the greater wing and the facial structures) will be expressing relative extension, while the posterior structures on the same side (the occiput and temporal bones) will be expressing relative flexion. The front of the cranium and the rear of the cranium on same side will seem to be held in paradoxically opposite phases of motion. The reverse pattern will be seen on the opposite side of the cranium.

It may be difficult to distinguish between a torsion pattern and a side-bending rotation pattern by simply looking at the front of the face. The way to differentiate between the two is that in the torsion pattern the front and back of the cranium on the same side seem to be in opposite phases of motion, while in side-bending the structures on the same side of the cranium express the same phase of motion.

NON-PHYSIOLOGICAL PATTERNS

In this section, we will explore patterns of motion that are not naturally allowable within the SBJ. *Non-physiological patterns* are considered to have more serious consequences than physiological ones because they may generate strong strains within reciprocal tension motion. The tissues are held in positions that may generate a strong resistance within natural inhalation-exhalation motions because the system is not designed to move in these ways. The distortion patterns generated in these non-physiological strains tend to be more extreme and intransigent, and symptoms also tend to be more extreme.

In physiologically allowable patterns the bones are said to rotate around their axes in opposite directions. In non-physiologically allowable motions the bones are forced to rotate in the same direction.

Non-physiological patterns commonly arise during pre-natal or birth processes when sutures are not yet formed. The vault bones have space between them, and the cranial base is flexible and resilient. The forces of birthing may compress and shear parts of the cranium. The bones don't rotate into sheared positions; they are literally forced into patterns of distortion by the shearing forces present.

The three non-physiological patterns are lateral shear, vertical shear and compression. In the two shearing patterns, the sphenoid and occiput seem to shear in opposite directions at the SBJ instead of meeting precisely in the middle. This can generate strong resistance to motion within the SBJ and strong backpressures throughout the system.

All non-physiological strain patterns are the result of strong, traumatic outside forces and must be approached with this understanding. This might include birth trauma, accidents, and falls. Compression patterns may be generated by emotional shock and are commonly associated with chronic states of hyper-arousal and stress.

SPHENOBASILAR LATERAL SHEAR

Lateral shear is said to occur around the same vertical axes as side-bending patterns. But here the rotation of the sphenoid and occiput is in the same direction. If the two bones are forced to rotate in a clockwise direction (viewed from above), the body of the sphenoid will shear laterally to the left side of the cranium relative to the occiput. If the two bones are forced to rotate in a counterclockwise direction around vertical axes, the body of the sphenoid will shear laterally to the right of the cranium relative to the occiput.

Lateral shear may generate a parallelogram shape in the cranium when viewed from above. This can most easily be seen in infants when the pattern arises due to birth trauma. The frontal bone/forehead may

be slightly shifted anteriorly on the side of the lateral shear. Visualize this as though the two bones are wagon wheels laid flat on the floor of the cranial base. As they are made to rotate in the same direction, they laterally shear at the place they touch. If lateral shear is present, you may sense that the greater wing of the sphenoid has shifted laterally to one side of the cranium (Fig. 8.12). As in all of cranial base patterns, these are actually patterns of distortion within the whole cranium and, indeed, within the whole body, not just two bones.

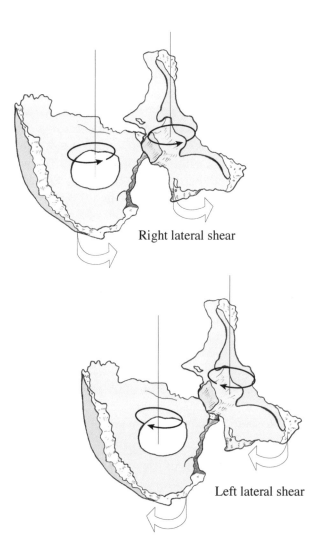

Right lateral shear

Left lateral shear

8.12 Sphenobasilar lateral shear

CLINICAL APPLICATIONS: SPHENOBASILAR LATERAL SHEAR

In the clinical application below, you will be inquiring into the possibility of lateral shear in both directions. As lateral shear is not a physiologically allowable motion, if there is no fixation present, the joint will not like to move in either direction.

1. Once again, negotiate your contact with your patient's system via the *vault hold.* Orient to the mid-tide. Again sense that you are holding a unified fluid-tissue field. A lateral shear pattern generates a parallelogram shape throughout the cranium. To ask the question, "Do you like right lateral shear/parallelogram shape?" momentarily shift your hands in a way that suggests or amplifies this form. In *Sutherland's hold,* the index fingers of both hands shift to the right, while the little fingers of both hands shift to the left. In *Becker's hold,* the thumbs of both hands shift to the right, while the little fingers shift to the left. The rest of your hand follows these motions. It is not a simple push on the sphenoid and occiput, but a motion of your whole hand in relationship to the tissues of the cranium. To ask, "Do you like left lateral shear/parallelogram shape?" shift your index fingers or thumbs gently to the left as you shift your little fingers to the right. See which direction, if any, the cranium as a unified field prefers.

2. Listen to how far the tissues float into the lateral shear pattern. If there is a right lateral shear, the sphenoid will tend to shift towards your right hand. If there is a left lateral shear, the sphenoid will tend to shift to the left. Note which side the sphenoid tends to prefer (Fig. 8.13).

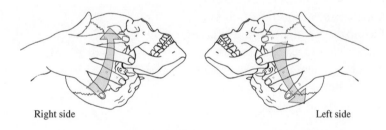

Right side　　　　　　　　Left side

Left lateral shear

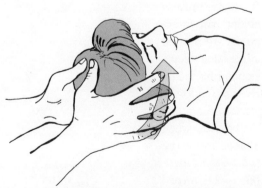

8.13 Palpation intention in lateral shear

Lateral shear is named according to the side of the sphenoid's movement. If the sphenoid is held laterally to the right side of the cranium, it is called a *right lateral shear* and if it is held to the left it is called a *left lateral shear*. If no lateral shear is held at the SBJ, you will not sense much tendency to shift to either side. It will feel balanced with little movement towards either direction.

Facilitation of Sphenobasilar Reorganization of Lateral Shear

1. If you sensed a tendency to laterally shear to one side, then again suggest motion to that side. This time follow the lateral shift, give it time to clarify, and help the system access the state of balance. At most, slow the motion down without grabbing on to the tissues in any way. This is a negotiation into the possibility of a state of dynamic equilibrium within all of the forces and effects present.

2. Within the state of balance listen for expressions of Health. If the inertia within the SBJ is very dense, direct fluid towards the SBJ or use lateral fluctuation. You are waiting to sense a softening and expansion, and a reorientation of the tissues to Sutherland's fulcrum and the midline within Becker's three-phase awareness.

Sphenobasilar Vertical Shear

In vertical shear the sphenobasilar junction becomes sheared in a superior or inferior direction. Vertical shear contradicts the SBJ's basic flexion/extension movement. Instead of rotating in the opposite directions around transverse axes, the bones are pushed in the same direction of rotation. Vertical shear occurs when the body of the sphenoid has been forced to rotate either superiorly or inferiorly relative to the basilar portion of the occiput. This pattern commonly originates during later stages of the birth process when anterior-posterior pressures are placed upon the infant's cranium.

In superior vertical shear the sphenoid is forced into a relative inhalation-flexion position while the occiput is forced into a relative exhalation-extension position. Visualize this as though the two bones are vertical wagon wheels with their axles within the natural transverse axis of each bone. As the wagon wheels are made to rotate in the same direction, a vertical shear is generated where they touch.

Vertical shear is named after the position of the rear of the body of the sphenoid. Superior vertical shear is when the sphenoid is held in relative flexion while the occiput is held in relative extension and the rear of the sphenoid is forced superior relative to the basi-occiput. In inferior vertical shear, the sphenoid is forced to rotate into a relative extension position, while the occiput is forced to rotate into a relative flexion position. The body of the sphenoid is forced inferiorly in relationship to the basi-occiput (Fig. 8.14).

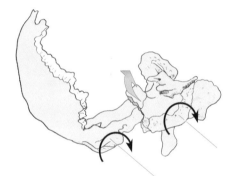

Superior vertical shear

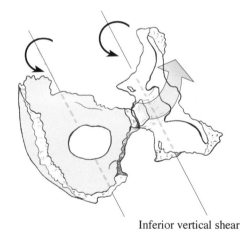

Inferior vertical shear

8.14 Sphenobasilar vertical shear

Clinical Applications: Vertical Shear

We will once again follow a two-step learning process. First you will ask the right questions and see what the preference of the tissues is. Then you will follow this preference into a treatment process.

1. Once again, negotiate your contact and orient to the mid-tide. Again orient to the cranium as a unified fluid-tissue field. See if you can sense the fluidity of the inhalation and exhalation motions as the SBJ rises and settles. See if you can sense the flower petals of the cranial bones opening and closing.

2. First inquire into superior vertical shear. Imagine that each hand is holding a wagon wheel with a transverse axle connecting their centers. To inquire into superior vertical shear, intend/suggest that you are rotating these wheels in an anterior-inferior direction. As your whole hand momentarily transfers the motion to the tissues, your index fingers or thumbs rotate away from you, while your little fingers rotate towards you. The fingers over the greater wings of the sphenoid intend/suggest a push in the flexion direction and the fingers over the occipital squama intend/suggest a push in the extension direction. Gently suggest this as a question and let the fluids take the tissues in that direction. After asking the question, listen to how far and how easily the tissues move in that direction. If the system likes to move into this direction, then the sphenoid is fixed in relative flexion, while the occiput is in relative extension. The body of the sphenoid will be held in a superior position relative to the basi-occiput.

3. Then inquire into inferior vertical shear. Again imagine that your hands are holding the two wagon wheels as above. To inquire into inferior vertical shear as a distortion pattern, intend/suggest that you are turning these wheels in a posterior-inferior direction. Your index fingers or thumbs rotate towards you, while your little fingers rotate away form you. The fingers over the greater wings of the sphenoid intend/suggest a push in the extension direction and the fingers over the occipital squama intend/suggest a push in the flexion direction. Listen and sense how far and how easily the tissues move in this direction. See which direction, if any, the unified field prefers. You are simply asking a question. Let the fluids take the tissues in that direction; do not try to guide them there. The intention is to sense which direction the system prefers (Fig. 8.15).

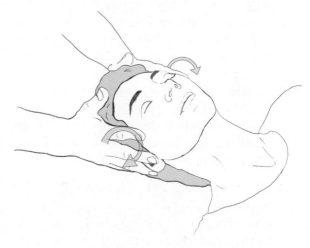

8.15 Palpation intention in vertical shear

If there is no vertical shear the system will not want to move into either direction very much and the possibilities will seem equal in both directions.

Facilitation of Sphenobasilar Reorganization of Vertical Shear Patterns

We will now explore the pattern of fixation that emerged in the above process.

1. If you sense a preference for a specific vertical shear pattern, again initiate the motion in that direction as above. This time, follow the tissues and help access the state of balance. Simply slow the motions perceived until a settling and stilling is sensed.

2. Once again, within the state of balance, listen for expressions of Health. You may sense heat, pulsation, and even a force vector literally leaving the system as a stream of energy and heat. Direction of fluid or lateral fluctuation processes can be used to encourage the expression of the potency of the system.

3. You are waiting to sense a softening and expansion, a reorganization of tissue structures, and a reorienting of the tissues to the midline and their natural fulcrums. You may also perceive a general sense of expansion within the cranium and the body as a whole.

Cranial Patterns in Vertical Shear

Superior Vertical Shear: As the sphenoid is held in relative flexion, the facial structures may follow this and have a widened, externally rotated look. In the extreme, this may yield a frontal bone with a prominent superior aspect, such as a bulging forehead. This is most prominent if the pattern is the result of birth trauma. At the same time, the occiput is held in relative extension and may have a narrowed look or feel. The temporal and parietal bones will follow the occiput in their expression of motion. Since the occiput is held in extension, the temporals and parietals will be held in internal rotation. Viewed from above, the person's face may seem wide while the back of the head seems comparatively narrow.

Inferior Vertical Shear: As the sphenoid is held in relative extension, the facial structures are held in an internally rotated position and may have a narrowed look. In chronic situations, the frontal bone may follow the greater wings posterior to the extreme and the forehead will look sloped at an acute angle, sometimes called a ski-slope forehead. This is obviously the reverse of the bulged look seen in the superior vertical shear pattern. At the same time, the posterior structures (occiput, temporal, and parietal bones) are held in flexion-external rotation and will have a widened, externally rotated feel to them. Viewed from the front, the

person's face may seem narrow while the back of the head seems comparatively wide.

COMPRESSION WITHIN THE SPHENOBASILAR JUNCTION

In compression, inertial forces within the SBJ close down the available space and generate density within the tissues of the joint. During the inhalation phase, space cannot be generated within the SBJ for smooth movement, reducing interosseous motion between the bones.

Compressive forces are always due to traumatic events such as birth process, accidents, overwhelming emotional shock, and blows to the head. SBJ compression can also be generated by other chronically compressed relationships along the structural midline within the vertebral column and pelvis. Specific areas commonly coupled with SBJ compression include compression at the O/A junction and at the lumbosacral junction, and intraosseous distortions of the occiput, such as condylar compressions and torsions. It is also common to see a telescoping of multiple structures in relationship to the SBJ. For example, the atlas, occipital squama, condyles, and basilar sections can all be compressed and telescoped together as part of large-scale axial issues along the midline due to birth trauma. These axial forces must be treated as a unit of function, and dealt with as a whole, before individual fulcrums can resolve efficiently.

Severe compression held within the SBJ and cranial base can generate inertial conditions within the system as a whole. As you listen to the dynamics within the SBJ, the cranium may seem very dense. The sphenoid and occiput may not be expressing much motion. In some chronic situations, it may feel like you are literally holding a very dense solid mass with little or no motion. The fluid system may also feel very dense and congested, as there may be much potency bound in centering the traumatic forces that generate the compressive pattern.

In the foundation training, we generally teach about SBJ compression before working with other patterns because it can mask or be coupled with other patterns. Symptoms can even be aggravated by following a torsion, side-bending, or shear pattern when these are coupled with SBJ compression. Compression may also be the most obvious pattern to manifest within the SBJ. It can override the other patterns, and call for treatment first.

Compression is different from the other patterns in that it is traditionally described as a gliding motion rather than a rotation.

Clinical Application: Compression, Disengagement, and Facilitation of Sphenobasilar Reorganization

Our inquiries into compression are essentially questions about space and disengagement. We use the principle of disengagement to ask the tissues, "Are there compressive forces present within the cranial base and can you access space there?" We pose the question through the tissues in order to initiate a conversation with the forces at the heart of the tissue compression. It is not just about tissue decompression. Relate to the forces at work, not just the effects they generate. There is always Health within the heart of the fulcrum organizing the compression. Disengagement is about accessing that Health, not about releasing a physical resistance. Resistance will resolve when the forces organizing it resolve.

1. Initially, it seems easier to learn this process using Becker's vault hold, with thumbs at the greater wings of the sphenoid bone. In the vault hold, orient to the mid-tide. Let the dynamics of the cranium come into your hands. Notice how the sphenoid and occiput express motility and motion. From here use an intention of disengagement and space to initiate a conversation about space with the potencies, fluids, and tissues.

2. Using your thumbs (or index fingers if you are in Sutherland's hold) in an inhalation phase, subtly intend the sphenoid anteriorly, away from the occiput and toward the ceiling. As you do this, also spread your other fingers apart. This is similar to the "Do you like Inhalation?" question above, but includes more of an orientation to the SBJ. If compressive forces are absent, the sphenoid will seem to float anteriorly, and inhalation within the tissue field will be sensed to be easy and open. If there is compression, you may sense pulling into the SBJ, density, or lack of motion, or a block-like resistance to your suggestion (Fig. 8.16).

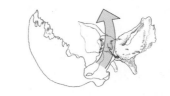

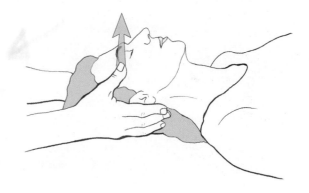

8.16 Intending disengagement
and space within the SBJ

3. If compression is present, at the beginning of inhalation, again intend an anterior lift at the SBJ and a spreading apart of your other fingers. You are asking the question, "Can you access the space in this relationship?" Listen for space to be accessed. There is always space present, even within the deepest compression.

147

4. When space is accessed, listen for an expression of potency. Potency may be sensed to build rhythmically within the relationship or to permeate the area in some way. Inertial forces may then be processed. Alternately, when space is accessed, you may sense a settling into a state of balance. Help the system attain this state if necessary. Listen for expressions of Health within its stillness. In either case, wait to sense an expression of potency within the compressive fulcrum. This may be sensed as pulsation, as a driving force within the fluids, or as a deeper, softer welling up and permeation of potency within the area.

5. As inertial forces are resolved, the sphenoid bone may be sensed to float anteriorly as part of a softening and expanding in the whole cranium. Wait for a reorganization of the fluids and tissues to midline functions such as Sutherland's fulcrum, the fluid tide, and the primal midline. When the compressive forces are truly resolved, you may sense a strong expansion throughout the cranium and the system as a whole.

Clinical Highlight: Pseudo-Flexion-Extension

In extreme situations when little or no motion is allowed, you may sense what has been called *pseudo-flexion-extension*. In these cases, no motion can be expressed between the two bones, and in an attempt to express natural flexion-extension, they rock as a unit first in one direction, then in the other. This will feel like alternating superior and then inferior vertical shear as the two bones are forced to rock back and forth. Sometimes, in severe compression as described above, the vault bones make up for the resistance in the cranial base by expressing excessive motion. It may feel as if you are holding a soft rubber ball that is expressing extreme motion, but they are really just compensating for extreme compression.

As an example, I was once confused by a patient who had severely chronic sacroiliac pain, a very depleted system, and suffered from depression. When I palpated her system, I sensed a very forceful interosseous motion at the parietal bones. It felt like I was holding a dense rubber ball that was strongly changing shape under my hands. In inhalation it felt like this rubber ball was filling my hands. The bones seemed to be expressing a huge motion. On further exploration, I discovered extreme compressive forces within the SBJ and throughout her midline. Her whole vertebral axis was locked up. Extreme pressures were driving the parietals and affecting her whole articular-membranous-fluid system. It was as if they were being "blown up" by the severe pressures within her fluid system. It was almost like a safety valve at work. The forces generating these axial compressions were birth related, and needed attention over many sessions. Eventually her potency was able to come through and the Inherent Treatment Plan was able to engage at a deeper level. I saw her over a period of six months, more or less weekly. By the end of this time, her symptoms were greatly alleviated, her system had a much stronger expression of potency and tidal motion, and her depression had lifted. I referred her to a psychotherapy colleague, as she was very interested in her early childhood experience and its connection to her original symptomology.

Clinical Application:
Axial Compressive Issues

Our inquiry into compression at the SBJ can be extended to a wider application, especially in the case of axial compression, or compression all along the midline axis of the body. Compressive forces can impact whole areas of the midline all at once. Working with axial compression is not a question of locating individual fulcrums, but of relating to whole areas of compressive force. Birth trauma is the most common source of axial compression.

1. Once again place your hands in Becker's hold. Let your hands float on the tissues and orient to the biosphere and the mid-tide level of perception. Hold the whole body and the field around it within your awareness.

2. As you view the whole system, sense the tissues as a unified tensile field of action. Allow a more specific awareness of the midline to arise within your perceptual field. With a subtle intention of inquiry, intend a cephalad lift at the greater wings of the sphenoid. The intention is to bring a conversation about space and disengagement, not just to the SBJ, but rather to the whole midline axis. Have a sense that you are bringing this intention to the whole tensile tissue field and its midline axis. Very subtly intend space through the midline axis (Fig. 8.17).

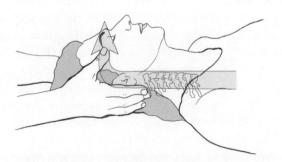

8.17 Intention of disengagement and space through the axial midline

3. Maintaining the intention of disengagement and space, facilitate a state of balance. Notice the tendency to settle into stillness and assist it by suggesting a slowing down of movements. Again listen for expressions of Health, the action of potency, and the processing of inertial forces.

4. Resolution of axial compression may feel as if hydraulic forces from within disengage the midline compression. Have patience with what happens next, as a series of fulcrums may now present. These more discrete fulcrums have been generated by the axial force you have engaged. Having resolved the overall axial compressive pattern, its sub-patterns have space to be resolved individually.

EXPLORING THE SYSTEM IN TRIADS

Working in groups of three is a great way to learn and explore SBJ patterns. Two students are in the roles of practitioner, and the third person takes the role of patient. The intention is to explore the work as a shared experience, as all three report their perceptions and give feedback throughout the session. One practitioner holds the cranium via the vault hold and the other holds the sacrum. The practitioner at the cranium follows the motility and motion around the SBJ, and the practitioner at the pelvis follows the motility and motion within the sacrum and pelvis. The intention here is to explore how the superior and inferior poles of the system reflect each other's shape and process.

Each practitioner may notice that the poles of the system are moving around similar or different fulcrums. Each practitioner tries to work with the shapes and fulcrums in a way that is coordinated with the other practitioner. Sense the system working as a whole, and notice changes as the state of balance is accessed. The practitioner at the vault hold may sense and follow the SBJ patterns that have been described above, while the practitioner at the sacrum does the same in relation to the pelvic structures. A continuing dialogue between the three participants can greatly aid the learning process. End the session with some integrative work, such as stillpoints at occiput and sacrum.

FORCE VECTOR ISSUES

A *force vector* is a category of biokinetic force introduced into the body via a traumatic experience such as an accident or fall. As these forces are introduced into the body, they take discrete pathways. A vector pattern is set up within the body as the potency acts to center and contain the traumatic force encountered. This generates tissue strain and contraction along the path of the force vector. This strain will orient to the inertial fulcrum generated by the encounter.

In preparing these books, I decided to wait until this chapter to discuss force vectors because they are very common in cranial base patterns. You may have already noticed this in your clinical sessions. Within a state of balance, the biokinetic forces within a fulcrum may be perceived to dissipate. As these forces are resolved, you may have sensed a streaming of a force from the fulcrum area out of the body. The traumatic force being processed usually leaves along the same pathway it took to enter the system. If you sense a force vector being processed, there is generally not much you have to do except appreciate it.

It sometimes helps to direct fluid and potency behind the vector toward the direction it is moving. For example, let's say you are working with a torsion pattern, and the fulcrum for this pattern is within the right temporal bone. The system enters a state of balance and you sense potency welling up within the bone. Then you sense a streaming of force from the area. Perhaps you sense this as a stream of heat or energy of some kind. Let's say it is streaming out of the temporal bone from deep within it, along its petrous ridge and out of the body. You could direct fluid from behind the streaming with your left hand. In this case you might change your hand position to the opposite side of the frontal bone to get as much fluid as possible between you and the force being processed. You might then direct fluid from here in the direction the force is streaming. You are directing fluid and potency from "behind" the force vector towards its exit pathway.

The direction the force vector takes may change as it flows along its exit pathway. This pathway may not be straight. In a traumatic experience like an accident, the body may move in all sorts of directions and patterns, and the biokinetic force introduced into it may then change its direction of motion. This process can be applied anywhere within the body. As a perceived force vector is discharged within a state of balance, you simply direct fluid behind it towards the direction it seems to be taking.

Clinical Application:
The Inherent Treatment Plan

Motion testing as described above orients you to the patterns allowed within the dynamics of the SBJ. After you have learned the details of SBJ patterns, including all the biomechanical terms, the time comes to shift to a more intuitive and less mechanistic approach. Torsion or side-bending patterns do not really happen in isolation as pure forms; they occur in the context of the whole person. Once we are quite comfortable with the particulars and fully capable of visualizing the patterns accurately, we can step back and see the whole picture. This brings us back to the Inherent Treatment Plan at the heart of the craniosacral biodynamic approach. In this approach, rather than orienting to the motion allowed within the dynamics of a joint, you orient to the motion actually expressing within the phases of primary respiration.

In this clinical application, do not hold preconceived ideas of movement patterns or relationships. Don't ask questions or expect answers. Simply settle into a state of listening in which forces may call to you from within and communicate the priorities of the Breath of Life. As this inherent plan unfolds, you may sense SBJ patterns as distortions within a larger tensile tissue field. You will also begin to appreciate that these distortions will be shown to you in the precise order in which the healing process needs to unfold. The more you allow a wide, gentle, yet keenly aware field of listening, the more this will become apparent.

1. Make contact with the patient's system via the vault hold. Establish your practitioner neutral. Let your hands float within fluid. Widen your perceptual field to include the whole biosphere of the patient. As you listen, the slower 2.5 cycles per minute mid-tide may come to the foreground. Give it time. Let yourself come into relationship to the tidal potencies. You may begin to sense the whole tensile tissue field expressing a unified inhalation and exhalation as cycles of surging and settling. This tensile motion may also be perceived to move in relationship to a locus of potency ideally found at Sutherland's fulcrum. Simply orient to motility and motion within the phases of inhalation and exhalation.

2. Take at least ten minutes to settle and let the system begin to show you its priorities. Do not chase compensatory patterns. Wait for the holistic shift discussed in Chapter 1. It will seem like the system shifts to its resources, primary respiration clarifies, and the body is a truly unified field. Sense the cranium to be like a flower opening and closing its petals within a fluid field. As the SBJ rises, the flower opens, and as it settles, the flower closes. As you orient to this, is space accessed within the sutures? Which sutures seem inertial, unable to access space? What patterns are organized around this?

3. Have patience and wait for something to engage from within. An inertial pattern may begin to clarify within the larger tensile field of action. You may sense patterns similar to those of the cranial base previously explored, but now these patterns are expressed within a unified tensile tissue field. Potency, fluids, and tissues are really perceived as a unified field of action. Wait for a settling of this whole field. As a particular inertial pattern clarifies, perceive that cranial base pattern as a wider tensile phenomenon. The whole cranium, indeed the whole body, may be perceived to express a tensile distortion as a whole. Tissues will be experienced as a true unit of function organized as a whole around both natural and inertial fulcrums.

4. The organizing fulcrum for the inertial pattern may now become clear, located within the cranium or remotely. Let this fulcrum come into your awareness. The whole tensile field may seem to distort around the fulcrum.

5. Give the Inherent Treatment Plan time to be expressed. Follow whatever inertial pattern comes to the forefront. Trust that the Intelligence of the system will communicate the Inherent Treatment Plan to you and will set its own priorities. Follow the potency into its direction of action. Help access the state of balance. Listen for Becker's three-phase healing awareness. Listen for the reorganization and realignment of potencies, fluids, and tissues to the midlines.

6. The work may also lead to other fulcrums that are related or next in line in the Inherent Treatment Plan. You may sense the potency shifting through the fluids to attend to other inertial issues.

THE LAYERING OF CONDENSED EXPERIENCE

The layering of our history is clearly seen within cranial base dynamics. For instance, a particular pattern may be accessed in one session, let's say a left torsion pattern. This torsion pattern and its organizing fulcrum may seem to resolve. Then, in a subsequent session, a new torsion pattern organized around a different fulcrum is perceived. These kinds of clinical experiences are expressions of layers of unresolved experience. The various life experiences and unresolved forces are held layered within our system, centered by the potency all at once, and available within the present moment for inquiry and healing.

Stanislov Grof has developed a beautiful way of discussing this kind of holistic process. He coined the term COEX matrix, or COEX system.[3] *COEX* means "condensed experience." In this idea, all of our history is held within present time in a layered and condensed fashion. The various layers of experience coalesce and generate various mind-body states and behavioral patterns. In the classic COEX system, a theme ties certain layers of condensed experience together. This theme has the quality of a life statement or life theme. For instance, various condensed experiences may resonate with a theme of abandonment, while another layering of condensed experience may resonate with a particular self-view, or sense of self-worth, and another may hold the sense of a loss in trust in intimacy and intimate relationships, etc. We may be holding numerous COEX systems within us, and they are, in turn, all coupled and condensed together as the Breath of Life acts to center all of our unresolved experience as a unified whole.

When a present experience resonates with a COEX system, a whole layering of life process, reactions, beliefs, and conditions will be activated all at once. Under stress or trauma of some kind, the whole system of coupled and layered experience arises together. It can be overwhelming when this occurs. It is the layering of fulcrums and the condensed experience they represent, that is crucial to understand. Thus, a car accident may resonate with a deep fear of loss and abandonment held from previous experiences. Many layers of unresolved experience may be activated by the accident. Patients may find themselves lost in seemingly unfounded emotional states; they may find that all sorts of symptoms arise, and they may make unskillful major life decisions in such a state.

I have worked with many people who have had recent experiences touch off layers of past history all at once. This is a common finding in session work. When this occurs, it is not just the present experience that patients are dealing with, but the whole of the coupled, condensed, layered and unresolved forces still active within their systems. It is like when striking the middle "C" on a piano, all other "C" notes vibrate.

I worked recently with a patient who was in a car accident. He was thrown out of the car; his clavicle hit the pavement and was fractured. He was fortunate that this was the only physical damage other than bruises. However, beyond the shock of the present experience, he found himself entering a deep depression. This was a familiar childhood state. In session work, we discovered that a deeply seated COEX system was activated that had layered fulcrums within the system and held a theme of abandonment that went right back to birth experience and early childhood. As we held the tissue patterning within his system, we were holding all of that.

The skill of the work is to help these condensed layers of experience uncouple and to work with one thing at a time. This is a natural process. Potency will tend to work with one issue at a time. If coupled fulcrums arise, then it is important to slow things down and orient to the most prominent fulcrum and action of potency at that time. The important thing here is that the Breath of Life acts to center all of our conditions as a whole, and the art of the work is to help uncouple these multiple fulcrums so that forces can be processed within the resources of the system.

CONDENSED EXPERIENCE AND CRANIAL BASE PATTERNS

This brings us to a wider view of the statements at the beginning of this chapter. As practitioners perceive a particular SBJ pattern, they are meeting a much wider and deeper orb of experience. The SBJ pattern perceived represents a whole psycho-dynamic-emotional-embodied experience, the wholeness of that person's life. Layers of condensed experience may be activated either by recent experience, or within session work. The physical symptoms they present may be generated by these patterns, yet even more poignantly, the pattern perceived is an expression of a unique life experience. Each torsion, side-bending, shearing, or compressive pattern is unique and coupled with wider issues. They are an expression of the wholeness of that person. Please do not forget this within your clinical practice.

As you relate to a cranial base pattern, it is still important to ask the question, "What organizes this?" Let the organizing fulcrum come into your hands and orient to the potency within the fluids and wider field. It is this potency that will be generated and focused in the session work. It will make the decisions. It is not uncommon for one SBJ pattern to clear and for another layer to surface. Have patience and allow the session work to unfold as the potency dictates. Once you have a clear relationship to these patterns, they will be communicated to you in a precise and organic way within the context of the Inherent Treatment Plan. If the resources are present, the system will orient to them, and the healing process will be precise and particular to a particular person's needs. All we then have to do is be present and support the unfolding process. As Becker advised, trust the tide and get out of the way!

Working with cranial base patterns can have vast repercussions in a person's life. The COEX matrix will be de-condensing and patterns will be uncoupling from each other. As particular patterns clarify, they are uncoupled and de-layered from all other patterns. The potency of the Breath of Life can orient to that one particular within the whole. Related life statements or themes may also arise. Sometimes a process of

insight ensues, within which clarity is attained and something let go of. Sometimes an emotional component will discharge and clear. Sometimes shock affects will be expressed, autonomic energies engaged, and traumatic cycling completed. The COEX matrix is de-layering and resolving its issues in a step-wise fashion. All of this can change a person's life. Remember to allow space, not to judge or have any needs around the session work, and to reverently hold that person within your field of awareness. Remember, it is not you who is doing the healing work. As Still stressed, this work, and the laws governing it, are not framed by human hands.

1. See Chapter 13 in Volume One, "Fulcrums and Forces."
2. This way of motion testing oriented to tissue field distortion around fulcrums was suggested by Mij Ferrett and Michael Kern, D.O.
3. Stanislov Grof, *The Holotropic Mind* (Harper's, San Francisco, 1993).

9

The Venous Sinuses

The venous sinuses provide fluid drainage for the cranium. While venous sinus issues often resolve by themselves in the course of general craniosacral biodynamic treatment, they may require more specific attention. Inertial forces may be located within a specific sinus area, and a direct contact can help the system dissipate and resolve these forces. In this chapter we will learn how to contact the form and function of the venous sinus system directly and comprehensively. The clinical intention is to facilitate fluid drainage and the general uptake of potency in the fluids. In standard Sutherland-style cranial courses, venous sinus release processes are commonly taught before learning to address cranial base patterns. Working with the venous sinuses can generate space within the fluid system and encourage fluid fluctuation, useful preparations for a journey into the life patterns held within the cranial base.

In previous session work you may have sensed sluggishness within a patient's fluid tide and an overall sense of low vitality even after stillpoints and other processes. Congestion within the venous sinuses may be a factor in this situation. Compressive forces, cranial base patterns, and dural strain patterns all affect the form and function of the venous sinuses, leading to stasis and a reduction of the system's capacity for vital circulation of fresh arterial blood and CSF to nourish the brain. All membranous articular stain patterns affect the venous sinuses in some way. Fluid backpressure and stasis within the system as a whole affects the quality of potency and drive of fluid fluctuation throughout the system.

In this chapter we will:

- *Describe the venous sinus system.*

- *Describe clinical approaches for improving venous outflow from the cranium.*

- *Describe specific clinical applications related to venous sinus congestion.*

THE VENOUS SINUS SYSTEM

The venous sinuses carry venous fluids and cerebrospinal fluid out of the cranium toward the heart. The venous sinuses are not true veins; they are cavities formed in dura that collect old blood and cerebrospinal fluid for recycling via the circulatory system. They are an integral part of the dural membrane system.

Cerebrospinal fluid is produced within the choroid plexuses that line the ventricles of the brain. After bathing the brain tissues, CSF moves into the venous sinuses via the arachnoid granulations, found especially in the sagittal sinus (Fig. 9.1). Venous blood and cerebrospinal fluid then flow by gravity pressure through the sinuses to the main outlets from the cranium, the jugular foramina and internal jugular veins, and on to the heart. Other smaller exit routes include the facial vein, the deep cervical vein, and the external jugular vein.

The major venous sinuses include the sphenoidparietal sinuses, the superior and inferior petrosal sinuses, the cavernous and intercavernous sinuses, the basilar plexus, the sagittal sinuses (superior and inferior), the straight sinus, the transverse sinuses, the occipital sinus, the marginal sinus, and the sigmoid sinus. Effective venous sinus treatment requires a thorough knowledge of their anatomy. I suggest that you trace or draw these channels in a number of views, to include the sinuses mentioned above (Fig. 9.2 a and b). This will give you a clear visual sense of their relationships.

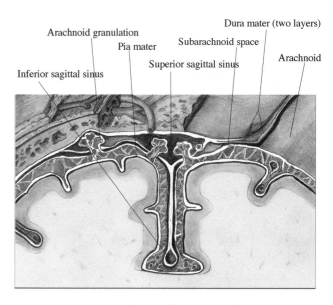

9.1 Section through the sagittal sinus showing arachnoid granulations

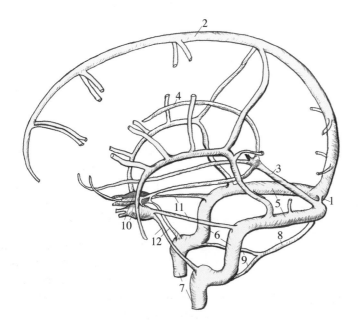

1. Confluence of sinuses
2. Superior sagittal sinus
3. Straight sinus
4. Inferior sagittal sinus
5. Transverse sinus
6. Sigmoid sinus
7. Internal jugular vein
8. Occipital sinus
9. Marginal sinus
10. Cavernous sinus
11. Superior petrosal sinus
12. Inferior petrosal sinus

9.2a Major venous sinuses and the venous system

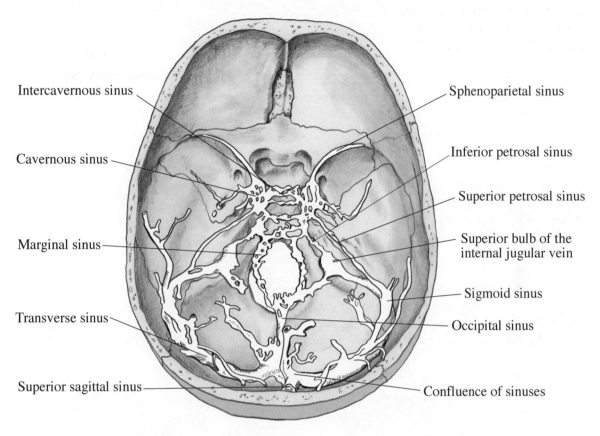

Intercavernous sinus

Cavernous sinus

Marginal sinus

Transverse sinus

Superior sagittal sinus

Sphenoparietal sinus

Inferior petrosal sinus

Superior petrosal sinus

Superior bulb of the internal jugular vein

Sigmoid sinus

Occipital sinus

Confluence of sinuses

9.2b Venous sinuses at the base of the cranial cavity, seen from above

Venous flow moves:

1. From the superior cranial fossa, the venous flow moves from the sphenoid-parietal sinuses toward the middle cranial fossa via the cavernous and intercavernous sinuses. It then flows via the basilar plexus to the inferior cranial fossa and then to the internal jugular veins via the jugular foramina.

2. The temporal area drains from the superior and inferior petrosal sinuses to the sigmoid sinuses and then to the jugular foramina.

3. The parietal areas drain from the superior and inferior sagittal sinuses to the straight sinus and to the confluence of sinuses, to the transverse sinuses, and then to the sigmoid sinuses and jugular foramina.

4. From the occipital sinus the venous flow moves inferiorly toward the marginal sinuses, the sigmoid sinuses, and the jugular foramina and will also leave the cranium via cervical veins (Fig. 9. 3).[1]

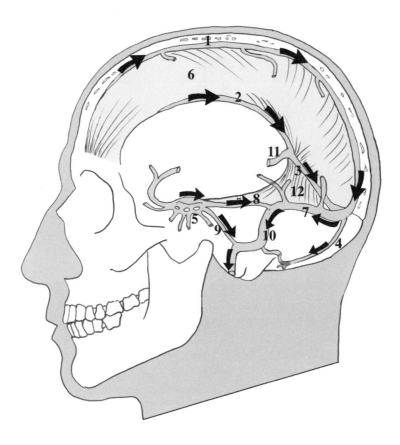

1. Superior sagittal sinus
2. Inferior sagittal sinus
3. Straight sinus
4. Occipital sinus
5. Cavernous sinus
6. Falx cerebri
7. Transverse sinus
8. Superior petrosal sinus
9. Inferior petrosal sinus
10. Sigmoid sinus
11. Great cerebral vein (Galen)
12. Tentorium cerebelli

Venous flow will seek the easiest way out of the cranium via these routes and always has an alternative route. Obstruction in one route can be partially accommodated by other routes.

9.3 Direction of flow in venous sinuses

INERTIAL ISSUES OF THE VENOUS SINUS SYSTEM

Venous sinus stasis is not uncommon. The fluids within the sinuses can become inertial due to biokinetic forces present and strain patterns in the dural system. Stasis within the venous sinuses can contribute to low vitality and poor ignition of potency within cerebrospinal fluid. Congestion within the sinuses can generate fluid backpressure within the cranium and inefficient drainage of blood, waste, and cerebrospinal fluid. As a result of this, fluid fluctuation and circulation in the skull can become sluggish, reducing the ability of the cerebrospinal fluid to become potentized. Venous sinus congestion can also generate tension and strain within the membrane system, hormonal imbalances, and pressure on cranial nerves, especially in the cavernous and intercavernous sinuses (Fig. 9.4). A cranium holding chronic fluid congestion and inefficient venous drainage may feel rigid and solid. Motility and motion of tissues and fluids may feel thick or dense as the potency becomes inertial and the fluid drive of the system is dampened down. This venous sinus drainage process encourages fluid movement throughout the cranium by decongesting the channels of flow that fluids must take to leave the cranium.

CRANIAL OUTLETS

Viewing the venous sinuses as the plumbing system of the cranium, it makes sense to start with the lowest level of blockage so that higher congestion has an exit route when it is resolved later. If the drain is blocked, fluids will back up through the rest of the plumbing system. Thus, we will work with the outlets of the cranium first and then continue from the bottom up.

The thoracic inlet is the first area to consider. Inertia here generates backpressure against venous flow. Pressure can be fed into the internal jugular vein and into the other venous outlet routes such as the external jugular vein, deep cervical vein, and the vertebral vein. Other potential relationships at the low end of the cranium that may generate backpressure include

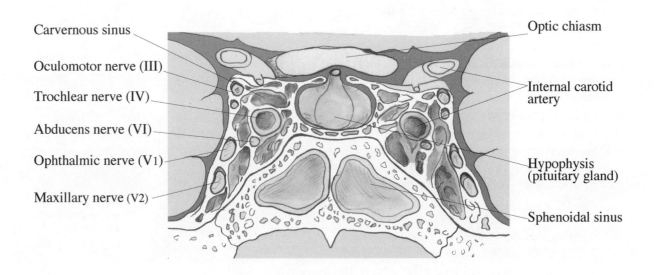

Carvernous sinus

Oculomotor nerve (III)

Trochlear nerve (IV)

Abducens nerve (VI)

Ophthalmic nerve (V1)

Maxillary nerve (V2)

Optic chiasm

Internal carotid artery

Hypophysis (pituitary gland)

Sphenoidal sinus

9.4 Section through the cavernous sinus

the cervical fascia, the occipital cranial base (including the axis, atlas, occipital condyles, foramen magnum and intraosseous occipital issues), cervical vertebra, and the jugular foramina.

THORACIC INLET RELATIONSHIPS

The main discussion of the thoracic inlet is in Chapter 13, in the connective tissue section. But if this area is not relatively free of inertia, work to encourage venous drainage above may result in discomfort for the patient instead of renewed circulation. Discomfort can take the form of a congested head, heaviness, spaciness, headaches, etc.

As you follow the shape and motion patterns of the tissues of the thoracic inlet, be sure to include the related vertebra, including the cervicals and upper thoracics. Vertebral fixations in this area can also affect venous and cerebrospinal fluid flow. Follow through with cervical vertebral restrictions using the spinal dynamics processes described in Chapter 5.

Clinical Application: Thoracic Inlet

A continuous, multifaceted set of relationships creates the opening from the neck into the torso. Key structures include the manubrium, clavicle and scapulae, and the inner circle created by the articulations of the first ribs with the manubrium and first thoracic vertebra. Many important structures pass through this opening, including the jugular veins and arteries, and the vagus and phrenic nerves.

1. Sitting at the side of the table, place your caudad hand under C7-T3, perpendicular to the patient's body. After establishing a relationship with the patient's system, place your other hand transversely over the patient's clavicles and upper sternum to make a sandwich over the thoracic inlet. Establish a relationship to the fluid tide and to tissue motility within the mid-tide in this position (Fig. 9.5).

2. Allow your hands to float on the tissues and follow motility and motion within the phases of primary respiration. Use all of the biodynamic skills here, such as disengagement and directing fluids. Wait until the system settles into a sense of wholeness and primary respiration clarifies. Wait until a particular pattern clearly emerges. Have patience, as this can take some minutes. Help access the state of balance. If the thoracic inlet is very congested and inertial, use lateral fluctuation processes to initiate motion and a seeking of the neutral. You can "push" fluid and potency from one hand to the other without changing your position. Another approach may be to deepen your contact with the tissues using a firmer touch until increased motion arises. This must be done in a subtle and negotiated way. Again, listen for Becker's three-phase awareness here.

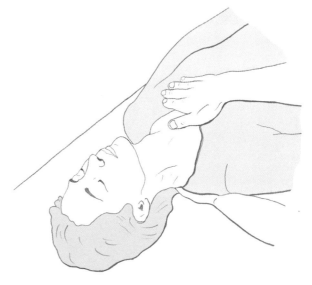

9.5   Thoracic inlet hold

OCCIPITAL BASE ISSUES

Next in sequence from the bottom up is the occipital triad area. Inertial issues here can strongly affect venous outflow. These issues may go back to birthing forces and birth trauma. If inertial issues are present here, explore the occipital triad as described in previous chapters. The occipital triad will directly affect the dynamics of the jugular foramina, internal jugular veins, external jugular veins and the deep cervical veins.

JUGULAR FORAMINA

The jugular foramina are the narrowest points in the drainage system. Located in the occipito-mastoid suture, between the occiput and temporal bones (Fig. 9.6), this important pair of openings is the path for the internal jugular veins, receiving the outflow of the major sinuses of the head. The transverse sinuses merge into the sigmoid sinuses as they pass through both jugular foramina to become the internal jugular veins. Obviously, compression or congestion within jugular foramen relationships can be a major factor in venous sinus congestion.

The jugular foramina are also important because they are passageways for important nerves: the vagus, glossopharyngeal, and spinal accessory nerves. Compression within jugular foramen relationships is commonly generated by birth trauma. Whiplash can also be registered here, leading to puzzling visceral symptoms. Inertia held here can generate digestive, respiratory, and sucking problems in infants, and digestive

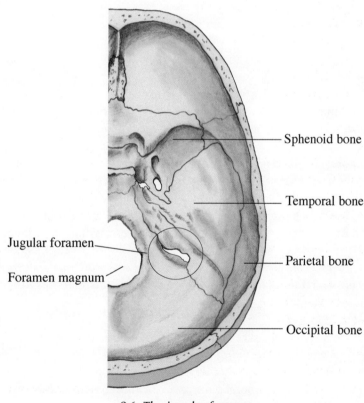

Sphenoid bone

Temporal bone

Jugular foramen

Foramen magnum

Parietal bone

Occipital bone

9.6 The jugular foramen

and respiratory issues in adults, as well as a wide range of other symptoms. Hypersensitivity or facilitation of these nerves often indicates impingement at the jugular foramina, and neuroendocrine effects may be far-reaching.

Clinical Application: The Jugular Foramen

In the following application, we will make a direct relationship to the jugular foramina via a new hold, the temporal-occipital hold. The intention is to facilitate the resolution of inertial forces by working with the principles of the state of balance and disengagement. The first step will be to listen in a vault hold and to see if we are drawn to work with either jugular foramen.

1. With the patient in the supine position, hold the cranium in the vault hold. Orient to the mid-tide. Sense the quality of the fluid tide and of tissue motility within the phases of primary respiration. Then orient to the jugular foramina using your knowledge of the area's anatomy. Let yourself be open to the possibility that you can sense these relationships. As the system settles, see if an inertial pattern or fulcrum clarifies. See if you can sense inertia within either jugular foramen. This may be sensed as a pull into the area or a motion dynamic organized around it. You may sense that the temporal bone and occiput move in a block-like fashion on the side of a compressive issue, without a sense of space or fluidity between them. See which jugular foramen you are drawn to first.

2. To relate directly to that specific jugular foramen, change your hand position. First place one hand under the occiput, cradling it in the palm with your fingers spread wide to give support. Be sure that the heel of your hand is not pressing against the patient's head. This hand position will stabilize the occiput as you cradle it. Place your other hand at the temporal bone in the *temporal bone hold*. Here your middle finger is curved and

placed lightly in the patient's ear canal. Your index finger rests anterior to the ear at the zygomatic process while your ring finger rests posterior to the ear over the mastoid portion of the temporal bone. Your index and ring fingers make a solid contact, though the pressure is very light. You now are in relationship to the two bones bordering the jugular foramen. In this position, see if you sense the jugular foramen (Fig. 9.7).

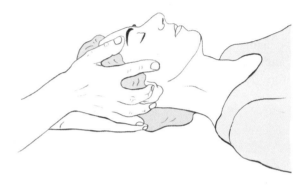

9.7 The temporal hold

3. Again orient to the mid-tide. Sense the motility and motion at both occiput and temporal bones. As the occiput and temporal bone express their inhalation motions, is there a sense of space generated at the occipito-mastoid suture? What inertial pattern clarifies? Help access the state of balance and listen for Becker's three-phase process. Within the stillness of the state of balance, listen for expressions of Health. Wait for a sense of softening and expansion within the tissues of the relationship.

4. From this position, change your temporal bone hand position to the temporal bone ear hold position. Here your fingers are holding the posterior aspect of the ear next to the cranium, while your thumb is placed at the ear canal. Notice any compressive forces at work within

the jugular foramen. You may sense a medial compression of the temporal bone on that side. If there is medial compression, use the conversation skills of disengagement to encourage space within the relationship. This involves introducing a gentle and subtle traction along a forty-five degree angle from the horizontal towards the treatment table. This is offered as a conversation, not as a demand or intention to release anything. There is always potential space, even in the most compressed relationship. There is always a kernel of Health at work within the densest inertial fulcrum.

5. Access the potential space until you sense potency coming into play and the first stage of Becker's three-phase awareness. The tissues will seem to be seeking a stillness, a state of balance within all of the force factors present. Help access the state of balance and listen for expressions of Health. Wait for a resolution of the inertial forces present. You may sense expansion and reorganization as the potencies, fluids, and tissues reorient to midline phenomena.

Clinical Highlight

Infants often present issues of the jugular foramen. I have attended to many infants with colic, related digestive issues, respiratory issues, sleeping issues and sucking problems, all due to the aftermath of the birthing process. As we will discuss in Chapter 16, infants must be approached with extra-sensitive negotiation and conscious contact. They will sense your intentions and will accept your contact if they feel safe and resourced in your presence.

Many years ago a young woman came to see me with chronic digestive issues including excessive acidity, headaches, and exhaustion. Her headaches had been a feature of her life from childhood onward and the hyperacidity was a relatively new symptom. Orthodox investigations did not reveal any physiological etiology. She was diagnosed as having anxiety states and psychological tension. Tranquillizers were prescribed by her physician.

We initially worked with stillpoints and resources because her system was very depleted and inertial. As she gained resources over a number of sessions, the Inherent Treatment Plan began to express itself. One of the main fulcrums that came to the forefront was an intraosseous distortion of the occiput and a very compressed jugular foramen on the right side. There were also temporal bone issues on this side. The suboccipital area was tender to the touch.

These issues were related to forces generated by birth trauma. There was also sympathetic autonomic nervous system activation and brain stem facilitation. As the forces resolved, sympathetic shock affects cleared through the fluids, and emotional edges of fear and sadness also arose. These seemed to give rise to her anxiety states, and the headaches were directly a result of these forces at work within her system. She was able to clear these emotional affects in a resourced and very present manner. The headaches were clearly related to the jugular foramen issue. Fluid backpressure was arising from the jugular foramen, and it was alleviated by venous sinus drainage. We worked with these issues over time. Once the jugular foramen and temporal bone issues resolved, her system began to come back to life. Resolving the inertial forces within the jugular foramen itself was a key to the alleviation of her symptoms.

Clinical Applications:
Venous Sinus Drainage

With the lower areas cleared, we turn our attention "upstream" to the actual sinuses. Particular hand positions allow you a direct relationship to some of the major sinuses. As we systematically work our way through the major venous sinuses, remember that although each sinus area has a particular name, you are really relating to a continuous space formed within the dural membranes. We will work with states of balance and intentions of space as we orient to each sinus.

Clinical Application:
Confluence of Sinuses

The confluence of sinuses is the meeting place of the major venous sinuses, including the sagittal, straight, transverse, and occipital sinuses. The confluence of sinuses can be found just anterior to inion, the external occipital protuberance.

1. With the patient in the supine position, let the external occipital protuberance (inion) rest on your two middle fingers. Place your two middle fingers together and then support them by placing your index and ring fingers under them (Fig. 9.8). Let the head rest on these two middle fin-

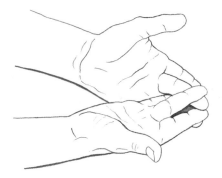

9.8 The confluence of sinus hold
and occipital sinus hold

gers, balanced on them by the thumbs and heels of your hands. Allow all the weight to be taken on your middle fingers. With the head's weight on your fingers, this contact becomes a new fulcrum for the patient's system. Once the contact is well established, visualize the anatomy of the confluence of sinuses anterior to your fingers.

2. If congestion is present, the occipital bone and the confluence may feel dense and rigid. The contact may feel sensitive or painful to the patient. Give the system space and facilitate the state of balance. Wait here until you feel a distinct softening and expansion of the area. As the confluence opens, you may sense a flushing through of fluid as the congestion resolves. The occiput will also soften locally, and the sensitivity that the patient first experienced will be alleviated.

Clinical Application:
Occipital and Marginal Sinuses

After this first process, start an exploration of the occipital and marginal sinuses. The occipital sinus lies below the confluence. It ends at the foramen magnum where it splits to form the marginal sinus around the foramen (see Figures 9.2 a, b and 9.3).

1. For the occipital sinus, maintain the same hand position as above and move one finger width inferior (caudad) along the mid-line of the occiput to form a relationship to the occipital sinus. If you sense density there, repeat the above process. If there is congestion at the level of your contact, the tissues of the occiput may feel dense and rigid. With the weight of the head on your middle fingers, again help access the state of balance and wait for a sense of softening and expansion and fluid movement.

2. Continue to move down the occipital sinus one finger-width at a time until you reach the foramen magnum. Whenever you sense density, access the state of balance and wait for a soft-

ening and expansion within the tissues. When you arrive at the foramen magnum, shift your intention from the occipital sinus to the marginal sinuses. At the foramen magnum, the occipital sinus divides into two sinuses on either side of the jugular foramen. To relate to these interior sinuses, use a condylar spread hand position similar to the one used for the occipital triad (Fig. 7.6 in Chapter 7).

3. Separate your middle fingers and point them toward the occipital condyles and foramen magnum. Your hands are slightly separated, and your middle fingers form a V-shape pointing towards the foramen magnum. The weight of the cranium is taken by the middle fingers and by your hands in general. Suggest a gentle spreading across the foramen magnum by bringing your elbows together, as you did in the condylar spread learned previously. This will place you in relationship to the marginal sinuses. See if you can sense them within the intention of your contact. Suggest spread to the boundary of the space accessed, facilitate the state of balance, and wait for a softening and spreading in the area (Fig. 9.9).

Clinical Application: Transverse Sinuses

Next we move superiorly, to the transverse sinuses. The two transverse sinuses move in opposite directions laterally from the confluence of sinuses across the occiput to merge with each sigmoid sinus. The sigmoid sinuses dive into the jugular foramina and are continuous with the internal jugular veins (see Fig. 9.2a). If you have a skull model, look at the inner surface of the occipital bone. You will usually see narrow indented areas fanning out on either side of the confluence of sinuses. Dural membranes peel off from the lining of the cranium at these raised areas to form the transverse sinuses.

1. Place your little fingers at the external occipital protuberance and line up the other fingers in a more or less straight line along the transverse sinuses. Your little fingers are touching along their outside edges. Your other fingers are touching each other and are lined up transversely under the transverse sinuses. Try to make your fingertips line up horizontally as much as possible (Fig. 9.10).

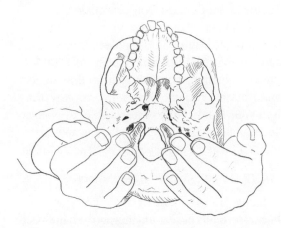

9.9 Marginal sinus hold

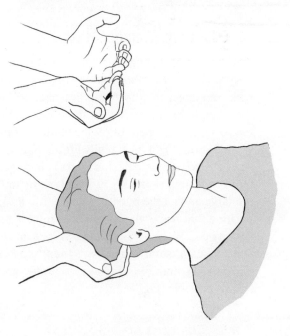

9.10 Tranverse sinus hold

2. Again, take the weight of the cranium onto your fingertips. You may have a sense that you are subtly balancing the sinus system upon your fingertips. As before, help facilitate the state of balance and wait until a softening and expansion within the tissues is felt. You may again sense fluids flushing through as the congestion resolves.

Clinical Application: Straight Sinus

The straight sinus starts at the confluence of sinuses, anterior to the external occipital protuberance. It then moves anteriorly at about a thirty-degree angle. The anterior aspect of the straight sinus is the ideal location for Sutherland's fulcrum, the suspended automatically shifting fulcrum for the connective tissues of the body. You can't physically have your fingers directly over the straight sinus because it extends interiorly from inion. In this process, you will have a relationship with its posterior pole via inion and will contact its most anterior pole through your intention. I will describe two processes; one is a traditional contact and the other is a modified version that may initially be easier to use.

First Hold for the Straight Sinus

1. Place your middle fingers at the external occipital protuberance as above, lift the patient's head with your fingertips into anatomical flexion (forward-bending), and place your thumbs on top of the patient's head near or on the midline of the sagittal suture. You must really lift the patient's head off the table into flexion to get your fingers in this position. Then let your hands settle onto the table and let the patient's head settle into a position that rests balanced on your middle fingers. You now have your middle fingers at the confluence of sinuses and your thumbs as far along the sagittal sinus, and as close to the midline, as possible (Fig. 9.11a).

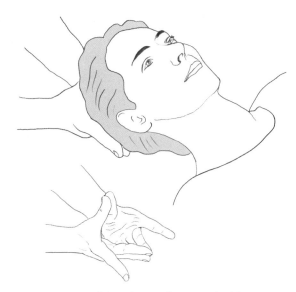

9.11a Traditional straight sinus hold

2. Project your intention from your thumbs to the anterior aspect of the straight sinus within the cranium, about one third of the way in from the posterior of the head. This will place you in relationship to the anterior pole of the straight sinus. The weight of the cranium should be mainly placed on your middle fingers at inion, while you balance the patient's head with the rest of the fingers of your hands. Don't create lateral pressure with your other fingers. When you find yourself in relationship to both poles of the straight sinus, it may feel like you are literally holding the straight sinus between your middle fingers and thumbs. You may also sense inion settling into your hands. Help access a state of balance and wait for a perception of softening and expansion. This may be perceived most clearly at inion.

Second Hold for the Straight Sinus

If your hands are too small, or if you find the above hold uncomfortable, here is an alternative hand position. I find that the first hold gives a clear sense of holding the sinus between the fingertips and is worth continuing effort even if it seems difficult at first. However, the second hold does work and is easier for people with small hands.

3. While cradling the occiput with one hand, place the middle finger of that hand at inion and take the weight of the cranium on that finger. With your other hand, place your thumb at the sagittal suture on top of the cranium. Use this thumb to project your intention inward (Fig. 9.11b). Using two hands separately to relate to the straight sinus, proceed as above.

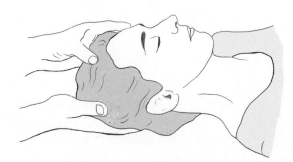

9.11b   Alternative straight sinus hold

A Third Alternative for the Straight Sinus

4. Another alternative is to use a V-spread at the straight sinus. While cradling the occiput in one hand, place a V-spread at inion. Use the index and middle fingers of the cradling hand to do this. Inion should be placed within the middle of your V-spread. Place the fingers of your other hand at the superior aspect of the frontal bone and sense the fluids from that contact.

5. Direct the potency of the fluid tide to the anterior aspect of the straight sinus. Sense, feel, and hear the response at the straight sinus. As inion begins to pulsate, subtly intend a spreading across the confluence until a state of balance is attained.

Wait for a sense of pulsation at inion and a fluid release from the straight sinus through the confluence of sinuses and transverse sinuses. The straight sinus generally drains more into the left transverse sinus, and you may thus sense more of a fluid release on that side.

Clinical Application: Sagittal Sinus

Next we move to the superior sagittal sinus. The sagittal sinus stretches from above inion to the superior aspect of the frontal bone at the metopic suture. We will gradually move along the sagittal sinus in an anterior direction, from just above inion to the beginning of the metopic suture, working in three steps.

Step One

1. Place the fingers of both hands together under the patient's head along the midline above inion. Your little fingers are just above inion, and your other fingers are oriented along the midline and almost touching. In other words, your fingers are vertically oriented on either side of the sagittal sinus (Fig. 9.12a).

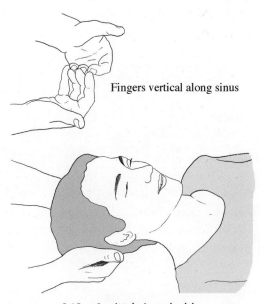

Fingers vertical along sinus

9.12a Sagittal sinus hold

167

2. Take the weight of the cranium on these fingers and, with all of the fingers at once, suggest a subtle lateral spreading of the sagittal suture. Facilitate the state of balance and wait for a softening and spreading of the sinus. When this occurs, move anteriorly one finger-width at a time along the sagittal suture with the same intention.

Step Two

1. When your hands come out from under the patient's head, cross your thumbs and place them on either side of the sagittal suture just anterior to where you were last working.

2. Intend a gentle transverse spreading across the sinus to the boundary of space accessed. Again access the state of balance and wait for a softening and expansion of the sinus. Continue by moving anteriorly one finger-width at a time along the sagittal sinus. Focus on the sagittal sinus areas that feel dense or congested. If the suture and sinus spreads easily, move to the next contact point. You can expect to have some areas feel congested while others do not (Fig. 9.12b).

Step Three

1. At the top of the forehead, we are in relationship to the metopic suture. This suture is still present in some form in about ten percent of the population. Change your hand position here by aligning your fingers closely together along the midline as we did in step one, on either side of the metopic suture. Again suggest a gentle lateral spreading across the sinus to the boundary of space accessed and wait for a sense of softening, expansion and spreading (Fig. 9.12c).

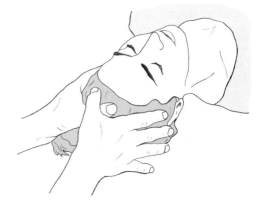

9.12b Sagittal sinus hold
(thumbs crossed)

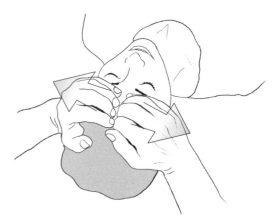

9.12c Metopic suture and most anterior aspect of sagittal sinus

Clinical Application:
Cavernous and Intercavernous Sinuses

The cavernous sinus and intercavernous sinuses are located in critical positions. The cavernous sinuses lie on either side of the sella turcica and the body of the sphenoid, and are connected by the intercavernous sinuses. They provide venous drainage for the pituitary gland area. Congestion within these sinuses can directly affect pituitary function. In addition, the internal carotid artery and its sympathetic nerve supply passes through the cavernous sinus. Cranial nerves also pass through the sinus, including the oculomotor, trochlear, opthalmic, and the maxillary branches of the trigeminal nerve. Congestion within the cavernous sinus can have direct effects on these nerves, causing entrapment neuropathy and nerve facilitation. We will use a contact with the greater wings of the sphenoid bone to engage these sinuses. If you look in a skull model, notice how the greater wings of the sphenoid merge with the lesser wings and take you to the sellae turcica and cavernous sinus. As you contact the greater wings, you have a direct entry to the cavernous sinuses.

Step One

1. These sinuses may be engaged via the sphenoid bone by using Becker's vault hold. Your hands are gently surrounding the ears with the thumbs lightly placed on the greater wings of the sphenoid. Orient to the membranous continuity from the greater wings, to the lesser wings, to the diaphragma sellae, to the cavernous sinus. Visualize the sinuses as you do this.

2. Use your thumb contacts to very gently intend the greater wings posterior. This is really an engagement of the membranes via the sphenoid to the cavernous sinus. As the sphenoid moves posteriorly, you are placing a subtle intention into these sinuses. This is an extremely subtle process and uses no force. It is an intention placed through the tissues. Avoid feeding compression into the SBJ. Access the state of balance, and again wait for a sense of softening and expansion in the area.

Step Two

1. After expansion, suggest a subtle anterior traction via the sphenoid. This is similar to the disengagement process of the SBJ discussed in Chapter 8. In this case, your intention is with the membranes and the cavernous and intercavernous sinuses.

2. Intend a very subtle anterior traction at the greater wings of the sphenoid bone until the membrane and sinus are engaged. Again facilitate the state of balance and listen for softening and expansion.

The CV4 Finish

Finish the venous sinus drainage work with a CV4 (Volume One, Chapter 16). CV4 helps to clear residual congestion through the sinuses and is helpful as an integrating process. Alternatively, you can facilitate a stillpoint via the sacrum.

Additional Considerations with Venous Sinus Processes

• *Low Blood Pressure*

Low blood pressure is a commonly discussed contraindication for venous sinus work.[1] I have not seen this as a major problem in the gentle, state-of-balance way we approach the work. However, this classic contraindication should be considered. In the reverse situation, high blood pressure, venous sinus drainage is positively indicated, along with CV4 and stillpoint processes.

• *Autonomic Effects*

With venous sinus processes, patients may experience autonomic effects such as nausea, other digestive symptoms, and heart palpitations. Unresolved jugular foramen compressive issues affecting the vagus nerve are the probable cause of these kinds of responses. Also, increased fluid flow can place temporary pressure on the vagus nerve, generating vagal responses from the viscera and elsewhere. Unresolved jugular foramen issues can also generate headaches and cranial nerve responses due to backpressure. Backpressure or change of pressure can even affect the orbital nerves passing through the cavernous sinus, leading to temporary visual distortions such as blurring. Autonomic effects may also relate to unresolved intraosseous occipital issues or nerve facilitation in brain stem autonomic nuclei that was activated and not resolved. All of these can be noted and treated in subsequent session work. Educate patients about these possibilities to help them understand their experiences.

• *Toxic Release*

Increased fluid fluctuation and fluid flow, and a related intensifying of potency within the fluids, may encourage the processing of toxicity. Cleansing of toxic material can temporarily give rise to nausea, joint pain, and digestive issues. Tell patients to drink eight glasses of pure water each day for at least three days after this work. Reducing toxic intake, such as cigarettes and alcohol, is highly recommended.

• *First Aid*

Venous sinus work, along with the use of stillpoints, is useful as first aid for acute episodes of migraine, vertigo, inflammation, and fever. These processes can also be an important part of igniting the potency within the fluid system generally, and the third ventricle specifically, as described in Chapter 3.

---

1. In American anatomy texts it is usually stated that the occipital sinus drains upwards into the confluence. In some European texts it states that the occipital sinus drains into sigmoid sinus below. For example, see Carmine Clemente, *Anatomy: A Regional Atlas of the Human Body,* 4th ed. (Williams & Wilkins, 2001), plate 768. My sense is that it can flow either direction and commonly drains inferiorly towards the sigmoid sinus during session work. I used that direction of flow here.

2. Thanks to Bhedrena Thussumi for reminding me of this.

10 Facial Dynamics

The next few chapters explore the relationships of the face, the hard palate, and the temporomandibular joints. Work in these areas is an extension of our studies of the cranial bowl and sphenobasilar junction, based on the same underlying concepts and using the same skills. The face and hard palate are not separate from the dynamics of the body as a whole, and they have direct connections with the cranial base and the cranial bowl in general.

In this chapter we will:
- *Explore the dynamics of the frontal and ethmoid bones and orbital structures.*
- *Learn specific clinical approaches to compressive fulcrums in these areas.*

INTRODUCTION

The bony structures of the face and hard palate can be considered to be hanging off the cranial bowl, suspended from the frontal and sphenoid bones. The bones of the face and hard palate will mirror the sphenoid bone in motion and positioning (Fig. 10.1).

The sphenoid, face, and hard palate are a unified field. Inertial patterns found within the cranial base and the cranial bowl generally will be reflected in the face and hard palate. Similarly, inertial patterns in facial and hard palate structures will also be mirrored

in the dynamics of the sphenoid bone and cranial base. There is a direct and interactive reciprocal relationship between the cranial base and the face and hard palate: what happens in one group can be palpated in the other. For this reason, understanding the cranial base is a prerequisite for approaching the face and hard palate.

To learn about the face and hard palate we will be using a series of clinical applications designed to give you a clear experience of the relationships involved.

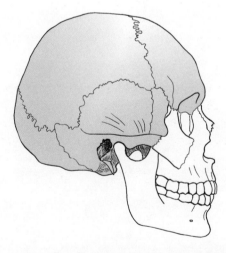

10.1 The facial structures are suspended from the cranial bowl

These are not treatment protocols; they are explorations set up as a learning process. As you build up experience and awareness of the system, you will discover that the Intelligence of the system itself will show you the Inherent Treatment Plan. Use these applications to learn the area and processes, but avoid excessively extending them into clinical practice.

DYNAMICS SUPERIOR TO THE HARD PALATE

We will first focus attention on the frontal and ethmoid bones. The frontal processes of the maxillae articulate with the frontal bone at the frontal-maxillary suture. The maxillae express their motility and motion as though they are hanging from the frontal bone (Fig. 10.2). The maxillae articulate directly to the ethmoid bone and indirectly to the sphenoid via their articulations with the palatine bones and vomer. Inertial fulcrums in superior structures may generate distortions within facial, hard palate, and TMJ relationships because the maxillae cannot hang freely. As we found in previous clinical applications, it can make sense to orient to inertial patterns in sequence, starting with the foundational factors, in this case the supe-

rior structures. If these structures hold inertia, the structures below might continue to fulcrum around the inertial issues above.

The relationships directly superior to the hard palate that can affect its dynamics include the sphenoid bone, reciprocal tension membrane, the frontal bone, the ethmoid bone, and orbital structures in general. We will first generally tune into the area above the maxillae. Then we will more specifically relate to the frontal bone, the falx cerebri, the ethmoid bone, and the orbital structures to get a clearer sense of their dynamics.

Clinical Application: Orbital Relationships

The intention in the following application is to tune into the motility and motion of the orbital region and begin to appreciate both its specific dynamics and its relationship to the hard palate below.

Each orbit of the eyes is composed of seven interrelated bones. These are: (Fig. 10.3):

Bone(s)	Orbital Area
Frontal	"Ceiling," or superior wall
Sphenoid	Back and lateral (outside) walls
Maxillae	Floor and part of the medial rim
Zygomatic	Parts of the lateral walls and floor
Palatines	Small part of the posterior floor
Ethmoid	Majority of the medial wall
Lacrimals	Part of the medial wall

Vault Hold

1. With the patient in a supine position, begin with the vault hold. Negotiate your contact and orient to the mid-tide level of action. Sense the fluid tide and its quality of drive.

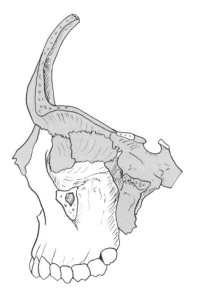

10.2 The maxillae hang from the frontal bone

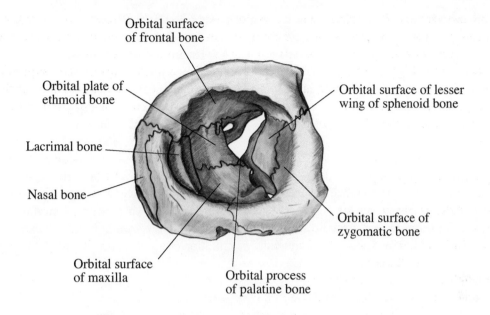

Orbital surface
of frontal bone

Orbital plate of
ethmoid bone

Orbital surface of lesser
wing of sphenoid bone

Lacrimal bone

Nasal bone

Orbital surface of
zygomatic bone

Orbital surface
of maxilla

Orbital process
of palatine bone

10.3 Orbital region

2. Then, include the tissues and their motility within your awareness. Become especially aware of the frontal and orbital areas anterior to your hold. Do not narrow your perceptual field as you do this. From this vantage point you may sense particular inertial fulcrums and their related tissue motility and motion.

Orbital Hold

1. From the vault hold change your hand position to an orbital hold to sense the general relationships of the orbital area and its expression of motility and motion. Still sitting at the head of the table, place your palms over the patient's frontal area and form a "V" with your thumbs gently touching the glabella area between the eyebrows. Spread your other fingers over the maxillae and zygomatic bones (the cheek bones) (Fig. 10.4).

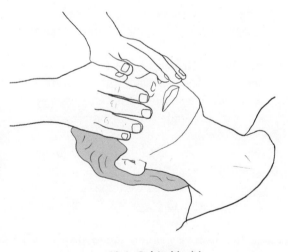

10.4 Orbital hold

2. From this vantage point notice the motility and motion of the tissues within the phases of primary respiration. As you listen, you may sense a general widening and narrowing of the orbits. As the sphenoid expresses its inhalation motion, the orbit widens obliquely and becomes more shallow. The opposite occurs in exhalation.

3. In the orbital hold, follow the motility of the tissues in the orbital area. Notice the general sense of inner breath. Can you sense the tissues literally breathing? Also notice the quality and shape of the motion of the orbit structures. Follow the motion within the phases of inhalation-exhalation. Notice any inertial issue that begins to clarify within your field of perception. Help access the state of balance and listen for Becker's three-phase healing process. Listen for expressions of Health within the stillness. Wait for a sense of softening and expansion of the relationships. Listen for reorganization of tissue structures and realignment to the primal midline and to Sutherland's fulcrum. Notice how the tissues now express motility and motion.

FRONTAL RELATIONSHIPS

The orbital hold can provide a wealth of information about the frontal area. General information can include overall relational symmetry and orientation to the midline and how the tissues are expressing their inner breath, or motility. More specifically, tissues may express a preference for inhalation or exhalation, or one side may express a different pattern compared to the other. Any pattern of expression not directly aligned to Sutherland's fulcrum and to the primal midline is organized around an inertial fulcrum of some sort. You may have noticed tissue pulls, or inertial patterns relating to other areas of the cranium, the hard palate, or the rest of the body. For example, the orbit may generally move around

a sutural relationship of the frontal bone due to a local compression between it and another bone.

The frontal bone expresses its motility and motion as though it is two bones, reflecting its state at birth. The suture between the two parts is called the metopic suture. This suture gradually fuses to form a single bone although the metopic suture is still partially or wholly present in some adults. In the inhalation phase, the frontal bone expresses an external rotation. Its lateral aspects move anteriorly while the glabella area moves posteriorly as though there is still a hinge at the fused metopic suture. Simultaneously but less obviously, the frontal bone can express the unified motion of a single bone. In inhalation you may sense an upward rotation around a transverse axis in a direction opposite to the movement of the sphenoid bone. (Fig. 10.5)

The frontal bone has a number of direct relationships that can affect hard palate dynamics. First among these is the articulation with the maxillae that is discussed above. The frontal bone also has a direct relationship to the ethmoid bone through the frontal bone's ethmoid notch. The ethmoid's crista galli anchors the

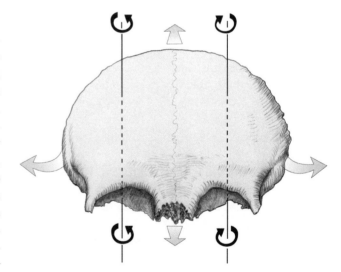

10.5 The motility and motion
of the frontal bone in inhalation

falx cerebri through this notch. This relationship makes a direct link between the structures of the face and the entire membrane system, and the link is reciprocal. Inertial issues and tension on either side can be transferred to the other. Both the frontal and ethmoid bones also articulate with the sphenoid bone. Their interrelationships are totally integrated with the hard palate. Because of this continuity of relationship, the dynamics of the frontal, sphenoid and ethmoid bones will directly affect the hard palate below (Fig. 10.6).

Indirect relationships will also be a factor for the face and hard palate. For example, strain patterns in other parts of the system, such as the occiput and membranes, can be transferred to the frontal bone in various ways. As with all areas, keep in mind the big picture of the whole system as a single unit of function.

As we approach the frontal/ethmoid area, hold respectful awareness for the rich implications of this region. Most prominent among these is the possibility of tissue memories of birth and even prenatal trauma. More subtly, the area between the eyebrows is esoterically considered to be related to the sixth chakra or *ajana chakra,* relating to self-understanding and spiritual manifestation. The pineal/pituitary axis through the third ventricle is just posterior to this area, so inertia here may extend into the neuro-endocrine-immune realm. The frontal cortex of the brain, just posterior to the frontal bone, relates to present time awareness and mediates sophisticated stress responses. Finally, this area is the terminus of the embryological longitudinal axis, and it is thought to be the site of tissue memories of implantation of the fertilized egg into the wall of the mother's uterus. For all these reasons, this is quite a sensitive area that deserves to be approached with respect and sensitive negotiation.

Clinical Application: Frontal Bone Relationships

Vault Hold

1. From the vault hold, orient to the mid-tide and sense the quality of the fluid tide and the potency expressed within the system. Then include the frontal and ethmoid relationships in your listening. Sense the motility of this area within the phases of primary respiration. From this vantage

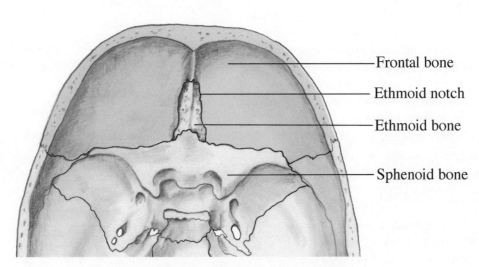

10.6 The relationship of frontal bone to the ethmoid and sphenoid in the cranial base

Frontal bone

Ethmoid notch

Ethmoid bone

Sphenoid bone

point, you may sense specific inertial fulcrums and related motion patterns in the area.

Frontal Hold

2. From the vault hold move to the frontal hold as previously learned in Volume 1. The hands are over the frontal bone with your thumbs crossed and your fingers are in gentle contact with the frontal bone's anterior and lateral aspects, with fingertips just overlapping the orbital ridge. Your thumbs are fulcrums for your palms and fingers, stabilizing each other where they are crossed and enabling both hands to act as one unit. Contact is all along the fingers and upper palm, not just at the fingertips.

3. Orient to primary respiration and the motility and motion of the frontal bone, the glabella area and ethmoid bone. Take time to allow things to settle and for the system to orient to primary respiration. See if any inertial patterns clarify involving any combination of frontal, ethmoid and/or falx cerebri.

4. Follow the motility and motion of the tissues as they manifest to you. Facilitate the state of balance. Listen for Becker's three-phase process. Again listen for expressions of Health within the stillness. Use any of your skills of conversation within tissues and fluids as appropriate. Wait for a sense of softening and expansion and note any changes to the dynamics in the area. Wait for the reorganization phase and note any new motion in relationship to Sutherland's fulcrum and the primal midline.

Clinical Application: Frontal-Occipital Hold

A frontal-occipital hold allows you to sense the continuity between the falx cerebri and its bony relationships. You may also see how membrane dynamics influence the frontal/ethmoid complex. If inertial patterns exist in the cranial membranes, they may be palpated as a pull in any direction, or a distortion affecting the cranial bowl generally. Resolving tension patterns in the falx may be another preliminary step before working with the face and hard palate.

General Frontal-Occipital Relationships

1. With the patient in a supine position, place your hands in a frontal-occipital hold. One hand balances the occiput, fingers spread and pointing caudad. Balance the occiput on your hand, without putting pressure on the occiput with the heel of the hand. The other hand goes over the frontal bone with fingers spread and also pointing caudad. Your fingertips are just below the orbital ridges of the eyes. Contact is all along the fingers, not just at the fingertips. Orient to the mid-tide level of action. First let the fluid tide come to you and then include the tissues in your awareness. Orient to the falx from the ethmoid all the way to the back and base of the occiput (Fig. 10.7).

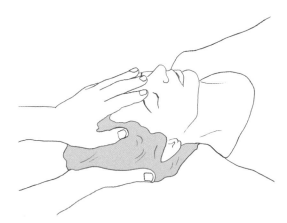

10.7 Frontal-occipital hold

2. From this vantage point, allow the reciprocal tension membrane to come into your awareness. Can you sense the reciprocal tension motion of the falx and the frontal and occiput bones? Do not over-focus; use a wide relaxed view and let these motions come to you.

3. Following the motions, notice the unity of bone and membrane. Does there seem to be a balanced motion between the bones and membrane system? Does there seem to be a balanced relationship to Sutherland's fulcrum? If an eccentric motion pattern clarifies, help access the state of balance. Within this state of balance, you are in intimate contact with the whole of the articular membranous pattern that connects the frontal bone and the occiput. Listen for expressions of Health and for a reorganization of the tissues and fluids to their natural fulcrums and the midline. Do you sense a shift to a more balanced relationship and motion around Sutherland's fulcrum? How has the fluid drive of the system responded to the work?

Frontal Spread

The next hand position offers a more specific awareness of the frontal notch of the frontal bone. The crista galli of the ethmoid passes through this opening to anchor the falx. If the falx is holding a contractive tension pattern, the ethmoid may be compressed into the notch. This may reduce the natural range of motion of both ethmoid and frontal bones.

1. In this hold, I find it easiest to work standing at the head of the table while stabilizing my body against the table. I also stabilize my arms by keeping my elbows in contact with my body. In this standing position, place one thumb over the glabella area, just above the nasal bones. Place your other thumb over the first with your fingers along the lateral aspects of the frontal bone (Fig. 10.8). Negotiate your contact with the patient's system and orient to the mid-tide. Allow the tissues to come to you. Sense their motility and motion. Let the dynamics within the ethmoid notch come to you.

2. Maintain a wide perceptual field and do not crowd the system. It is like standing on a vast beach and looking widely at the ocean in front of you. The

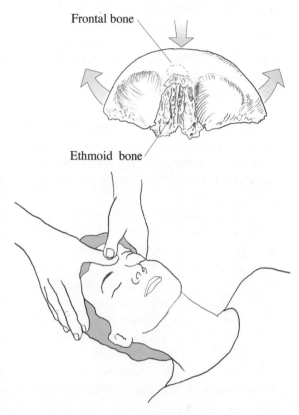

10.8 The frontal spread

waves, the tidal motion, the light sparkling off the water, even the salt air, all come to you. You do not have to go out to them to know them. In this process, you will use the intention of space and disengagement to initiate a conversation with the inertial potencies that are maintaining and centering the compressive pattern.

3. During inhalation, the frontal/ethmoid area will seem to drop posteriorly as the sides of the frontal bone flare out. During an inhalation cycle, follow the inward movement with your thumbs while also following the lateral aspects of the frontal bone anteriorly. Sense the ethmoid notch. Your thumbs suggest a deepening at glabella,

while your fingers suggest a lateral/anterior flaring and spreading of the frontal bone. This combination has the effect of suggesting space within the ethmoid notch. This intention begins a conversation with the inertial potencies that are maintaining and centering the compressive pattern. Do not lose a sense of the whole body as you do this, but continue holding the entire tensile tissue field within your perceptual field. Engage in this conversation very slowly and very gently. Remember that it is a conversation, not a demand.

4. As space is accessed within the relationship, listen for the expression of potency in the area. Help access the state of balance if appropriate. When the state of balance is attained, once again listen for expressions of Health. As potencies are expressed, you may sense a processing of inertial forces and an expansion across the ethmoid notch. You may also sense a freeing up of the relationship between the frontal bone and the ethmoid bone. This may be perceived as a softening and spreading of the ethmoid notch and a clearer ethmoid motion. If the compressive issue was very dense and chronic, the ethmoid bone may not have been expressing much motion at all. As it frees up, you may sense a powerful surge during the inhalation phase. Listen for a reorganization of the tissue elements and a more balanced motion in relationship to Sutherland's fulcrum.

RELATIONSHIPS OF THE ETHMOID BONE

Having explored wider relationships, let's now view the ethmoid bone more closely.

Located at the most anterior-superior aspect of the reciprocal tension membrane, the ethmoid has total continuity with the membrane system all the way to the sacrum and coccyx. Patterns anywhere in this continuum of bone, tissue, and fluid are directly conveyed to any other part of the whole system. Inertial fulcrums, such as compression between the ethmoid and frontal bone, or inertial patterns, such as torsion and side-

bending between ethmoid and sphenoid, can be transferred to the coccyx and sacrum. The ethmoid and coccyx are also paired embryologically as the two poles of the primitive streak and notochord, and energetically within Stone's "as above, so below" principle.

The ethmoid is also the site of unusual properties relating to directionality because it has one of the richest concentrations of biogenic magnetite in the body. This substance responds to electromagnetic fields such as the earth's magnetic field, and is thought to be a factor in orienting and homing instincts as well as sensitivity to electromagnetic fields.

In mystic traditions, the ethmoid bone is considered to have important esoteric functions. The ethmoid is a very light and airy bone. Its lateral masses contain spacious air cells that are considered to be an important interface between the energies of the outside world and the life force within. The outer breath of the air meets the inner breath of primary respiration within the ethmoid. This brings the *prana* within the air into relationship with the prana of the sixth chakra located within the third ventricle, just interior to the ethmoid. In many spiritual traditions, this area is a focus of meditative practices as a gateway to the soul. I point all this out to encourage you to treat this area with utmost respect and humility.

Traumatic force vectors generated by falls on the coccyx can be expressed as compressive patterns at the ethmoid. The trauma force is laterally transferred to the superior area via the continuity of fluid and tissue relationships.

Common inertial patterns include compression within the ethmoid notch of the frontal bone as explored above, compressive patterns in relationship to the sphenoid bone, the maxillae and vomer, and compressive orbital patterns. You may also sense patterns of torsion and side-bending in the ethmoid's relationship to the sphenoid bone.

ETHMOID DYNAMICS

In traditional terms, the motility and motion of the ethmoid bone are expressed as flexion-extension around a transverse axis. As with all midline bones, its rotational motion is considered to be opposite to that of the sphenoid. Its lateral masses and air cells express motility during inhalation by widening, while its anterior end shifts posteriorly as part of the general anterior-posterior shortening of the cranium (Fig. 10.9).

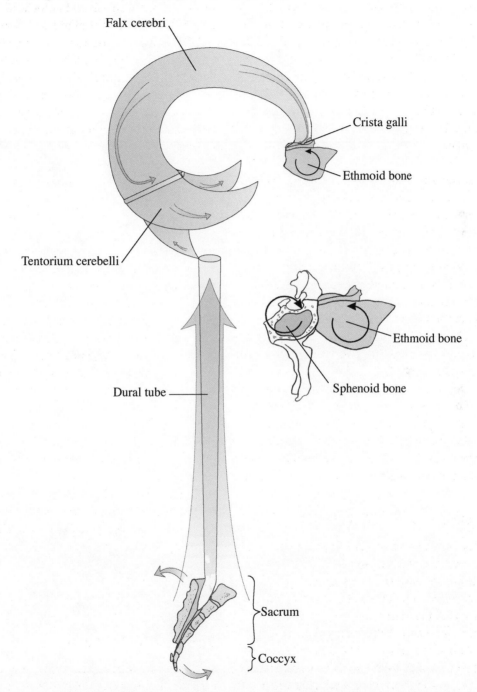

10.9 Relationship of the ethmoid bone to the reciprocal tension membrane in the inhalation phase

All the patterns of the cranial base (between the occiput and the sphenoid) can also occur between the sphenoid and ethmoid bone. To review, these include patterns of fixation in five categories:

- Compression occurs when the two bones have been forced together.

- Torsion occurs when two bones have rotated in opposite directions around an anterior-posterior axis.

- Side-bending occurs when the two bones have rotated in opposite directions around vertical axes.

- Lateral shear occurs when they have rotated in the same direction around vertical axes.

- Vertical shear occurs if the two bones have been forced to rotate in the same direction around vertical axes (Fig. 10.10).

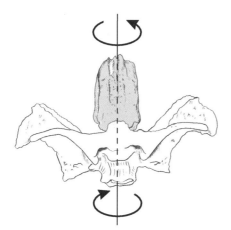

Torsion around A-P axis

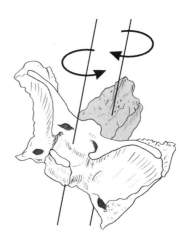

Side-bending around vertical axes

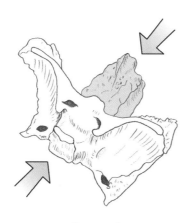

Compression

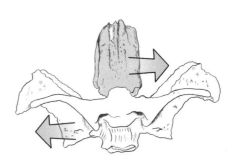

Lateral shear

10.10   Inertial patterns between the sphenoid and ethmoid bones

Patterns of the cranial base and patterns of the sphenoid/ethmoid are totally interrelated and may be treated as a single unit of function. Patterns expressed behind the sphenoid in relationship to the occiput can also be expressed in front of it in relationship to the ethmoid bone and to the hard palate as a whole. Patterns may develop in either direction, the ethmoid influencing the cranial base or vice versa. Approaches to sphenoid/ethmoid patterns follow the same basic principles as approaches to the cranial base patterns.

We are expanding our view of the ethmoid to embrace new relationships, including the maxillae and the nasal bones, in addition to continuing our interest in the frontal bone and the sphenoid. This area needs to be relatively fluid and free in its expression for the maxillae and the hard palate to hang with ease from the orbital processes at the frontal bone.

Clinical Application:
Frontal-Maxillae-Nasal
and Ethmoid-Sphenoid Dynamics

In the next processes, we will contact the nasal bones to explore the relationships between the frontal bone, maxillae, and ethmoid bone, as well as the relationship between the ethmoid, the sphenoid, and orbital structures generally.

Please remember that these are not treatment protocols. The intention here is to systematically become familiar with these relationships so that we can approach treatment creatively and knowledgeably. Our intentions are:

• Encourage ease between the maxillae and frontal bone so that the maxillae can hang freely from their orbital processes.

• Explore the medial relationships of the orbits of the eyes.

• Begin to explore the specific relationships of the ethmoid bone in relationship to the sphenoid bone.

First we will listen to the superior relationships between maxillae and frontal bone, then we will view the relationships in the medial aspect of the orbit of the eye. The medial orbit is composed of the orbital process of the maxilla, the lacrimal bone, and the orbital plate of the ethmoid bone.

1. With the patient in the supine position, begin with the vault hold. Viewing from the mid-tide level, negotiate contact with the system and listen to the relationships mentioned above. Orient to motility and motion within the phases of primary respiration. Take your time and see if any pattern of motion around the ethmoid clarifies.

2. Then change your hand position. Sit at the cephalad corner of the treatment table. Very gently contact the frontal bone at its lateral aspects with your thumb at one lateral aspect and the pads of the fingers of the same hand at the other. With your other hand's thumb and index finger, lightly hold the nasal bones near their articulation with the frontal bone. Elbow support can be very helpful for this (Fig. 10.11).

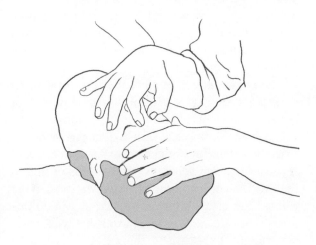

10.11 Frontal–nasal hold

3. In this position, listen to the motility and motion of these tissues. Sense the relationships between

the frontal bone, nasal bones and the orbital processes of the maxillae. As the frontal bone expresses its inhalation motion, you might also sense the nasal bones and maxillae doing the same. This may be sensed as a widening and filling in inhalation and the reverse in exhalation. Listen to any inertial patterns that clarify. Sense the priority arising from within the fluids and tissues. Facilitate the state of balance.

4. Listen for expressions of Health and become aware of how the system expresses its potency and Intelligence in that relationship. Wait for a sense of softening, spreading and reorganization of tissues and sutures in the area.

COMPRESSIVE ISSUES

The above process may be all that is needed to resolve inertial forces and re-establish an ease of motion and fluidity at the ethmoid. But particular compressive patterns may be resistant to change due to the depth of the forces held within the inertial fulcrum. There may not be enough space for the inertial potencies to be expressed. It may then become useful to initiate other conversations with the compressive forces within the inertial fulcrum. Let's look at each compressive possibility in turn.

Making the attention more specific and viewing particular compressive patterns brings up the risk of over-focus. As you initiate any conversations with the system in the work below, such as disengagement and space, do not narrow your perceptual field in any way. If you do, you may add to the compression or shift to the CRI level of action. Maintain an awareness of the whole body as a unified tissue field as you do this work. These are inquiries into the possibility of space, not attempts to release anything. Let the potencies do the work.

Superior-Inferior Relationships

Compression can occur within any sutural relationship, in this case including the nasal bones, the maxillae, and the frontal bone. You may sense this as a superior pull or as inertia or distortion between these bones. The area may seem to be jammed or very dense and resistant. You may also sense motility and motion organized around particular inertial fulcrums. In relating to these compressive patterns, we will use the same hand position and processes as described above; this exploration can be considered as being continuous with the previous work.

1. If you sense compression between the nasal bones, orbital processes of the maxillae and the frontal bone above, you can initiate a conversation with the inertial potencies by intending disengagement and space between the frontal bone and the structures below. To do this, gently stabilize the frontal bone with your cephalad hand and suggest space and disengagement by intending an inferior traction at the nasal bones with your lower hand. Intend this as a conversation about potential space and facilitate the state of balance.

2. When space is accessed, listen for the expression of potency and Health. Note the action of potency and facilitate the state of balance if appropriate. Wait for a softening and resolution of compressive forces within the state of balance and the functional stillpoint. You are waiting for a sense that the nasal bones are floating freely caudad, away from the frontal bone (Fig. 10.12).

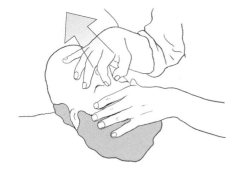

10.12 Frontal–nasal hold
and disengagement inferiorly

Anterior/Posterior Relationships

As you tune into the relationships in the hold described above, there may be a sense of a posterior pull or resistance arising from compressive forces within the medial aspects of the orbit. The nasal bones and maxillae may be held or pulled into one or both medial orbits. This indicates compressive fulcrums between the nasal bone, maxillae, lacrimal bones, and the orbital plates of the ethmoid bone on one or both sides. The compression may pull into the left or right orbit. Compression in both medial orbits is possible but there is usually greater compression on one side. Once again, initiate a conversation about space.

1. Again stabilize the frontal bone. As you become aware of a compressive pull into one orbit, suggest a disengagement of the structures involved. To do this, very subtly traction the structures anteriorly via the nasal bones. This will bring the conversation about space to the orbital relationships (Fig. 10.13). You may sense osseous fulcrums within the medial orbit as you do this. This includes the sutural relationships of the nasal bones, maxillae, lacrimal bones, ethmoid, sphenoid and zygomatic bones.

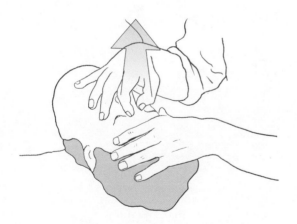

10.13 Frontal-nasal hold
and disengagement anteriorly

2. Once space is accessed, listen for the action of potency and help access the state of balance if appropriate. Listen for expressions of Health within the stillness. Wait for a softening and resolution of the sutural relationships and inertial forces. You may sense the sutures releasing in a ratchet-like way as first one sutural compression resolves, then another.

The above process encourages ease in the articulations around the nasal bones and allows you to use the nasal bones as handles into the medial aspects of the orbital area. It helps open the relationships between the frontal bone and the orbital processes of the maxillae and further encourages freedom of movement between the frontal, ethmoid, and sphenoid bones.

Clinical Application:
Sphenoid and Ethmoid Dynamics

In this process we will be exploring the specific relationships and patterns of the ethmoid bone in relationship to the sphenoid bone.

1. Gently place the thumb and index finger of one hand on either side of the nasal bones near their articulation with the frontal bone. Place your other hand over the lateral aspects of the greater wings of the sphenoid bone. If your hand is too small to actually reach the greater wings, you can still perceive the greater wings via the lateral aspects of the frontal bone. Negotiate your contact and listen within the mid-tide level of action.

2. In this position, orient to the motility and motion of the sphenoid and ethmoid bones within the inhalation-exhalation phases of primary respiration. Settle into your listening and allow things to clarify.

3. You may notice one or more of the patterns mentioned above, including compression, torsion, side-bending, and shear. When a particular pattern clarifies, facilitate a state of balance via your contact with the nasal bones. Within the state of

balance, listen for expressions of Health. You may sense the transmutation of the potency from stillness to fluids to cells and tissue. Listen for expressions of potency and fluid within the state of balance. Wait for a sense of softening and expansion. Note the realignment of the tissues to their natural fulcrums and the midline, as the inertia is resolved. You may sense the ethmoid expressing a deeper and clearer motility and motion.

Clinical Application: Ethmoid Disengagement.

If the biokinetic forces maintaining a compressive pattern are very dense, initiate a further conversation with the potencies, through disengagement. To do this, we will again stabilize the sphenoid bone while subtly intending the ethmoid bone anteriorly.

1. Maintaining the same hold as above, gently stabilize the sphenoid bone. This intention to stabilize implies a deeper quality of contact, without grabbing on to the tissues or holding with any force. If you cannot reach the greater wings, project your intention from the lateral aspects of the frontal bone. While stabilizing the sphenoid bone, suggest an anterior traction into the ethmoid bone via the nasal bones. This will initiate a conversation about space into the relationship between the sphenoid and ethmoid bones (Fig. 10.14).

2. When space is accessed, listen for the action of potency and facilitate the state of balance if appropriate. Listen for expressions of Health. Wait for a sense of softening, disengagement, and expansion in these relationships. The ethmoid may be sensed to float anteriorly toward the ceiling.

3. If the ethmoid seems chronically compressed and congested, you may sense a sudden surge of motion at the ethmoid and a sense of greatly improved motility and motion throughout the system. The patient sometimes perceives that a long-term sense of pressure is being released. This can have a revitalizing effect on the whole system due to the ethmoid's strategic position at the anterior-superior pole of the membrane system and the primal midline.

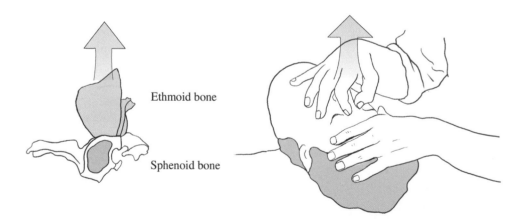

Ethmoid bone

Sphenoid bone

10.14 Disengagement of the sphenoid and ethmoid bones via the frontal-nasal hold

11

The Hard Palate

Having explored the relationships superior to the hard palate, we are ready to approach the vomer, maxillae, and palatines. The maxillae make up the front of the hard palate and the palatines the rear. The sphenoid bone, vomer, maxillae, and palatine bones are an integrated unit of function. The phrase *sphenoid-maxillary complex* is often used to acknowledge this unified quality.[1]

In this chapter we will:

- *Explore the general dynamics of the sphenoid-maxillary complex.*
- *Explore compressive issues and specific inertial patterns in the hard palate area.*

THE MOTION DYNAMICS OF THE SPHENOID–MAXILLARY COMPLEX

The maxillae and the palatine bones articulate with the sphenoid at its pterygoid processes. The vomer articulates with the body of the sphenoid above and the maxillae below (Fig. 11.1a and 11.1b). The palatine and vomer contacts with the sphenoid are gliding articulations, protecting the cranial base from impacts of biting, chewing, and talking. Sutherland called the palatines and the vomer *speed reducers* because of this function. Think of them as *amplitude*

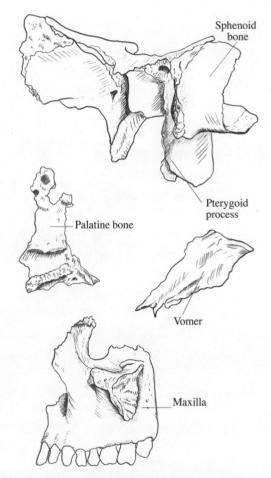

11.1a Sphenoid bone, palatine bone, vomer, and maxilla (disarticulated)

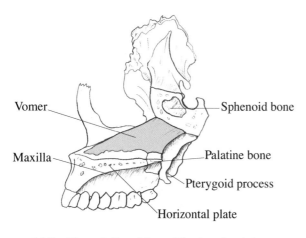

11.1b The relationships of the hard palate

reducers, as they reduce the forces generated by the physical motion of the mouth (Fig. 11.2).

A craniosacral biodynamic understanding recognizes that the potency of the Breath of Life is moving, organizing, and integrating everything in the human system as a whole, all at once. The motion patterns of the sphenoid bone, maxillae, palatines, and vomer are part of this whole. They express an inner motility driven by potency within the system. As everywhere else in the body, these structures express their motility like kelp beds at the bottom of the sea, moved by the tidal potencies within the fluids as a unified tensile field.

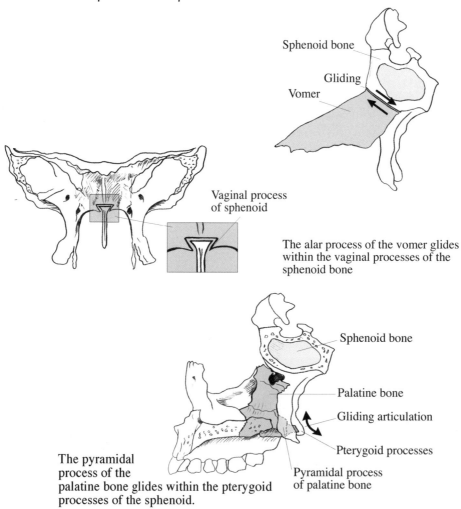

The alar process of the vomer glides within the vaginal processes of the sphenoid bone

The pyramidal process of the palatine bone glides within the pterygoid processes of the sphenoid.

11.2 Speed reducers

The actual motion of tissue structures such as the facial bones and hard palate is thus organic and fluid. This is clearer within the mid-tide where the surge of the tidal potencies is more evident and available for perception. It is not that one bone moves another, or that the membranes move the bones, but rather that everything moves simultaneously as a unified tensile field.

Descriptions of individual bony motion are at best approximations of reality, giving practitioners a chance to break down a unit of function into manageable parts. Traditionally movements of this area have been described in terms of each bone's "axis of rotation" in flexion and extension phases. But bones don't really move around axes of rotation; they express a unified intraosseous and interosseous widening and a unified narrowing within the phases of the tide. The relatively free or restricted quality of interosseous motion is a function of the space generated within sutures and joints in the inhalation phase as potency is surging within the fluids. As the sphenoid expresses its flexion-motion in inhalation, the following interdependent motion patterns occur. (Figs. 11.3 and 11.4)

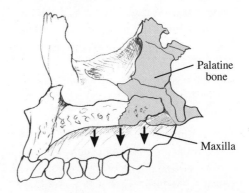

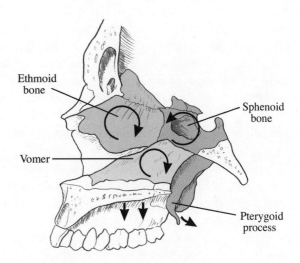

The Maxillae

If all articular relationships around the maxillae are relatively free, the maxillae will express their motion as though they are suspended from the frontal bone. In inhalation, the horizontal plates of the maxillae

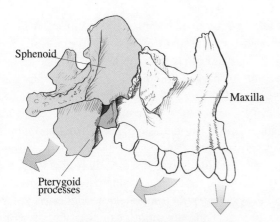

11.3 Movement of the hard palate in the inhalation phase

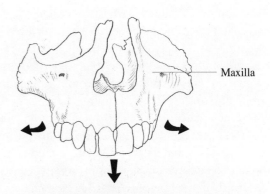

11.4 Movement of the hard palate in the inhalation phase, continued

drop inferiorly as the rear of the vomer descends at the interpalatine suture. The arch of the hard palate flattens and widens in external rotation. The palatine bones mirror this as they move inferiorly and laterally at their horizontal plates.

The Palatines

The palatine bones lie between the pterygoid plates of the sphenoid at the rear and the maxillae at the front. The anterior aspects of their horizontal plates overlap the horizontal plates of the maxillae in shelf-like articulations. Posteriorly, their pyramidal processes articulate with the pterygoid processes of the sphenoid bone. Each palatine rests in the groove between the medial and lateral pterygoid plates. In the inhalation phase, the pterygoid processes widen apart and rotate in an inferior/posterior direction. As this occurs, the pyramidal process of the palatine bones glide between the pterygoid processes and move inferiorly and laterally as part of the lowering of the hard palate in external rotation. The inhalation motion of the palatine bone is integrated with that of the vomer as it descends inferiorly onto the hard palate.

The gliding action of the palatine bone between the pterygoid processes of the sphenoid is extremely important. Compressive issues between the pyramidal processes of the palatines and the pterygoid processes of the sphenoid can compromise the amplitude reduction inherent in the joint. This will generate inertial distortions directly affecting the cranial base.

The Vomer

The vomer articulates with the maxillae, the sphenoid, and the ethmoid bones. The alar surface of the vomer is flared open and articulates with the rails of the vaginal processes of the sphenoid. As the sphenoid expresses inhalation, the vomer rotates in the opposite direction in a gliding action. Chewing motions are absorbed and dispersed similar to the palatine/pterygoid process action. In inhalation, as the vomer rotates in the opposite direction to the sphenoid bone, its inferior/posterior aspect descends inferiorly at the rear of the hard palate. As the sphenoid expresses its inhalation-flexion motion, the inferior-posterior aspect of the vomer descends towards the hard palate as the horizontal plates of the maxillae and palatines lower and widen transversely.

CONTACT AND INTIMACY IN INTRA-ORAL WORK

Working with the hard palate may involve finger placement inside the patient's mouth. Here we are literally entering the patient's body. We are venturing into an extremely sensitive psycho-emotional area, and due caution is needed. The mouth directly registers our experiences of getting our most fundamental needs met. Termed *oral needs* by some psychologists, these arise within the womb and are highlighted immediately at birth with the baby's securing of maternal bonding and protection through nursing. The baby may perceive lack of contact and bonding after birth as life threatening, so the oral impulses have a tremendous emotional urgency from the very beginning. Taste and smell are strong senses at birth, and babies will constantly place things into their mouth as they explore their world. The experience of oral needs continues throughout life with essential nourishment both physically and emotionally.

The mouth is our life-preserving interface with the outside world, first with mother and with food as we get older. The mouth also plays a survival role as the vehicle for verbal communication, the baby's primary way to alert caregivers of needs and later the medium of social communication. Later the mouth plays crucial roles in eating for comfort, expression of feelings, and sexual contact and gratification. Problems with expressing our needs and emotions can show up as tension in the mouth area. Oral needs can become so charged that the issues involved may lead to eating disorders such as anorexia, bulimia, and obesity. The mouth is extremely sensitive, with a highly disproportionate supply of sensory and motor nerves in its tissues and correspondingly in the brain. Several psychology systems, especially neo-Reichian forms, note the reflex relationship between the mouth and the pelvis, a view also advanced in Stone's Polarity Therapy. Thus, the mouth can also hold tensions relating to sexuality, including traumatic experiences.

I know from clinical experience that issues of abuse,

abandonment, and rejection can all generate tissue tensions and psycho-emotional charge in the mouth area. Tissues of the hard palate and jaw can hold memories of experiences that may not be directly related to the physical dynamics of the mouth. These include a whole range of factors that all relate to our ability to get our needs met and our sense of safety with intimate contact and close relationships.

Dental experience is another reason to approach intra-oral contact cautiously. Many people have had dental experiences that are unpleasant and even traumatic. These can be restimulated by having a practitioner's fingers inside a patient's mouth.

When you need to place your fingers in a person's mouth, the first priority is to communicate what you are doing and why it is necessary. Approach the work delicately, with respect and slow pacing. Give the patient power and control in the situation. Explain the work to the patient before doing it and give a clear sense of choice and options. I also work out a code, such as a hand signal, so the patient can easily indicate when to stop. The important thing here is to be conscious of the issues and to approach things slowly with awareness of the full implications. As in all of our work, we are not imposing our will onto a person's system, but rather we are initiating conversations and helping to open doors and windows that have perhaps been forgotten.

Surgical gloves or finger cots are used in all intra-oral work, including every application in this chapter. These are widely available at drug stores or medical supply companies.

TUNING TO THE DYNAMICS

In the first exercise we will simply listen to the motion between the sphenoid bone and the hard palate to see if we can sense sphenoid/maxilla and sphenoid/vomer dynamics. We will use two different holds to approach these. The intention is to become familiar with this area generally, before moving to specific structures or motion patterns. Repeated practice is highly recommended, using numerous study sessions to develop the capacity to accurately palpate and visu-

alize this fairly complex set of interrelationships. By having lots of practice with this sensitive area, the practitioner will be able to more comfortably hold a neutral space for clients in actual clinical practice.

The Sphenoid-Maxillary Hold

1. With the patient in the supine position, place one hand over the frontal bone so that your thumb is over one sphenoid greater wing and your index or middle finger is over the other. If you cannot reach the two greater wings, you can still sense them from the lateral aspects of the frontal bone. Place the palmar surfaces of the index and middle fingers of your other hand so that they are touching the biting surfaces of the upper teeth. Be sure that you are over the rear molars. Your fingers form a V-shape as they span the alveolar arch. Place them as far back as possible without eliciting a gag response (Fig. 11.5a).

2. Orient to the biosphere and mid-tide. See if you can sense the motility of the sphenoid and the maxillae as a unified and integrated dynamic. Review the descriptions and illustrations on the motions of these bones so that you have a sense of what to expect. In inhalation, the hard palate lowers and the alveolar arch widens apart. You may sense this as a widening between your fingers as they contact the upper teeth. Maintain a wide perceptual field as you listen to motility. Do not narrow your intention; let the tissues and their motions come to you.

3. As an inertial pattern clarifies, see if you can help access a state of balance. Listen for expressions of Health and for the reorganization of tissue structures to the midline.

The Sphenoid-Vomer Hold

1. The patient is in the supine position as above. Place one hand over the frontal bone and greater wings as described above. This time, place the index finger of your other hand over the midline of the hard palate, touching the underside of the interpalatine suture. The inferior end of the

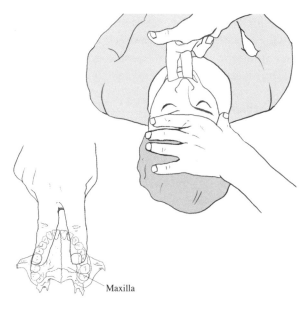

11.5a Sphenoid–maxillary hold

vomer is directly above your contact. Some people have a bump at the roof of the mouth, where the vomer is pressing upon the suture. This is an expression of compressive forces and implies restricted motion (Fig. 11.5b).

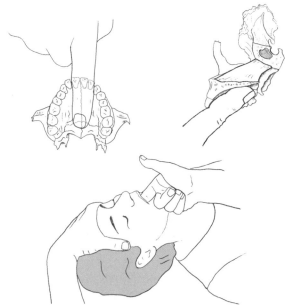

11.5b Sphenoid–vomer hold

2. Orient to the mid-tide. See if you can sense the unified and integrated tissue motility and motion of the sphenoid bone and vomer. In inhalation, the vomer descends upon the rear of the hard palate as the alveolar arch widens. You may sense this as a subtle pressure on your finger. Maintain a wide perceptual field as you do this. Do not narrow your intention; let the tissues and their motions come to you.

3. As an inertial pattern clarifies, see if you can help access a state of balance. Listen for expressions of Health and for the reorganization of tissue structures to the midline.

COMPRESSIVE ISSUES IN THE HARD PALATE

We will explore compressive forces first because they can mask other inertial patterns such as torsion or shear and bind them into fixed relationships. Compressive issues can also fix the amplitude reducers so that forces of eating and chewing directly impinge upon the cranium.

Compression within the sutures of the hard palate is quite common and usually generated by trauma. Origins can be diverse, from birth processes to dental work, impact shock from accidents or sports, various forms of abuse, or other causes. Properly negotiate entering the mouth of the patient in all of these intra-oral sessions. Work slowly and give patients the option of not doing the work if it is initially too charged for them. All our skills for working with trauma that were presented in the first volume, such as slow pacing and cultivation of resources, come into play when we work in this area.

Key Relationships In Hard Palate Compression

- The relationship of the inferior aspect of the vomer with the interpalatine suture
- The maxillae, vomer and sphenoid relationships

190

- The relationship between the maxillae, palatines and pterygoid processes of the sphenoid.

COMPRESSION IN VOMER–INTERPALATINE RELATIONSHIPS

First we will explore the inferior surface of the vomer as it rests on the interpalatine suture. The vomer can become compressed inferiorly into the interpalatine suture, generating inertia within hard palate dynamics and affecting the cranial base and the whole system. Compression in the interpalatine suture is often coupled with compression between the alar surface of the vomer and the rostrum of the sphenoid. The two maxillae may also be compressed medially into each other at the interpalatine suture, transferring inertia to the vomer (Fig. 11.6).

Clinical Application: Interpalatine Compression

First we will listen for motion and ease at the interpalatine suture and relate to compressive forces found within the specific relationship between the vomer and maxilla.

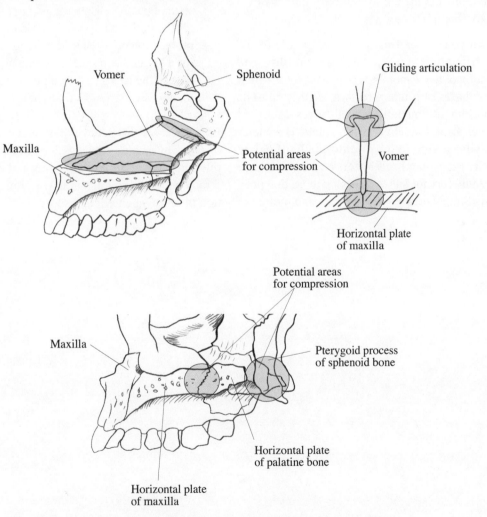

11.6   Sutural relationships and potential compression sites

1. Begin with a vault hold. Negotiate your contact and orient to the mid-tide field of action. Become aware of the fluid tide and the resources of the system, and then include the tissues in your field of awareness. See if you are drawn to the hard palate in any way.

2. Moving from the vault hold, sit or stand at the head of the table. Place both index fingers side-by-side on the roof of the patient's mouth, one on either side of the interpalatine suture. I find the most comfortable position to be standing at the head of the table with my body braced on the table and my elbows supported by my own body (Fig. 11.7).

3. With your index fingers on either side of the interpalatine suture, sense the motility and motion of the vomer and the two maxillae within the phases of primary respiration. Listen to its unfoldment. Inhalation ideally gives a sense of lowering and widening of the palate. The vomer may be sensed to lower onto the hard palate while the palate itself lowers and widens. Give this time; do not follow the first pattern that presents. Simply orient to the motility and motion of the tissues as a unified field of action within the phases of primary respiration.

4. See if an inertial pattern clarifies. You may sense distortions of motion and structure within the tissue relationship, eccentric motions, tissue strains and pulls, general congestion, or even very little motion at all. Notice the inertial fulcrum that seems to organize this. Is there a specific sutural relationship that is involved? Do not narrow your perceptual field; let the tissues and their history come to you.

5. Help facilitate the state of balance. Within the state of balance, listen for expressions of Health, for the initiation of inertial potencies and for the permeation of potency into the relationship. Wait for a general sense of softening and expansion. Notice the reorganization phase and new alignment to Sutherland's fulcrum.

In many cases this may be all that is needed to help the system resolve compressive issues within these relationships. If there is still a sense of compression, it may be useful to engage in the clinical conversation of disengagement and space.

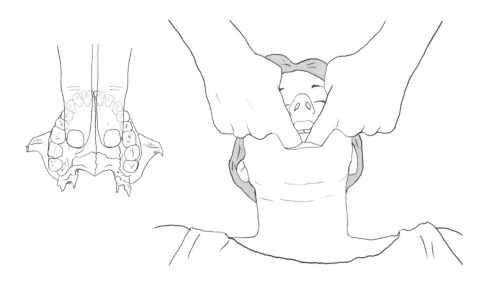

11.7 Interpalatine hold

Clinical Application: Disengagement and the Interpalatine Suture

Next we will explore the possibility of medial compression between the two maxillae within the interpalatine suture. The vomer and the two maxillae can become compressed or jammed together. The intention here will be to engage in a conversation about space, and the possibility of disengagement, not just of the tissue structures involved, but of the forces that generate their compression.

1. In the same position, very gently spread your two fingers apart laterally in a rolling fashion (Fig. 11.8). You are suggesting a lateral spreading apart of the two maxillae at the interpalatine suture. This disengagement process is traditionally called an intermaxillary spread. We are initiating a conversation about space. How much space is possible here?

2. Once space is accessed, listen for the action of potency and facilitate the state of balance if needed. This shifts the focus of conversation to

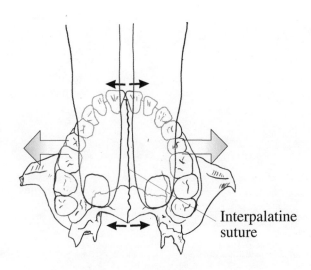

11.8 Disengagement in the interpalatine hold

Interpalatine suture

the Health that is centering the biokinetic forces maintaining the compression. Listen for expressions of fluids, potency, and the processing of biokinetic forces. You may sense heat, pulsation and force vectors. Wait for a sense of softening of sutural relationships. As usual, listen for reorganization and the evolution of a new motion dynamic.

Clinical Application: Compression within Sphenoid-Vomer-Maxillae Relationships

As you were listening at the vault hold, you may have sensed a strong force pushing against the inferior aspect of the sphenoid. This indicates that the sphenoid and vomer may be in compression. It may also indicate that the multiple sutural relationships between the sphenoid, vomer, and maxillae are all holding compressive issues (i.e. sphenoid-vomer and vomer-maxillae). As seen above, the vomer can also become compressed into the interpalatine suture; this compression can also be transferred into the dynamics of the cranial base as a strong pressure against its normal movement.

In this next application, we will explore this three-part relationship (sphenoid-vomer-maxilla). The vomer forms an angle of approximately thirty degrees between the sphenoid and maxilla. We will engage in a conversation about space and disengagement along this thirty-degree angle to the horizontal plane of the hard palate.

1. Stand or sit at the side of the treatment table. If you choose to sit, be sure your hands and arms are comfortably supported. If I sit, I tend to rest my elbows on small cushions so that tension doesn't build in my hands as I work. Creating elbow support also clarifies my contact with the patient's system and gives the patient's system stable reference points.

2. Place one hand at the greater wings of the sphenoid via the lateral aspects of the frontal bone. Your thumb is in relationship to one greater wing and your index finger is in relationship to the

other. Your other hand is placed at the inferior pole of the relationship with your thumb externally on the midline of the upper lip at the alveolar ridge and your index finger of the same hand on the alveolar ridge internally behind the upper teeth. Your internal finger is on the midline of the hard palate. You are now holding the superior pole of the three-part relationship at the sphenoid and the inferior pole at the maxillae (Fig. 11.9).

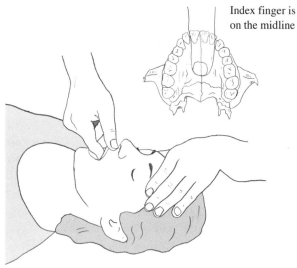

11.9 Disengagement hold for the sphenoid-maxillae–palatine bone relationship

3. In this position, you may sense a compressive pull superiorly along an angle of approximately thirty degrees, your lower hand being drawn toward your upper hand. Alternatively, you may sense very little motion at all, or a block-like locking between the structures as they express their motility. As you sense this, your intention will be to invite a conversation about disengagement and space within the sutural relationships.

4. Gently stabilize the sphenoid at the greater wings with a gentle suggestion, not by grasping the sphenoid with any force or pressure. After stabilizing the sphenoid, intend space into the relationships by your contact with the maxillae at the alveolar arch. Very subtly suggest traction along the thirty-degree angle of the vomer footward until a sense of space is accessed. Maintain a clear, gentle intention of space and disengagement along the thirty-degree axis (Fig. 11.10).

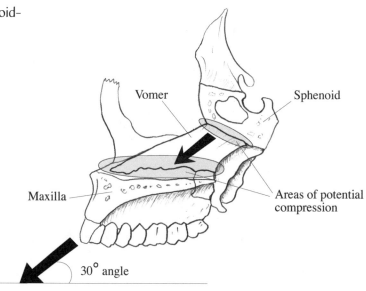

11.10 Direction of sphenoid-vomer-maxillary disengagement

5. Once space is accessed, listen for the action of potency and facilitate the state of balance if appropriate. Listen for expressions of Health within the stillness. Be especially aware of expressions of potency and fluid drive within the sutural relationships. Wait for a sense of softening and space to arise within the sutural relationships.

6. You may sometimes sense the forces present within the sutures releasing in a ratchet-like fashion. Different inertial fulcrums may resolve within the different sutural relationships at different times. You are ideally waiting to sense the maxillae floating with ease in an anterior and inferior direction. Listen for reorganization and realignment to Sutherland's fulcrum and the primal midline.

Clinical Highlight

Compression in sphenoid-vomer-maxillary relationships can have many clinical repercussions. Inertia can be transferred throughout the hard palate, generating malocclusion and other dental problems. Compressive forces can also be transferred to the cranial bowl above. Compression between the vomer and the sphenoid bone is especially contentious, directly affecting the cranial base generally and the relationship between the sphenoid and occiput more specifically. I have worked with many cases of cranial base congestion and related tension headaches that originated in the hard palate. I have even seen neuroendocrine issues arise due to the backpressure generated in the hypothalamus and pituitary area by a severely compressed sphenoid-vomer sutural relationship.

A number of years ago, a patient was referred to me by her dentist. The patient was experiencing trigeminal neuralgia coupled with low energy and exhaustion. After a number of sessions, the relationship between the sphenoid bone, vomer, and maxillae came to the forefront. A strong inertial force was present that seemed to have its origin in an accident which impacted these relationships. It generated fulcrums within the field around her body, and vortex-like motions could be palpated around her cranium. This inertial issue was intensified by the dental extraction of two upper molars. The intensification of these forces affected the trigeminal nerve and seemed to generate inertia within the cavernous sinus that, in turn, affected pituitary function. Her energy dropped and this also affected her motivation and self-esteem. The compensations that were maintained by her system in relationship to the earlier accident had been overwhelmed by the added forces introduced in the dental sessions.

These forces resolved over a three-month period. In one session I worked more directly with disengagement in the sphenoid-vomer-maxillary relationships as described above. As space was accessed within the relationships, I directed fluid and potency towards the area. A deep state of balance ensued. The vortex-like fulcrums within the field around her cranium seemed to still, and a gentle vibration or energetic interchange could be sensed. When the primary compressive force of the accident finally resolved, a force vector literally streamed out of her body. This occurred in a very resourced manner, and the patient commented that her whole body seemed to soften and relax. In subsequent sessions, the venous sinus system resolved its inertial issues, and her potency seemed to reignite within the fluid system. Her sense of vitality was greatly enhanced and upon palpation the fluid tide certainly seemed fuller and more present. She did not get tired as before and sessions were ended at this point.

COMPRESSION IN SPHENOID–PALATINE–MAXILLAE RELATIONSHIPS

Next we will explore the relationship between the sphenoid, palatine bones, and maxillae. As noted above, the sphenoid articulates with the palatines via its pterygoid processes. The relationship between the two is a gliding one and, like the vomer, also acts as speed or amplitude reducer. The force of chewing and talking is softened as the pyramidal processes of the palatines glide between the pterygoid processes of the sphenoid. If this relationship becomes compromised, then the gliding action is lost and these forces are directly transferred to the sphenoid and cranial base. As with the vomer and sphenoid above, this will affect the whole of the system. Anterior to that articulation is the relationship between the palatine and the maxilla. The palatine articulates with the maxilla, and its horizontal plate rests on the horizontal plate of the maxilla in a shelf-like fashion. The palatine rests on the shelf of the maxilla.

There are thus two sutural relationships to be aware of here. The first is the gliding relationship between the pyramidal processes of the palatines and the pterygoid processes of the sphenoid. The second is the articulation of the shelf of the horizontal plate of the palatines with the horizontal plate of the maxillae. Compression in any of these relationships may be sensed as a posterior pull into, or as an anterior-posterior jamming between hard palate relationships. Alternatively, you may not sense much motion at all.

Clinical Applications: Sphenoid-Palatine-Maxillae Compression

As you were listening at the vault hold, you may have perceived a sense of inertia, or backpressure, below the sphenoid. This can be generated by the presence of compressive forces between the pterygoid processes of the sphenoid bone and the pyramidal process of the palatine bone. Compression here can cause the bones to express their motion in a block-like manner. You may not be able to sense the individual interrelated motions of each bone. Furthermore, the gliding motion between the pterygoid processes of the sphenoid bone and the pyramidal processes of the palatine bones may be compromised, affecting amplitude reduction.

1. Place your hands in the same positions as in the sphenoid-vomer-maxillae disengagement application above (see Fig. 11.9). In this process you will be relating to the structures involved in an anterior-posterior plane rather than in a thirty-degree plane. Settle into your fulcrums, negotiate your contact with the system, and orient to the mid-tide. Allow the motions of the maxillae, palatines, and sphenoid bone to come into your awareness. Orient to their motility and motion within inhalation and exhalation.

2. As you do this, you may sense a posterior compressive pull, or a general sense of inertia. The conversation skill of disengagement can be used to relate to the inertial potencies maintaining and centering the compression. To do this, gently stabilize the sphenoid bone and intend space and disengagement via the maxillae. Intend an anterior suggestion of traction through the structures until space is accessed (Fig. 11.11).

3. When space is accessed, listen for the action of potency and facilitate a state of balance if appropriate. As you do this, you are engaging in a conversation with the inertial potencies and forces maintaining the compression through the tissues. As potency is expressed in some way, you may sense resolving of the compressive biokinetic forces involved, with the tissues softening and expanding either bilaterally or more on one side than the other. The sutural relationships may seem to expand in a ratchet-like fashion. The compression on one side of the hard palate may resolve before the other, and one articulatory relationship on the same side may soften before the other. Remember that on each side of the palate there are two separate articular relationships that may be compressed (i.e., pterygoid-palatine and palatine-maxilla on each side).

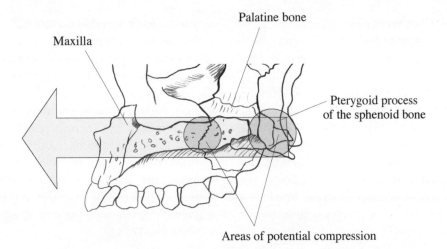

Maxilla

Palatine bone

Pterygoid process
of the sphenoid bone

Areas of potential compression

11.11 Direction of sphenoid–palatine–maxillary disengagement

4. Ideally you are waiting to sense the hard palate softening as a whole and floating anteriorly with ease (towards the ceiling with the patient in the supine position). Listen for the reorganization process. You may sense that the potency, fluids, and tissue elements reorganize in their relationship to the midline. Is there a greater ease and balance of motion within these relationships now?

CLINICAL REPERCUSSIONS OF COMPRESSION

Unilateral compression between one set of pterygoid processes and its related palatine bone can generate torsion patterns within the cranial base. Bilateral compression (between both sets of pterygoid processes and both palatine bones) can generate either inhalation or exhalation patterns within the cranial base, depending on the forces present.

Compression between the pterygoid processes and the palatine bones can also generate entrapment neuropathy issues. The sphenoid-palatine ganglia rest within the sphenoid-palatine fossa on each side of the midline and pterygoid/palatine compressive issues can directly affect these ganglia. The maxillary branch of the trigeminal nerve may be especially affected by pressure on this ganglion. Sensory facilitation of this

nerve may result in sensitivity in the maxillary sinuses, the maxilla generally and the upper teeth. Trigeminal neuralgia can result (Fig. 11. 12).

Birth trauma is a common origin of compression for either the sphenoid-vomer-maxillae or sphenoid-palatine-maxillae groups. Thumb sucking can alleviate a sense of compression and jamming within these

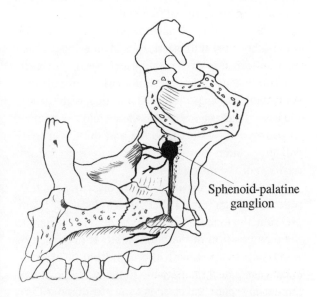

Sphenoid-palatine
ganglion

11.12   The sphenoid–palatine ganglion

sutural relationships, especially with sphenoid-vomer compression. In treating infants and young children for these issues, relate to their system as if they are a membranous-fluidic body, not firmly formed like adults. Base the work on perceiving the infant as a fully conscious being, and negotiate your contacts accordingly. Intentions of space, fluid skills, and disengagement of the sutural relationship are the primary focus. After a sense of space is established, move on to potency and fluid drive as the intention of treatment. Direction of fluid and potency can also help the infant mobilize inertial potencies within the compressive relationship.

Temporomandibular Considerations

In the above work, you helped the system resolve compressive issues within the maxillae and hard palate. As these issues resolve, the position and motion of the hard palate may also be affected. The resolution of posterior compression in the pterygoid-palatine-maxilla relationship can allow the maxilla to shift anteriorly. The resolution of superior compression in the sphenoid-vomer-maxilla relationship can allow it to shift in an inferior-anterior direction. As these forces resolve, the maxillae may reorient to the midline and their natural positions. When this occurs, they may shift inferiorly and anteriorly, affecting the occlusion of the biting surfaces of the teeth. The upper teeth may shift anteriorly and inferiorly. As you are working within the mid-tide, with the tensile tissue field as a whole, the whole field will respond to your work, so the mandible and the lower teeth will also realign to come into relationship to the new position of the maxilla.

However, if other fulcrums are affecting the temporomandibular joints (TMJ), such as local TMJ compression, the mandible may not be able to reorient to the new position of the hard palate. It may then be important to work with the mandible in order to encourage a new relationship to the maxillae above. Supporting space and disengagement within the TMJs and generally encouraging the mandible anteriorly

can restore comfortable occlusion.

The motility and motion of the mandible is closely associated with the temporal bones. In the inhalation phase, the temporal bones seem to rotate around an axis through their petrous portions. The squama widen laterally and inferiorly, and their mastoid portions move medially and superiorly as they come closer together. The temporomandibular fossae follow this motion, rotating inferiorly and widening apart. The mandible also follows this motion and, in inhalation, moves inferiorly as its legs widen apart laterally. It has a natural orienting fulcrum along the midline at C2 (see Fig. 12.2).

Clinical Application: TMJ Disengagement and Anterior Realignment

In this application, we will make our first contact with the mandible and the TMJs. We will go into TMJ dynamics in great detail in Chapter 12. Consider this application a very basic introduction that will give an initial feel for the TMJs and their inertial issues. The intention here will be to explore space within the joint dynamic and to encourage a resonance between the new position of the hard palate and the mandible in general.

The state of balance

1. Place the fingers of both hands just above the angle of the mandible (Fig. 11.13a). Negotiate your contact and synchronize your perceptual field with the mid-tide. Let the palm of your hand rest over the temporal bones and TMJs. In this position, let the motility and motion of the mandible come into your awareness.

2. Beyond their normal motions, the TMJs and mandible may express almost any possible motion pattern including compressive issues, circular motions, shearing motions, pulls in different directions, etc. As a pattern clarifies, help access the state of balance. Be patient. Don't rush this. Orient to primary respiration and let the tissues communicate their experience. Let the pat-

tern clarify from within. Listen for Becker's three-phase healing awareness. Wait for a sense of softening of tissue elements and realignment to the midline.

Disengagement and space

1. Once you sense softening and reorganization, very gently engage the tissues of the mandible via traction in an inferior direction. This encourages a conversation about disengagement and space within the TMJ joint relationships. Remember that the idea of disengagement processes is to access the potential space within the joint dynamic. It is really about disengagement of the biodynamic and biokinetic potencies and forces present.

2. As space is generated, listen for the action of potency and help access the state of balance if appropriate. Listen for expressions of Health and a change in the potency within the fulcrum and fluid-tissue field.

3. Listen for the joint relationship to soften and for the mandible to float inferiorly. As this occurs, add an anterior component and suggest a forward rotation of the mandible by rolling your hands anteriorly as the joints begin to float inferiorly. This encourages realignment of the biting surfaces of the upper and lower teeth. Access a state of balance here until a softening of the area is perceived and a clear sense of a general reorganization arises within the area as a whole (Fig. 11.13b).

SPECIFIC PATTERNS WITHIN HARD PALATE DYNAMICS

Now we will explore other inertial patterns of the sphenoid-maxillary complex. This integrated group of structures can express any of the patterns found in the cranial base (flexion-extension, torsion, side-bending, and lateral shear), and can even mirror cranial base dynamics. In a traditional context,

sphenoid-maxillary patterns are said to occur around the same rotational axes as the cranial base patterns. sphenoid-maxillary patterns can also be reflections of pelvic relationships. The head and pelvis are two ends of a unified tissue system. We have seen that the sacrum and occiput can reflect each other's patterns. In addition, the temporal bones can reflect the patterns of the ilia, the TMJs can reflect those of the

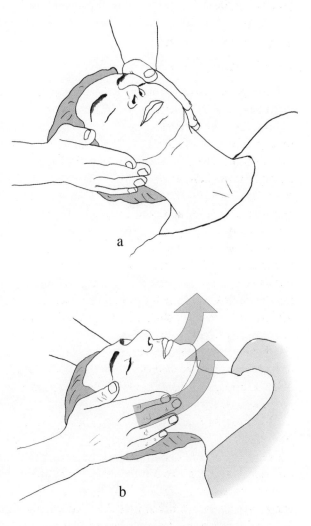

11.13 a and b   Mandible hold

acetabula (the hip joints), and the occipito-mastoid sutures can reflect those of the sacroiliac joints.

We will describe these motion dynamics in text and diagrams, but working with models is also a great way to become really familiar with the possibilities. The more familiar you are, the more accurately you can visualize, the more you can recognize in your listening process.

I am describing the clinical processes below in a way that encourages an intuitive relationship to these patterns. The patterns just show themselves as part of the treatment plan at work. It is simply a matter of recognizing them and responding appropriately. In basic courses I no longer teach motion testing for these structures.

Inertial patterns within the hard palate are a uni-fied function between the sphenoid bone, vomer, palatine bones, and maxillae. Birth dynamics often generate compression, torsion, side-bending or shearing patterns in the hard palate that will in turn be reflected within the cranial base. Imagine that the sphenoid bone is a transition point for cranial bowl-hard palate patterns (Fig. 11.14). Patterns behind it (i.e. sphenobasilar patterns) will reflect patterns in front and below it (i.e. face and hard palate patterns) and vice versa. The following sections describe dynamics in the sphenoid-maxillary complex in which the structures are fixed in relationship to each other in various ways. Remember that these patterns are not simply rotation patterns, but are literal distortions in the fluid-tissue field. The nomenclature and axes of rotation used are consistent with that of cranial base patterns

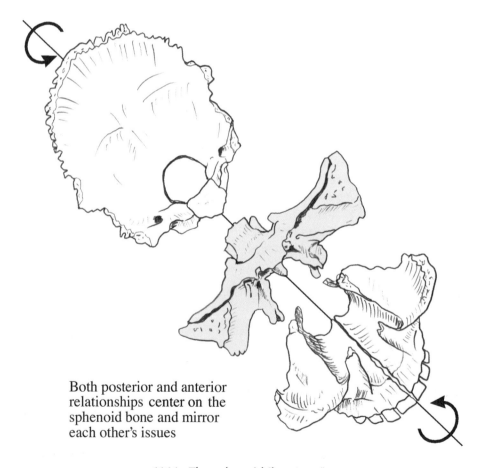

Both posterior and anterior relationships center on the sphenoid bone and mirror each other's issues

11.14   The sphenoid "keystone"

described previously. This is so that you can appreciate how the cranial base and the sphenoid-maxillary complex is a unified field of action.

Inhalation-Exhalation Patterns

In an inhalation pattern, the sphenoid bone is held in an inhalation-flexion position along with all of the other sphenoid-maxillary structures. The greater wings may seem to be rotated inferiorly. If you are also holding the vomer with a finger on the midline of the interpalatine suture, its posterior aspect will seem to be inferior, exerting a subtle pressure on your finger. The hard palate may seem inferior and wide. Holding the maxillae via the underside of the teeth as described above, you may sense that the arch of the palate is wide and the maxillae are externally rotated (see Figs. 11.3 and 11.4).

The extension-internal rotation position presents the opposite of all these positions, with the sphenoid bone relatively superior at its greater wings while the arch of the hard palate seems narrowed and high.

Torsion Patterns

Torsion is a relatively common sphenoid-maxillary pattern. Torsion occurs around an anterior-posterior axis, just as it does within the cranial base. In torsion, the sphenoid bone rotates in one direction around an A-P axis as the maxillae are rotated in the opposite direction. As you hold the sphenoid bone at its greater wings, and the maxillae at the upper surfaces of the teeth, you may sense a torsioning between them. The sphenoid tends to rotate one way around an imaginary A-P axis as the maxillae rotate in the opposite direction. The vomer may become twisted in the direction of the torsioned maxillae, but may also be bent in a C-curve (Fig. 11.15 shows left torsion).

Side-bending Patterns

Side-bending is also a common sphenoid-maxillary pattern. As with the cranial base, side-bending occurs around vertical axes, the sphenoid bone rotating one

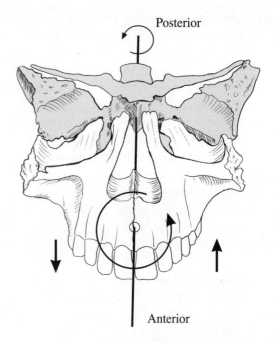

Left torsion: maxillae rotate around A-P axis, left maxilla is high

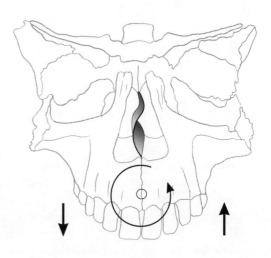

In left torsion of the spheno-maxillae complex the vomer commonly becomes twisted

11.15 Torsion of the hard palate occurs around an anterior–posterior axis way while the maxillae rotate in the opposite direction. This rotation can be felt as you hold the sphenoid bone at its greater wings, and the maxillae at the upper surfaces of the teeth. Side-bending is identified by the side that is bulging, so right-side-bending means the maxillae rotate away from the right side of the face. In side-bending the vomer usually becomes bent in a C-curve between the sphenoid bone and maxillae, but may also become twisted or torsioned between the two. (Fig. 11.16 shows left side-bending.)

LATERAL SHEAR PATTERNS

In lateral shear, the sphenoid bone has been forced laterally in one direction, while the maxillary complex shifts laterally in the opposite direction. Shear is palpated by holding the sphenoid bone at its greater wings and the maxillae at the upper surfaces of the teeth. Shear is named for the direction of movement, so right lateral shear means the maxillae are shifted to the right side of the face. The vomer is bent in an S-curve between them. (Fig. 11.17 shows left lateral shear.)

Clinical Applications: Exploration of Specific Sphenoid-Maxillary-Vomer Patterns

In these explorations, we will be using both the *sphenoid-maxillary* and *sphenoid-vomer holds* learned above. You will first sense whatever patterns arise within your sphenoid-maxillary hold, work with the dynamics that arise, and then follow the pattern through the sphenoid-vomer hold. We will use the examples of a flexion or extension pattern and then of a torsion pattern to give examples of following through a pattern within all of the relationships present.

The intention will be to let the pattern take its shape as you hold a wide and still perceptual field. Let the tissues communicate their history to you. It will take practice to really hear this story and to allow the treatment plan to make itself known. Give yourself the luxury of listening and the space to explore and learn.

From the *vault hold,* sense the quality of the fluid drive and potency of the system. Then sense into the hard palate below your hold. From this vantage point

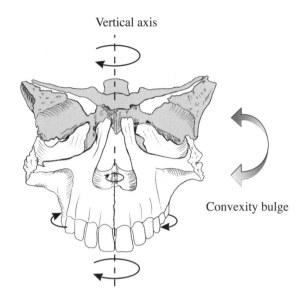

Left side-bending: maxillae rotate around a vertical axis, creating a convexity (bulge) on the left

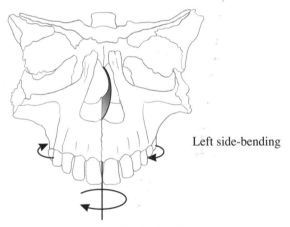

In side-bending the vomer bends into a "C" shape

11.16 Side-bending of the hard palate occurs around a vertical axis you may sense specific inertial fulcrums around which the system has had to organize. You may sense motions or distortions that relate to the patterns described above, such as torsion or side-bending. On a deeper level, you may perceive the inertial potencies that are organizing the tissue patterns.

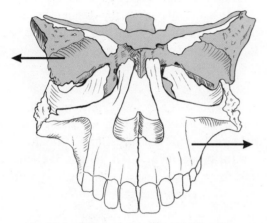

Left lateral shear: maxillae side-shift to the left

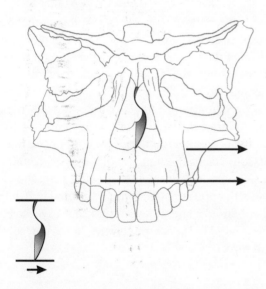

In lateral shear the vomer bends in an "S" shape

11.17   Lateral shear
of the sphenoid-maxillary complex

Sphenoid-Maxillary Patterns

Example: An Inhalation or Exhalation Pattern

1. Use the *sphenoid-maxillary hold* described above. Orient to the biosphere and mid-tide, holding a wide and still listening field. Listen for the inhalation and exhalation motions of the sphenoid-maxillary complex. You may sense the alveolar arch widening transversely in inhalation as the sphenoid expresses its inhalation-flexion motion. Listen to motility and motion within the phases of primary respiration. Spend some time listening; don't immediately engage a pattern. Notice if the system prefers one phase of motion to the other. Wait for something to engage from within and for a pattern to clarify.

2. If the system prefers one to the other, for example if it prefers inhalation, follow the tissues in that direction. If it prefers a torsioned motion, one maxilla will be sensed to be superior, so follow in that direction. For side-bending you may sense a rotation of the maxillae to one side or the other. For lateral shear, the maxillae seem shifted to one side or the other. Follow whatever pattern clarifies. Help access the state of balance. Simply slow things down if necessary. Listen for expressions of health within the stillness. Listen for the reorganization of tissue, fluids, and potencies during the third stage of Becker's three-phase awareness process. Do not narrow your perceptual field as you attend to these patterns.

3. Listen for the return of motion and motility. How do the tissue elements now express inhalation and exhalation? What is the fluid drive of the system like now?

Sphenoid-Vomer Patterns

1. Change your hand position to the *sphenoid-vomer hold* described above. Again orient to the mid-tide. Simply listen to motility and motion

within inhalation and exhalation. See if one phase is preferred. See if an inertial pattern clarifies.

2. Help access the state of balance and wait for a settling into stillness. Listen for expressions of Health and for the processing of inertial forces and force vectors. These may be sensed as a release of heat, streaming of energy or force, or expansion. Use conversational skills that may be helpful here such as direction of fluids, lateral fluctuation, or disengagement. Listen for reorganization of the tissue elements and for realignment to the primal midline. Pay attention to the quality of the fluid tide and the drive of potency within it.

The tissues may also show you one of the other inertial patterns described above. Let's use torsion as an example.

Example: Sphenoid-Maxillary Patterns in Torsion

1. In the *sphenoid-maxillary hold,* orient to the mid-tide. Let the fluid tide come into your awareness. Sense its quality and drive. Then listen to the dynamics of the motility and motion of the tissues.

2. The maxillae may indicate that the hard palate is in a torsioned position relative to the sphenoid bone. Torsion is named after the high side of the maxillae. For a left torsion pattern the left side of the hard palate is higher than the right side. You may also sense rotation of the hard palate around an anterior-posterior axis relative to the sphenoid bone.

3. Let the overall sense of this pattern come into your hands. Let its form, shape, and motion present themselves to you. Help access the state of balance. Listen within the stillness. Listen for expressions of Health such as potency and fluid motions, tissue expansion, etc. Again, bring in any conversational skills that may be helpful here. Listen for the new organization and for the fluid tide to reassert itself. What are the quali-

ties of tissue motion like now? How does the fluid tide express its potency?

Sphenoid-Vomer Patterns in Torsion

1. Now change your hold to the *sphenoid-vomer hold* as described above. Again orient to the mid-tide. Let the motion of the tissues come into your awareness within the phases of primary respiration. In a torsion pattern, the vomer is twisted as it follows the maxillae, but it may also have been forced into a C-curve with the concavity towards the high side of the hard palate.

2. Listen for Becker's three-phase awareness again. Follow the form and motion of this pattern to its boundary. Help access the state of balance. Listen for expressions of Health. Listen for reorganization of the tissue elements and for a new sense of motility and motion within the relationships.

OTHER CONSIDERATIONS

The torsion pattern may reflect a similar cranial base pattern, or it can be the reverse. For example, a right torsion of the hard palate may reflect a right torsion within the cranial base. The maxillae may follow the sphenoid and be high on the same side that the sphenoid's greater wing is high. A torsion pattern may seem to move through all of the structures at once, with the origin in either the sphenoid or the maxillae. Conversely, the high maxilla may be found on the side opposite to the high greater wing, showing torsion in opposite directions behind and in front of the sphenoid bone. I have found that reverse patterns of this kind are almost always due to unresolved birth forces.

Palatine Relationships

The palatine bones are connecting links between the pterygoid processes of the sphenoid and the maxilla. If palatine relationships are compressed, the gliding action within the pterygoid processes is lost, and motion and motility dynamics can be severely affected. We have already explored compressive issues between the sphenoid bone, palatine bones, and maxillae. Sometimes inertial forces are so strong and tissue effects are so ingrained that the pyramidal process of the palatines can become chronically impacted into the pterygoid processes, and the previous work may not fully resolve the compression. It may then be useful to make a more specific relationship to the palatine and its dynamics. In this next application, we contact the palatine bone and work with the state of balance in its relationship to the pterygoid processes of the sphenoid.

Clinical Application: The Specific Relationships of the Palatine Bone

Vault Hold

1. Begin this application in a *vault hold.* Orient to the mid-tide. Sense the quality of the fluid tide and the drive of the potency within it. Get a holistic sense of the cranium and its membranous-articular dynamics. Then allow the hard palate to come into your field of awareness. Tune into this area without narrowing your field of attention and without over-focusing on the details of the patient's system. Allow a sense of the structures below your hands to clarify.

2. Specific inertial fulcrums may become apparent. Tissue compression between the pterygoid processes and the palatine bone may feel like a strong pull into that relationship. The sphenoid bone may seem pulled inferiorly into the pterygoid/palatine area. Alternatively, you may sense a strong resistance or backpressure coming from the pterygoid area on one side or both sides. Compression may severely restrict the sphenoid bone and generate a torsion pattern within the cranial base as the greater wing of the sphenoid is pulled down on the compressed side. Start with the side that you sense to be most resistant.

Review the clinical issues described above, especially the possibility of entrapment neuropathy of the sphenoid-palatine ganglion.

The Sphenoid-Palatine Hold And The State Of Balance

3. With the patient in the supine position, sit or stand at the side of the table. Place one hand on the greater wings of the sphenoid as learned previously. Place the index finger of your other hand over the horizontal plate of the palatine bone at the rear of the hard palate. To do this, slide your gloved or cotted index finger along the upper molars past the last molar. Then slip your finger just medially to the rear of the hard palate. You are now on the horizontal plate of the palatine bone. Be sure that your elbows are comfortably supported on the table or on cushions, or stabilized on your own body (Fig. 11.18).

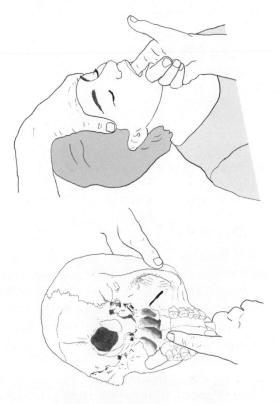

11.18 Sphenoid–palatine hold

4. In this position, you are in direct relationship with the sphenoid and palatine bones. Again orient to the mid-tide. Allow the motion dynamic of the two structures to come into your awareness. See if you can sense independent motion as they express their motility. If the motion seems block-like and rigid, there may be compression within the sutural relationships. The intention is not to decompress anything, but to resolve the forces that are maintaining these effects.

5. In this position, follow the motility and motion within primary respiration. See if a particular inertial pattern clarifies over time. Follow this dynamic however it is expressed and help access the state of balance. Bring in conversational skills as needed. Within the stillness of the state of balance, listen for expressions of Health and for a resolution of the forces involved. Listen for reorganization and realignment to the midline. You may sense a greater ease and independence in the motion between the two bones and better motility being expressed.

This may be all that is needed to help the system resolve the compressive forces involved. If resolution does not feel complete, the maxillae-palatine-pterygoid disengagement process described above can be used. This process can bring a conversation about space to the gliding articulation between the sphenoid and palatine bones.

ZYGOMATIC BONES

The last facial bones to explore are the zygomatic bones. These connecting links fill the spaces between the sphenoid, frontal, maxillae, and temporal bones. They allow these bones to have an indirect relationship and function as a structural and motion link for the area. The zygomatic bones allow for the complex set of motility and motions between the sphenoid, frontal, temporal, and maxilla bones to be reconciled as a unified system. The zygomatic bones also act as speed reducers and perform a protective role for facial structures similar to the functions of the vomer and palatines. Inertial issues within the relationships of the zygomatic bones can therefore strongly affect the whole system. Fixations within the sutural relationships of the zygomatic bones are generally due to physical trauma such as accidents, falls, and blows to the face (Fig. 11.19).

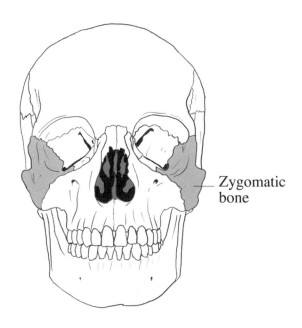

Zygomatic bone

11.19 Zygomatic bones in skull

MOTILITY AND MOTION

In the inhalation phase, the zygomatic bones express a transverse widening by rolling anteriorly and laterally along an imaginary oblique axis. This is classically called external rotation. This rolls the orbital border laterally and increases the superior/medial-inferior/lateral diameter of the orbit (i.e. the diagonal line from the superior medial aspect of the orbit to the inferior lateral aspect). This is part of the overall transverse widening of the orbit in the inhalation phase (Fig. 11.20).

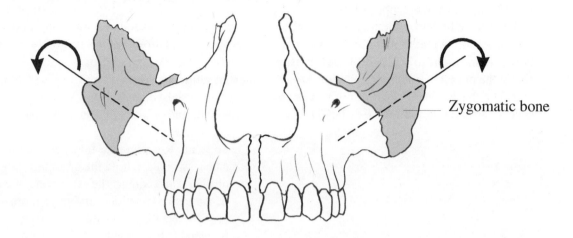

Zygomatic bone

In inhalation the zygomatic bone widens
transversely around an oblique axis.

11.20 Motility and motion of zygomatic bones

PERCEIVING ZYGOMATIC PATTERNS

Inertial issues within the sutural relationships of the
zygomatic bones are usually perceived by sensing the
motion of the bones that articulate with it. You may
sense density or backpressure from a particular articular relationship, or a tissue pull into one of its sutural
relationships. Alternatively, you may sense that the
motility and motion of another bone is organized
around an inertial fulcrum related to the zygomatic
bone or one of its sutures. The zygomatic bone may
seem to be moving in an eccentric or block-like way
in conjunction with one of its articulating bones. The
sense of fluidity and continuity with the unified tissue field may seem to be lost.

Clinical Application:
General Zygomatic Hold

1. Start in the vault hold. Orient to the biosphere
   and mid-tide. Hold a wide perceptual field and
   sense the quality of the fluid drive and potency
   of the system. Then allow the zygomatic area to
   come into your field of awareness. Let the tissues of this area come to you within the wide
   perceptual field rather than narrowing your
   attention down to the area. From the vault hold,
   orient to the motility and motion being expressed
   within the phases of primary respiration. See if
   eccentric tissue motions and/or fluid motions are
   organized around any of the zygomatic sutural
   relationships clarify.

2. Place the index finger and middle finger of each hand spread obliquely over the zygomatic bones in a V-shape with fingertips pointing medially and inferiorly. In this position see if you can perceive the motion and motility of the zygomatic bones. First orient to the motility and motion within the phases of primary respiration. Do any inertial patterns clarify? Are you drawn to any specific sutural relationship? (see Fig. 11.21.)

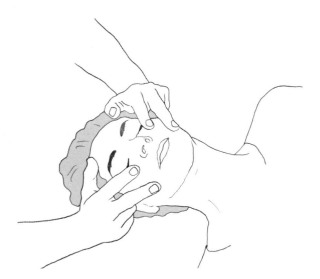

11.21 Zygomatic hold

3. Follow the patterns and shapes of the motions that you sense and help access the state of balance. As always, listen for expressions of Health and for the processing of any inertial forces present. Use any other skill that is appropriate here. Listen for softening and expansion of the tissues and for a reorganization and realignment to the midline. These motions are not new patterns being expressed, they are the system's attempt to realign to natural fulcrums.

Clinical Application: Specific Relationships of the Zygomatic Bones

As we become aware of specific sutural resistances in zygomatic relationships, we can relate to them in specific ways. The first approach is to V-spread the inertial suture. For instance, if the frontal-zygomatic suture is inertial, you can place a V-spread over it and direct fluids and potency to it as we discussed earlier.

1. To relate to an inertial fulcrum in a more specific way, you can hold the zygomatic bone with one hand and contact the other bone of that particular sutural relationship with your other hand. First contact the zygomatic bone. After you identify what suture to work with, place your cotted index finger in the patient's mouth external to the maxilla and as far posterior as possible, between the flesh of the cheek and the zygoma. Hold the zygoma with this index finger internally and with the thumb of the same hand externally. All the suggestions about sensitivity and negotiation apply here (Fig. 11. 22).

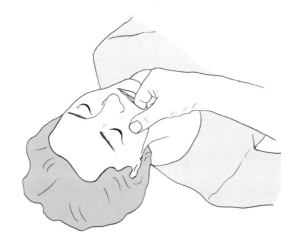

11.22 Internal zygomatic hold

2. Then place the index and middle fingers of your other hand over the other bone (the sphenoid, frontal, maxilla, or temporal bone) involved in the sutural relationship, near the suture with the zygoma. Orient to the mid-tide. Listen to motility and motion within the inhalation and exhalation phases. See if an inertial pattern clarifies. Help access the state of balance. Again listen for expressions of Health, for the processing of inertial forces, for the softening and expansion of the tissue elements, and for the reorganization of potencies, fluids, and tissues to the midline.

Clinical Application: Disengagement of Zygomatic Sutural Relationships

If this process or the V-spread does not fully resolve the inertial forces, a suggestion of disengagement and space may be useful. For example, let's say that you sensed an inertial fulcrum between the zygomatic bone and frontal bone.

1. Place one hand holding the zygomatic bone as described above and place the index and middle fingers of the other hand on the lateral aspect of the frontal bone near its articulation with the zygomatic bone. You are now in relationship to the two poles of the inertial pattern.
2. In this position, gently stabilize the zygomatic bone and suggest a subtle traction across the suture. This is a gentle intention placed on the frontal bone to float away from the zygomatic bone. It is a suggestion of space between the zygoma and frontal bone. When space is accessed, listen for the action of potency and help access the state of balance if appropriate.

1. I believe that this term was coined by John Upledger, D.O.

209

12

The Temporomandibular Joint

The intention of this chapter is to explore the temporomandibular joint (TMJ) and its dynamics. This will complete our tour of the face and hard palate and will also finish this volume's overview of the cranium.

In this chapter we will:

- *Introduce the dynamics of the temporomandibular joints.*

- *Discuss connective relationships and TMJ function.*

- *Explore the specific ligamentous relationships of the joint.*

- *Explore compressive issues unilaterally and bilaterally.*

THE TEMPOROMANDIBULAR JOINT AND THE UNIFIED TISSUE FIELD

As we have seen, the body is a physiological unit of function. Inertial dynamics within any of its parts will affect the whole field in some way. The temporomandibular joints are part of this unified field and will influence, and be influenced by, all other parts of the system. Inertial forces and related tissue problems found anywhere in the body, may affect temporomandibular joint function in many ways.

Understanding the TMJs' multiple relationships begins with their immediate location adjoining the temporal bones. Temporal bone issues can manifest immediately in the TMJs. A direct connection also exists with the membrane system of the cranium because the tentorium is continuous with the temporal bone; therefore, the TMJs can be affected by membranous strains elsewhere in the body.

This TMJ/temporal/tentorium complex responds to gravity along with the pelvic diaphragm, sacral base, the respiratory diaphragm, and the shoulder girdle. These structures work together to express balance and compensation in relationship to gravity. For instance, the body will respond to a side-bent sacrum by balancing all other horizontal structures in relationship to it. The shoulders may compensate by slanting in the opposite direction, the atlas and cranial base may also shift in response to the sacrum, and the tentorium and temporal bones will follow by adjusting their position and mobility (Fig. 12.1). Stone noted that the hip joints and TMJs have direct energetic, gravity line, and fascial resonances. He also noted that patterns involving the pubic arch and pubic symphysis would also be directly expressed in TMJ function and balance.[1] Nearby structures are also interdependent with the TMJs. For example, inertial issues within the face, hard palate, or cranial base can generate, or be affected by, TMJ patterns.

Muscular structures are particularly relevant to the TMJs. Chronic contraction of any of the muscles that

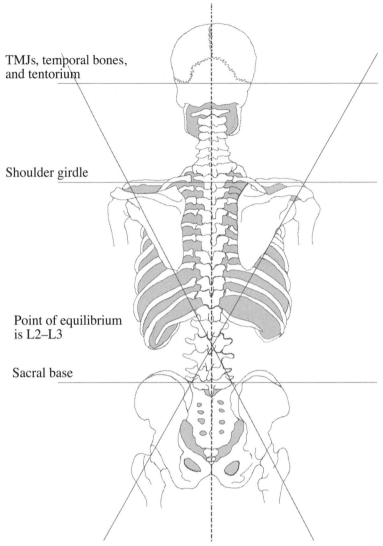

TMJs, temporal bones,
and tentorium

Shoulder girdle

Point of equilibrium
is L2–L3

Sacral base

12.1 TMJs and horizontal gravity lines

move the mandible can generate inertia in TMJ function and can affect the motion and motility of the temporal bones and mandible. This is especially true of the temporalis muscle, which is very responsive to stress. Chronic tension within its anterior fibers can be transferred to the sphenoid and frontal bones, immobilizing the sphenoid bone and holding the condyle in a superior/posterior position. Chronic tension within its middle fibers can affect the temporal-parietal suture, generating an internal rotation of the parietal bone and mimicking an extension-type pattern. Chronic tension within the posterior fibers of the temporalis muscle can place traction on the lateral inferior-posterior aspect of the parietal and temporal bones, generating an inhalation-external rotation pattern and maintaining an inhalation pattern within the cranium as a whole. Chronic temporalis tension can also generate compression within the TMJ itself, holding the condyle in a superior/posterior position and thus affecting TMJ function.

The TMJs can also reflect emotional tension. The TMJs often become tense when there is a need to hold back expressions of suffering or emotion that would be too dangerous or painful to allow. As noted in a previous chapter, the TMJs are part of the oral segment. This is a horizontal band that includes the upper cervical area, occiput, the TMJs and mouth. This whole segment can hold tension related to unresolved oral needs issues. These needs are commonly thought to derive from early childhood. They focus on the use of the mouth and jaw to get nutritional, nurturing, and contact needs met. In the adult, the oral segment may relate to generally getting one's needs met, as well as relating to sexual contact and sexual need and to comfort needs, such as eating and drinking.

Similarly, the TMJs may express nervous system activation. The trigeminal nuclei have connections to the sympathetic nervous system. Chronic tension and autonomic activation may be physiologically reflected at the TMJs, and anything that helps down-regulate CNS activation, such as stillpoint work, may provide TMJ relief.

Because the TMJs have so many interrelationships encompassing the entire body, holding a wide view of the whole system is particularly important. Do not narrow your perceptual field when working with the TMJ area; hold an awareness of the whole even while you are also simultaneously attending to local tissue details. The effectiveness of this approach depends on the ability to perceive the Inherent Treatment Plan. Fulcrums organizing TMJ motion and position may be located anywhere in the body, so treating TMJ issues may involve work elsewhere, as well as work with stress reduction, relaxation and trauma counseling.

The Motion and Motility of the Mandible

In the inhalation phase, the mandible expresses external rotation by following the temporal bones, rotating inferiorly and widening transversely. The temporal bones are said to rotate around an axis through their petrous portions as they express external rotation in inhalation. As this occurs, their squama widen laterally and inferiorly and their mastoid portions move medially and superiorly as they come closer together. The temporomandibular fossa follow this motion, moving inferior-laterally and widening apart. The mandible also follows this pattern and tips inferiorly as its legs widen apart in the inhalation phase (Fig. 12.2). Ideally, the condyles of the mandible should be floating within the synovial fluid of the temporomandibular fossa's joint capsules with an easy and balanced motion.

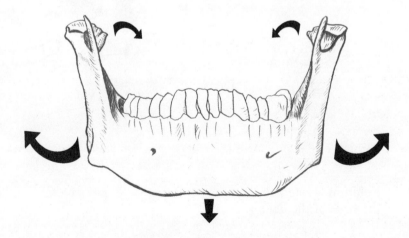

12.2 The motion of the mandible in inhalation

Like all connective tissue forms within the body, the TMJs naturally relate to Sutherland's fulcrum as a suspended automatically shifting fulcrum. This fulcrum orients them to the primal midline and midline functions in general. The TMJs have a further orienting fulcrum within the system. According to Guzay's theorem, the fulcrum for ideal mandibular motion is located at the base of the dens of the second cervical vertebra. Guzay described this fulcrum in relationship to opening and closing the mouth, but it is equally true for mandibular motility within the phases of primary respiration. As the mouth is opened, the mandible maintains its balanced relationship to C2. The temporomandibular fossa on each side shift in position, but the relationship to the fulcrum at C2 is stable. The mandible should ideally express its motility and motion as if the second cervical vertebra is an automatic shifting fulcrum or balance point.[2] (Fig. 12.3)[3]

The position of the mandible reflects the position of the temporal bones. Hence, the mandible will directly express its motion and motility in relationship to the temporal bones and their motion and motility. The mandible will obviously also express its motion dynamics relative to the nature of the forces within the TMJs. The mandible will tend to shift towards the externally rotated temporal bone. This will be overridden by compression within the TMJ, as the mandible will tend to pull towards the temporomandibular joint holding the most compression.

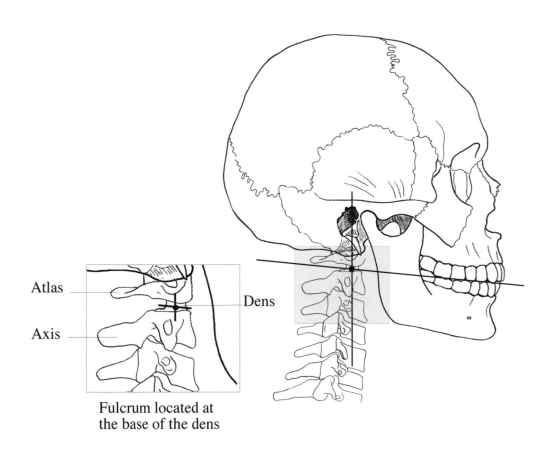

Atlas

Axis

Dens

Fulcrum located at
the base of the dens

12.3 The fulcrum for mandibular motion

Hence, the patient's chin may be seen to deviate towards an externally rotated temporal bone or the most compressed TMJ.

Basic Anatomy and the Articular Motions of the TMJs

The TMJs are the most used joints in the body. They are paired joints composed of the relationship between the temporomandibular fossae of each temporal bone and the two condyles of the mandible. The TMJ is the only synovial joint in the cranial bowl, and it is actually a double synovial joint with a disc separating the two compartments (Fig. 12.4).

Considering each compartment as a separate functioning unit, the upper compartment has a mainly gliding action and the lower compartment has a mainly hinged and rotational action. When the mouth opens, the mandible moves away from the upper jaw (maxilla) and the disc is drawn anteriorly. This is a gliding action as the disc and the condyle move forward on the mandibular fossa. The joint surface formed by the temporomandibular fossa and its articular eminence is an "S" shape. The shape of the disc follows this and has a biconcave configuration. The first movement in the joint as the mouth opens is an anterior and inferior gliding action with some rotation in its upper cavity between the disc and the fossa.

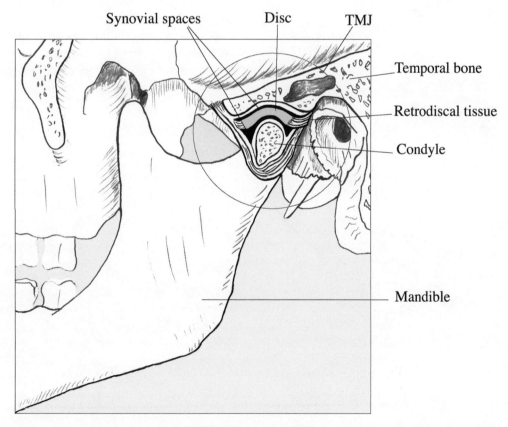

12.4 The anatomy of the TMJ

The disc/condyle complex is drawn anteriorly and inferiorly as a unit.

As the mouth opens further, the condyle then moves on the disc with a hinge-like motion. Thus, the disc becomes stabilized on the fossa and the condyle rotates on the disc like a hinged joint. The axis of rotation for this motion is located at about the center of the ramus of the mandible. The mandible is depressed (the mouth opens) by the lateral pterygoid muscles, aided by the digastric, mylohyoid, and genio-hyoid muscles. The mandible is elevated (the mouth closes) by the temporalis, masseter, and medial ptery-goid muscles (Fig. 12.5).

DISC AND LIGAMENTS

The disc, or meniscus, of the TMJ is an oval plate that sits between the condyle of the mandible and the tem-poromandibular fossa. It is thicker in its posterior aspect and can have a biconcave configuration that follows the "S" shape of the joint fossa. It is laterally attached to the joint capsule by connective tissue. Anteriorly it is attached to the tendon of the lateral pterygoid muscle and posteriorly to the elastic retrodiscal tissue (Fig. 12.6). As the mouth opens, con-traction of the lateral pterygoid muscle moves the disc and condyle anteriorly. This is opposed by the retrodiscal tissue posteriorly and by the thickened aspect of the disc itself. As the mouth closes, the lat-eral pterygoid relaxes and the retrodiscal tissue pulls the disc and condyle posteriorly. The disc and condyle function as one unit.

The important ligaments of the TMJ include the capsular ligament, the temporomandibular ligament, the sphenomandibular ligament and the stylo-mandibular ligament. Inertial issues relating to either the temporal bones or sphenoid bone can be trans-

A   Mouth closed

B–D   Progressive motions
as the mouth opens

12.5 Motion of the TMJ as the mouth opens

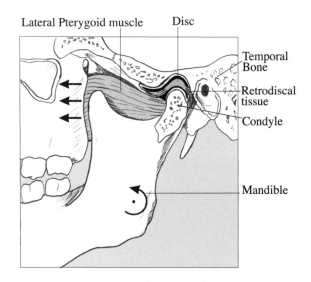

12.6 The lateral pterygoid muscle
opens the mouth

ferred to the TMJs via these ligamentous relationships. Likewise, inertial patterns and compressive issues within TMJ function can be transferred to either the temporal bone or sphenoid bone. These ligaments can individually generate various TMJ issues and will be clinically explored later in this chapter (Fig. 12.7).

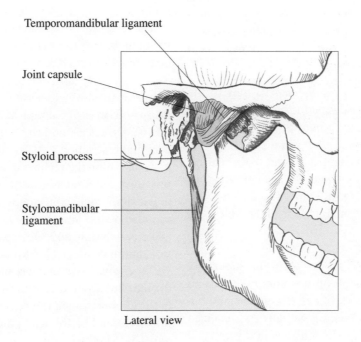

Temporomandibular ligament

Joint capsule

Styloid process

Stylomandibular ligament

Lateral view

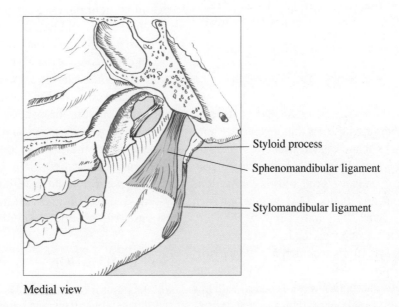

Styloid process

Sphenomandibular ligament

Stylomandibular ligament

Medial view

12.7 Ligaments of the TMJs

- *Temporomandibular Ligament:* Attaches to the lateral surface of the zygomatic arch and then divides into two portions, one connecting to the lateral surface of the condyle and the other to the lateral surface of the upper aspect of the ramus of the mandible. The first portion prevents posterior dislocation of the condyle in the fossa and the second portion aids in the anterior movement of the condyle when the mouth opens.

- *Sphenomandibular ligament:* Attaches to the spine of the sphenoid superiorly and to the medial (inner) aspect of the ramus of the mandible. It commonly has some fibers that penetrate the petro-tympanis ligament and attach to the malleus of the ear. Tensions held in the ligament can thus give rise to hearing problems and tinnitus. The ligament generally stabilizes the mandible in its actions.

- *Stylomandibular Ligament:* Attaches superiorly to the styloid process of the temporal bone and inferiorly to the posterior aspect of the mandibular angle. This ligament is actually a specialized band of cervical fascia; tensions in the cervical area can be transferred to the TMJs here. It stabilizes the joint and helps prevent anterior displacement.

TMJ SYNDROME AND DYSFUNCTION

TMJ syndrome is a general term that is used to describe a number of symptoms that involve the temporomandibular joint and related structures. This syndrome includes pain within the TMJs, facial pain, pain around the ears, pain in the skull, burning sensations in the nose, throat, and tongue, TMJ dysfunction such as lack of mobility, clicking noises, and swelling, ear symptoms such as ringing, hearing loss, and dizziness. Other common symptoms include painful chewing, clicking, and/or popping sounds when opening and closing the mouth, zigzag motions associated with jaw action, malocclusion, other ear symptoms such as pressure in the ears, ringing, or pains in the facial area,

skull, or even in the cervical area. TMJ syndrome may arise from the TMJs themselves, or the TMJ issue may be organized by patterns from almost anywhere in the body. As you can see, the term TMJ Syndrome includes a huge range of symptoms and functional problems.

The temporal bones and tentorium are usually contributing factors in TMJ problems. Ease in temporal bone function and balance in their positions are critical for properly functioning TMJs. TMJ function can also be affected by tension patterns in the cervical fascia and cervical muscles, in the muscular and connective tissues around the hyoid bone, cervical and occipital restrictions, atlas and axis fixations, strain patterns within the reciprocal tension membrane system (especially the tentorium), and respiratory and pelvic diaphragm contraction. Hard palate patterns can also be fed into the TMJs and generate inertial issues and dysfunction. Obviously there are many factors that may affect TMJ function.

Trigeminal neuralgia has similarities to TMJ syndrome and their origins may be interrelated. In trigeminal neuralgia the trigeminal nerve is hypersensitive, leading to facial pain, burning sensations, and TMJ symptomology. The common features of trigeminal neuralgia are severe lancing or burning pains in the face and jaw areas that may be initiated by chewing, talking, and cold weather. Trigeminal facilitation can also give rise to chronic tension within facial and temporalis muscles and this may also generate TMJ symptoms. Furthermore, as noted above, there are collateral links between the nuclei of the sympathetic nervous system and the trigeminal nuclei. General sympathetic hypertonis and related stress issues must be addressed in cases of trigeminal neuralgia. Hyperarousal states within the neuroendocrine system due to traumatization and chronic stress responses can generate trigeminal neuralgia.

TMJ EVALUATION

When a patient arrives with TMJ symptoms, it can be useful to establish a clinical baseline by assessing TMJ joint function to check the progress of treatment. Are compressive forces at work within the joint, and are external patterns affecting its function? The following is a traditional approach to analyzing TMJ function. For our purposes here, the evaluation is mainly to support initial learning, because it helps demonstrate effectiveness. Later, in a clinical setting, the evaluation process yields to a more direct holistic perception of the patient.

- *General alignment of facial structures:* Note any deviation from a straight line in the front of the face, running from the midline of the frontal bone, nasal bone, nose, and chin.

- *Alignment of teeth:* Open the patient's lips without physically opening the mouth. Look at the base of the teeth where they join the bone at the midline top and bottom. See if the lower and upper teeth line up at the midline or if there is a deviation.

- *Deviation from the midline:* Ask the patient to place the teeth "face to face." Again note any deviation from the midline at the roots of the teeth.

- *Deviation in motion 1:* Ask the patient to protrude the mandible forward as you watch the midline of the teeth. Note any deviation from the previous position during this movement.

- *Deviation in motion 2:* Ask the patient to slowly open the mouth wide. Notice how the jaw moves. Is there any deviation from a straight route? Does the jaw take a circuitous route? Is there a jumping motion in the movement? As the patient opens the mouth, are there audible clicks? Is there a jumping motion as the mouth opens?

- *Space expressed when mouth is open:* Ask the patient to open her mouth wide and see how many of her own knuckles can be fit in with the hand in a fist. A width of three to four knuckles is a normal range. If there is difficulty getting three knuckles into the mouth, there is a definite mobility restriction.

- *Posterior protrusion of condyles:* With the patient in a sitting position, place your little fingers into the ear canals (external auditory meatus). Draw your fingers anteriorly in the canals. Ask the patient to open and close the jaw. You can feel the condyles of the mandible in this position. As the patient opens and closes the mouth, note synchrony of motion side-to-side. As the mouth is closed, do the condyles protrude posteriorly and press on your fingers? This indicates a compressive pattern in the joint capsule.

- *Hypertonicity in muscles:* Check for tension/ hypertonicity in the lateral and medial pterygoid muscles by feeling around and under the mandible, from its angle to as far superior as you can feel. Feel for hypertonicity in the temporalis muscle above the joint and around the ears.

This procedure will give you a general clinical baseline and sense of the biomechanics of the TMJs. Remember that this picture may be arising due to intrinsic forces within the joint, or due to extrinsic influences from other parts of the cranium and body.

RELATIONSHIPS INFERIOR TO THE MANDIBLE

Structures immediately below the mandible can affect TMJ function, especially the relationships of the hyoid bone and related connective tissue tracts. It is also useful to explore the relationships of the occiput, atlas, and axis, and the cervical area in general. Inertial forces and related tissue conditions, such as compression and adhesions, may generate connective tissue tensions that can affect cranial base, hyoid bone, and mandibular function.

HYOID BONE RELATIONSHIPS

The hyoid bone is a floating bone that acts as a compression strut between the muscles and connective tissues of the anterior cervical area. There are important relationships above and below the hyoid that can directly affect the temporal bone, the mandible, and the TMJs. The hyoid is connected via muscles and connective tissues to the mandible, the temporal bone, the sternum, and the scapula. It is also directly connected to the cartilage of the thyroid gland and to the styloid process of the temporal bones via ligaments.

Superiorly, the hyoid is connected to the mandible via the geniohyoid and mylohyoid muscles. It is connected to the temporal bones via the stylohyoid muscle and the stylohyoid ligament. The digastric muscles and their fascia connect the mandible to the temporal bones via a ligamentous loop at the hyoid bone.

Inferiorly, the hyoid bone is connected to the cartilage of the thyroid gland via a membranous sheet of connective tissue and via the thyrohyoid muscle. It is connected to the sternum via the sternohyoid muscle and via the sternothyroid muscle, whose connective tissues are continuous with the thyrohyoid muscle mentioned above. Finally, the hyoid is connected to the scapula via the omohyoid muscle (Fig. 12.8).

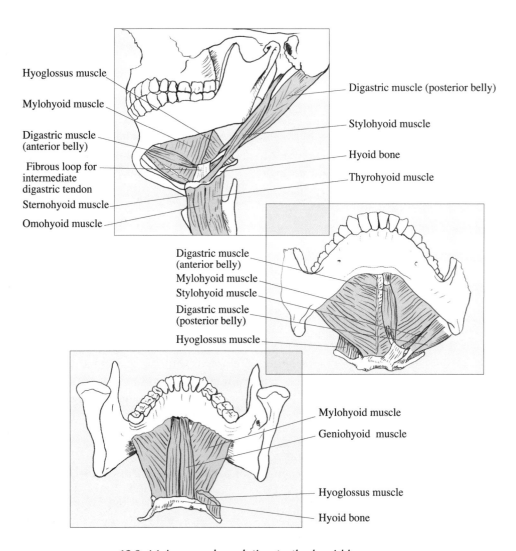

12.8 Major muscles relating to the hyoid bone

Tension and contraction within any of these structures will affect the position, motion, and motility of the hyoid bone, the mandible and TMJ above. See Fig. 12.9 for a diagram of some of the possible patterns of tension affecting the hyoid bone and its relationships. These tension patterns may include the hyoid bone's relationship to the mandible, the temporal bones, the sternum, and the scapula. All of these relationships are continuous with the inferior aspect of the cranial base; the deeper vertical fascial tracts of the body literally hang from the cranial base (Fig. 12.9).

Clinical Applications

The following clinical applications explore the dynamics around the hyoid bone. First you will use a particular hold to generally follow the dynamics between the temporal bones, the TMJs and the hyoid below. We will then approach the whole of the dynamic between the hyoid bone and its superior and inferior relationships. In the second application, you will learn how to approach the specific tension dynamics between the hyoid bone and the structures that directly connect to it.

Clinical Application: Temporal Bone and Hyoid Hold

1. Place your hands in relationship to the temporal bones and the hyoid bone by putting your palms over the temporal bones, your fingers over the mandible, and your fingertips on either side

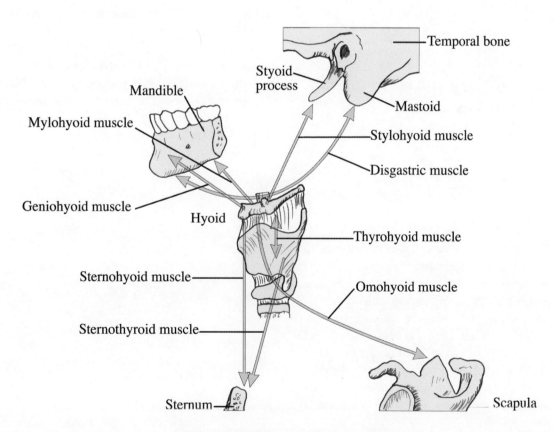

12.9 Tension patterns in hyoid dynamics

of the hyoid bone (Fig. 12.10). Orient to the mid-tide level of action. Let the motion dynamics of these tissue relationships enter your field of awareness. As an inertial pattern clarifies, help access the state of balance via Becker's three-phase healing awareness. Listen for expressions of Health, manifestations of potency, and for reorganization of potencies, fluids, and tissues to the midline.

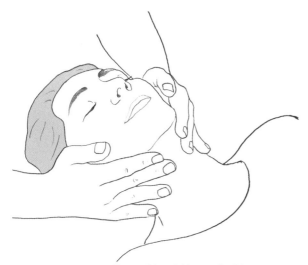

12.10 Bilateral hyoid bone hold

2. If tension patterns are still present, bring the conversation of traction and disengagement to the relationships. Still within the mid-tide, suggest/intend the hyoid bone inferiorly (caudad) while subtly stabilizing the temporal bones and mandible. When space is accessed, listen for the action of potency and help access the state of balance when appropriate. Again listen for expressions of Health, manifestations of potency, and for reorganization of potencies, fluids, and tissues to the midline.

Clinical Application: Specific Relationships

You may have perceived particular tension patterns between the hyoid bone and one of the structures with which it is connected. The hyoid bone sits under the mandible like a strut in a suspension bridge. It helps to balance all of the various tension patterns and pushes and pulls of the muscles and connective tissues in the anterior cervical area. The major relationships to think about include those of the hyoid bone to the mandible and temporal bone above (especially via the styloid processes) and to the sternum and scapula below. It might also be necessary to work with the cervical area and C2 and C1 more directly.

1. If you become aware of any specific connective tissue tensions or pulls around the hyoid bone, you might want to make a specific relationship to them. Place the index and middle fingers and the thumb of one hand over the lateral aspects of the hyoid bone (Fig. 12.11). Place the other hand over any of the structures that you are drawn to. These may include the mandible, the temporal bones, the sternum, the scapula, or the cervical area.

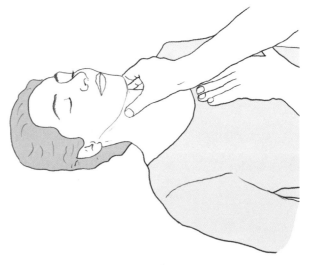

12.11 Hyoid bone
connective tissue hold

2. For instance, if you sense a tension pattern that relates to the mandible, you might hold the hyoid bone as described above and place your other hand cupped over the mandible. If a tension pattern relates to a temporal bone, then the other hand can be placed over the temporal bone on that side. If it is the sternum or scapula, place the other hand there. Finally, if it is the cervical area that you are drawn to, cup the area posterior to the hyoid bone in a general sense, or place the index finger and thumb of the other hand around a particular vertebra.

3. In any of the relationships above, the process is similar to what you have already learned. Wait for a tissue pattern to clarify and help access the state of balance. Listen for expressions of Health and for the processing of any biokinetic forces present. Wait for the reorganization of the tissue relationships and a reorientation to the midline. Do this via your contact with the two poles of the pattern. For instance, if you are holding the hyoid and the sternum, follow the motion between them and help access the state of balance.

4. Alternatively, you can bring an intention of traction and disengagement to the relationship. You can encourage space within the tension pattern by subtly tractioning the hyoid bone away from the other structure. For instance, with the hyoid and sternum, subtly stabilize the sternum with one hand and very gently traction the hyoid away from it until space is accessed. This is offered as a conversation about space and not as a technique to release anything. Again, when space is accessed, listen for potency and help access the state of balance if appropriate.

Specific Approaches to TMJ Dynamics

In this section we will begin to focus our attention more specifically on local dynamics within the temporomandibular joint. Please review the TMJ anatomy and motion dynamics sections above. First we will review the clinical applications outlined in the hard palate chapter because these are good general approaches to TMJ issues.

Clinical Application: Bilateral Contact, the State of Balance and the TMJs

In this application, make a bilateral contact with the mandible and the TMJs. In the first process, simply listen to the movements as they unfold within your contact, working to access a state of balance. In the second process, explore the space within the joint via a conversation about disengagement. This is for your learning process; it is not meant to be a treatment protocol.

The State of Balance

1. Place your hands in a *bilateral mandible hold* (see Fig. 11.13a). Place the fingers of both hands just above the angle of the mandible. Negotiate your contact and orient to the mid-tide. Let the palm of your hand rest over the temporal bones and TMJs. In this position, let the motility and motion of the mandible come into your awareness.

2. Beyond their normal motions, the TMJs and mandible may express almost any possible pattern. This may include compressive issues, circular motions, shearing motions, or pulls in different directions. Help access the state of balance within whatever pattern begins to clarify. Be patient. Don't rush this. Let the tissues communicate the experience they are holding. Let the pattern clarify from within. Listen for Becker's three-phase healing awareness. Wait for a sense of softening of tissue elements and a realignment to the midline.

Disengagement and Space

3. Maintaining the same hold, once you sense a softening and reorganization, very gently suggest the tissues of the mandible via traction in

an inferior direction. This encourages a conversation about disengagement and space within the TMJ joint relationships and the potencies and forces present.

4. As space is accessed, the tissues may naturally seek a neutral. This will feel different from an inertial pattern. It may seem as if the tissue and fluid elements are rocking and fluctuating like a teeter-totter around an organizing fulcrum. Maintain a wide perceptual field and subtly slow these motions down. Listen for the settling into the state of balance. Listen for expressions of Health and a change in the potency within the stillness.

5. Alternatively, as space is accessed, you may sense some kind of action of potency building within the area. Sometimes, like a groundswell, a welling up of potency and fluid within the area can be experienced. Sometimes there is a sense of a drive of potency into the space accessed. As inertial forces are processed, the natural disengagement of the joint in inhalation is re-established. This may occur without a sense of a state of balance needing to be attained. When space is accessed, there is a natural tendency for potency to express itself.

6. Listen for a processing of compressive forces and for a softening of the joint relationship. As the biokinetic forces within the joint are processed, the tissues may expand. You may sense that the mandible floats inferiorly. Notice the new orientation to the midline and automatically shifting fulcrums.

DIRECTION OF FLUIDS

The major ligaments around the joint respond to compressive forces by contracting. In this next section, we will direct the potency within the fluids to the ligamentous relationships around the joint and to the head of the sternocleidomastoid muscle. This is a traditional starting point for the specific TMJ work outlined below. A chronically contracted sternocleidomastoid muscle can lock the temporal bone in internal rotation and affect TMJ function. The intention of fluid direction work is to bring the potency within the fluids to an area that may have become very inertial and to tissue relationships that may have become contracted in response to the forces present.

1. Start from the vault hold and see if you can sense the most compressed and inertial TMJ. You may have already determined this via the analysis of the TMJs as described earlier, or via the process above. Alternatively, see if you can sense the more contracted joint from a vault hold. You may sense a pattern of tissue organization around it, a tissue pull towards one TMJ, or fluid fluctuation that leads you to it. Start this process with the most dense and inertial joint.

2. Place your index and middle finger in a V-spread. One finger is on the ramus of the mandible just anterior to the TMJ and the other finger is in the hollow just posterior to the mastoid process of the temporal bone. The V should be placed at a right angle to the cranium and neck (i.e., the fingers are at right angles to the head and neck, and the fingertips are touching the tissues as described above) (Fig. 12.12).

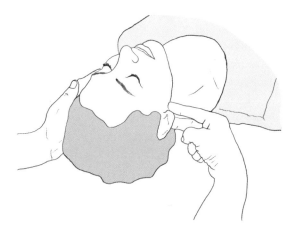

12.12 V-Spread of TMJ ligaments

3. Place the palm of your other hand on the opposite parietal bone. From this position direct fluids toward the V-spread. The potency within the fluids is being directed toward the ligaments of the TMJs and the superior aspect of the sternocleidomastoid muscle. Wait for a pulsation of potency within the area and for a sense of softening and expansion of connective tissues. Wait for reorganization and a return to a clear sense of motility. From here, we will start an exploration of the specific ligaments and the joint capsule of the TMJ. We are now at the heart of the dynamics of the TMJ.

Clinical Applications: Specific Ligamentous Work

In the following section we will directly relate to the major ligaments of the joint and to the joint capsule itself. We will work unilaterally, that is, with one joint at a time. We will explore the sphenomandibular, stylomandibular, and temporomandibular ligaments and joint capsule, relating to each joint and each ligament separately. You will be using the conversations of traction and disengagement to directly relate to the tensions and forces within each ligamentous dynamic. Before and after this specific work use the bilateral hold because it gives an overall sense of the joint dynamics and can help to balance TMJ function after specific unilateral work.

The Sphenomandibular Ligament

The sphenomandibular ligament attaches to the spine of the sphenoid bone superiorly and to the medial (inner) aspect of the ramus of the mandible (see Fig. 12.7). Its fibers have a roughly vertical (superior-inferior) orientation. Contraction within sphenomandibular fibers can also generate a dragging force on that side of the sphenoid via its pterygoid processes. This can, in turn, generate a torsion pattern within the cranial base. The fulcrum for this pattern will be found within the dynamics of the TMJ.

1. Sitting to one side of the patient's head opposite to the TMJ being treated, place your gloved or cotted thumb on the surface of the last molar tooth of the mandible. Place the fingertips of that same hand outside the mouth over the inferior aspect of the mandible. Rest your elbow on the table or on a cushion on the table so that the hand can float lightly on the tissues. Place the thumb or the index and middle fingers of your other hand over the greater wing of the sphenoid bone on the same side. Your arm goes around the superior aspect of the patient's head, and your fingers rest on the greater wing at the temple.

2. Settle into the mid-tide and hold a wide perceptual field. Try to get a sense of the motion and motility within the structures being palpated. Do not narrow your perceptual field as you do this. Try to let the tissue and fluid come to you. Do not look for anything. You may simply work with the state of balance here, or add the skill of traction and disengagement as described below.

3. The skill of traction may be useful to engage in a direct conversation with the tissues. When you intend traction into a tensile field, that field responds to your presence and communicates its history to you. The intention is to start a conversation with these tissues about their history and Health. To do this here, place a very subtle inferior traction on the sphenomandibular ligament by gently introducing a caudad pressure on the last molar. You are subtly intending the mandible inferiorly. Be sure that you have a clear knowledge of the anatomy and can sense the specific engagement of the sphenomandibular ligament. If the sphenomandibular ligament is holding inertial forces and is contracted, you may sense that the greater wing of the sphenoid bone moves superiorly as you intend traction. With normal tissue resilience you would not feel this. Note how inertial forces and contraction within this ligament can lock the sphenoid on that side

225

into a superior position. It may be perceived to be like a torsion pattern if it is unilateral, and like an extension pattern if bilaterally equal.

4. If tension is present, use the following process to encourage a resolution of the forces. This time, very subtly stabilize the greater wing of the sphenoid with your fingers, encouraging a stillness within the sphenoid rather than exerting a physical pressure. With the greater wing stabilized, again apply a subtle traction to the mandible with your thumb, until space is accessed. This is a conversation about space and the disengagement of the potencies and forces present. Help access the state of balance and listen for expressions of potency and for the resolution of the inertial forces involved. Wait for expansion and softening and for reorganization and realignment to midline phenomena (Fig. 12.13).

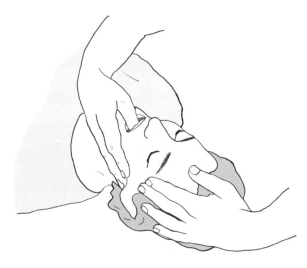

12.13 Sphenomandibular hold

The Stylomandibular Ligament

The stylomandibular ligament attaches to the styloid process of the temporal bone superiorly and to the posterior aspect of the mandibular angle (see Fig. 12.7).

1. Maintain the same contact as above on the mandible via the last molar tooth. Cradle the patient's head with your other arm and place your other hand at the temporal bone in the temporal ear canal hold (i.e. index finger over the zygomatic arch, middle finger in the ear canal and ring finger over the mastoid area). You are now in relationship to the two poles of the stylomandibular ligament. You may simply listen to the dynamics that evolve and help access the state of balance. Alternatively, you may want to engage the tissues in a more direct conversation with an intention of traction (Fig. 12.14).

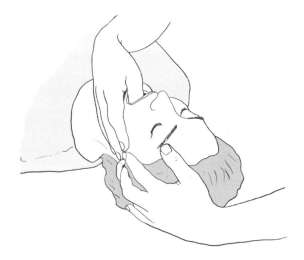

12.14 Stylomandibular and temporomandibular hold

2. As above, subtly suggest an inferior/anterior pressure on the mandible via your thumb at the last molar. This will be at an angle of approximately thirty degrees from horizontal. This follows the angle of the stylomandibular ligament and places a gentle traction on the ligament. Know your anatomy and be sure that you are engaging the ligament. Again the intention here is to begin a conversation with the tissues involved. This conversation will hopefully bring you into relationship with the forces maintaining the contraction

in the tissues. If the ligament is contracted, you will sense traction or pulling on the temporal bone. It will follow the mandible inferiorly. Under normal conditions the tissue of the ligament is resilient and will not influence the temporal bone in this way.

3. If tension is present, use the following process to encourage a resolution of the forces. As above, first stabilize the temporal bone. Again, this is an intention of local stillness more than it is a physical force. Then subtly suggest an inferior/anterior traction on the stylomandibular ligament via your thumb on the last molar. Intend this in an approximately thirty-degree angle to match the angle of the ligament as it meets the mandible. You are subtly intending the mandible inferiorly at this angle. Traction until space is accessed. Help access the state of balance and listen for expressions of potency and for the resolution of the inertial forces involved. Wait for expansion and softening and for reorganization and realignment to midline phenomena.

Temporomandibular and Capsular Ligaments

The temporomandibular ligament attaches to the lateral surface and inferior border of the zygomatic arch superiorly and then divides into two portions inferiorly. One attaches to the lateral surface of the condyle of the mandible and the other connects to the upper aspect of the ramus of the mandible (see Fig. 12.8). The joint capsule is continuous with the temporomandibular ligament and forms two compartments above and below the disc.

1. Maintain the same hand positions as with the stylomandibular ligament work. One hand is holding the mandible and the other the temporal bone as you listen to the local dynamics of the temporomandibular ligament and the joint. Here you are in direct relationship with the inner anatomy of the TMJ itself. Review the TMJ anatomy as needed. Simply listening to the dynamics that unfold and helping access the state of balance may be sufficient (see Fig. 12.14).

2. It also may be appropriate to engage in a conversation with the temporomandibular ligament and joint capsule via traction. To do this, subtly suggest traction directly inferior via a thumb contact on the first molar tooth. Do not restrict the motion of the temporal bone. If there are inertial issues, compressive forces, and compressed tissues present, the condyle of the mandible may seem compressed within the TMJ. If this is the case, the temporal bone may appear to be pulled inferiorly with your traction intention. This will also indicate the presence of compressive forces and tissues within the joint itself.

3. If inertial forces and tensions are present, encourage resolution of the forces involved with the following process. Maintaining the same position, stabilize the temporal bone. Again, the contact is more like a local stillness than a physical force. Then very gently traction the mandible directly inferior via the last molar and use your other fingers cradling the mandible to help maintain the inferior direction of the traction. Again, intend this until space is accessed and help facilitate a state of balance. Listen for expressions of potency and for the resolution of the inertial forces involved. Wait for expansion and softening of the tissues, and for reorganization and realignment to the midline.

4. After the above processes it is useful to again make a bilateral contact to both TMJs via the temporal bone-mandible hold as in the bilateral contact section above. This can help you gain an overall sense of the joint dynamics and sense any changes resulting from the session work.

Clinical Application: C2 and the TMJs

If there were not any inertial forces affecting TMJ motion and function, the mandible would naturally float within the synovial fluid of the TMJ joint capsules. Furthermore, the motility and motion of the mandible would naturally be expressed as though it was floating within the TMJs around a fulcrum of motion located at the second cervical vertebra (see Fig. 12.3). The upper cervical area and the mandible are in close proximity and intimately related. Remember that the stylomandibular ligament is a specialized band of cervical fascia and its relationships can be traced to the upper cervical vertebrae. C2 can be considered to be the location for a suspended automatically shifting fulcrum that orients the mandible and the TMJs to the midline. This is a concentration of potency, not just an anatomical location.

Here we will explore the relationship of the second cervical vertebra to the TMJs and mandible. This process can help the TMJs orient to the primal midline and also help resolve forces affecting their motion dynamic.

1. With the patient in the supine position, place your hands in a modified occipital cradle. Place your ring fingers over the transverse processes and articular masses of C2, your little fingers at the base of the occiput, and your thumbs over the mandible (Fig. 12.15). Orient to the biosphere and mid-tide. Hold a wide perceptual field.

2. In this position, follow the motion dynamics of the mandible in its relationship to the upper cervical vertebrae. Hold the whole of the tissue field, the occiput, the cervical vertebrae, and the mandible/TMJs within your awareness. Do not narrow your perceptual field as you do this. Be aware of Becker's three-phase healing awareness. Listen for a settling into stillness, the expression of potency, and the processing of inertial forces. Sense for a reorganization of the tissues and for a new relationship of the mandible to C2, the midline, and to Sutherland's fulcrum.

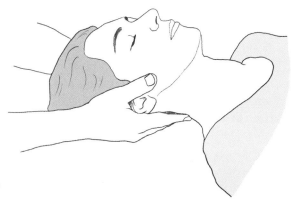

12.15 Modified occipital cradle hold (for orientation of mandible to C2)

1. Randolph Stone, *Polarity Therapy, Volume One, Books I, II, III; Volume Two, Book IV.*
2. See Hugh Milne, *The Heart of Listening* (North Atlantic Books, 1995).
3. Illustration based on Milne.

13

Connective Tissues and Joints

Bone, membranes, fascia, and all other connective tissues are a functioning whole. They are totally interconnected and express motility and motion as a unified tensile field. As we hold the body and maintain a wide perceptual field, we may sense organization arising around a particular issue. For instance, you may be holding the head or the feet as you listen within the mid-tide. As you patiently listen, something may engage from within and the whole unified field may begin to distort around a particular fulcrum. You may sense a tissue strain right through the field toward that fulcrum. You may sense a drive of potency towards a fulcrum, a shift within the fluctuation of fluids, and a distortion of the tissue field around this fulcrum. This is the treatment plan beginning to manifest at this level of action. We can sense this because the body is whole. The connective tissues within the body are a true unified field, and information will be holistically communicated to the sensitive listener.

In this chapter we will:

- *Discuss the nature of connective tissues.*
- *Explore the transverse relationships of the body.*
- *Explore the vertical connective tissue tracts.*
- *Learn therapeutic approaches for the connective tissue and fascial field.*
- *Introduce approaches to joints and their dynamics.*

CONNECTIVE TISSUES AND LIQUID LIGHT

Connective tissue structures include fascia, ligaments, tendons, membranes, and bones. There are even connective tissue components within each cell, called microtubules. Connective tissue is composed of hollow collagen tubes and other fibers intermeshed in matrices and sheets. These are held within a fluidic ground substance that has varying qualities dependent on the nature of the particular connective tissue. The ground substance is a viscous fluid that also surrounds all of the tissues and cells of the body. Thus, we are basically fluidic beings. Ground substance can vary greatly in quality and density, from a watery state to a more gel-like state, to a solid hardness. A wide variety of tissue types can manifest, depending on the fluidic nature of the ground substance, and on the quantity and arrangement of the collagen fibers (Fig. 13.1). Fluid is also found within the hollow collagen fibers themselves, so connective tissues are essentially fluid passageways. The composition of the fluid in collagen tubes is essentially the same as cerebrospinal fluid. Fluid is also found between fascial sheets. Sheets of fascia are lubricated by serous fluid and can glide in relationship to the surrounding tissues.

The organization of connective tissue is basically energetic in nature. Recent research shows that the fluids within collagen fibers are connected by hydrogen bonds that create a unified and cohesive fluid field. Collagen fiber itself is made up of triple helix tripeptides. The peptides are wound around each other

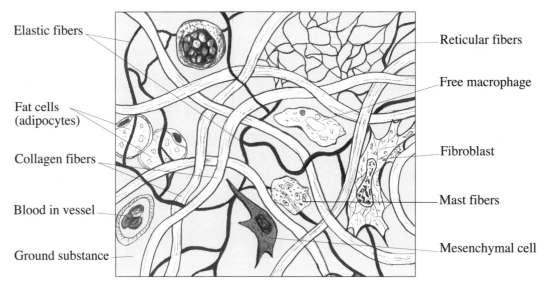

Elastic fibers

Fat cells
(adipocytes)

Collagen fibers

Blood in vessel

Ground substance

Reticular fibers

Free macrophage

Fibroblast

Mast fibers

Mesenchymal cell

13.1 Components of connective tissues

in a helical manner. There is clear evidence that the fluid within the collagen fibers forms coherent molecular bonds with these peptides. The fluid–cellular matrix that results forms a unified and ordered field throughout the body (Fig. 13.2). Collagen fiber and its ordered fluid field have been likened to liquid crystal.

The fibers assemble into coherent sheets that form an open, liquid crystalline fluid-tissue meshwork throughout the body. This meshwork has been found to be a unified whole. There is also evidence that this fluid-tissue matrix is a field of rapid communication, much faster than the nervous system, and that this

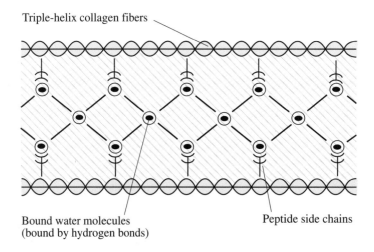

Triple-helix collagen fibers

Bound water molecules
(bound by hydrogen bonds)

Peptide side chains

13.2 The collagen fluid-tissue matrix

occurs within a coherent, quantum-level bioelectric field of action. Communication throughout this field is organized as a whole in coherent quantum waveforms, perhaps at near the speed of light![1]

There is also evidence that cerebrospinal fluid contains a high charge of light photons. Russian scientists discovered that light photons are concentrated within the cerebrospinal fluid and move in coherent waveforms throughout the fluid system. This includes the fluid-collagen matrix. An extremely rapid communication occurs throughout the body via coherent waveforms of liquid light within its cerebrospinal fluid and the fluid-collagen matrix! Sutherland's perceptual insight is being borne out by scientific inquiry.

There is thus a unified liquid crystal matrix expressed as a whole throughout the body. This matrix is a unified field of communication. It has been postulated that states of consciousness are quickly communicated throughout the body as coherent waveforms that mobilize the cells for various kinds of activity. In essence, there is a quantum level unified field of action that organizes form and allows for rapid communication throughout the body. There is a unified and coherent bioelectric, fluid, and tissue field, a true unit of function. We have the three fields of potency, fluids, and tissues, so central to the practice of craniosacral biodynamics, being discussed in scientific circles as a unified field of action!

The three unified fields are:

- Potency: the potency of the Breath of Life, expressed as a subtle ordering field around and within the body, and as an embodied force within the fluids.

- Fluids: the unified fluid matrix.

- Tissues: the unified tensile tissue field.

All of this has huge implications for the healing arts, no matter what framework or modality. In craniosacral biodynamics we consciously work with this unified bioelectric, fluid, and cellular matrix. This is one of the strengths of our work.

CONNECTIVE TISSUES AND STRESS

Connective tissues all have tensile capacity, reflecting reciprocal tension in response to pressure or load from any layer. Even relatively inelastic bone and membrane have this ability. The whole potency-fluid-tissue matrix has tensile qualities within the cycles of primary respiration. Each inhalation and exhalation cycle is registered and reflected in all three layers as reciprocal, interactive and palpable movement, so when we sense the tidal movement in any layer we are experiencing direct access to the original Health of the system in that layer as part of an interdependent whole.

This unified field responds to any stressor that impinges on its action. One way to imagine this is to visualize two sheets of transparent plastic film or wrap. Between these sheets, imagine water with colored oil mixed in it. Imagine that these sheets are taut or tense, and that the oil and water mixture is in some way bound to the sheets, like the peptide-hydrogen bonds mentioned above. As you press on the sheets, they distort and the colored water-oil shifts and responds to your touch. As you remove your touch, the sheets return to their original position, as does the water-oil field between. As long as your touch continues, the transparent sheets with their water and oil will respond to your force in some way.

As a force impinges on the potency-fluid-tissue matrix, that matrix responds. The fluid-tissue matrix is organized by quantum-level fields and the whole of that matrix responds to stressors. This information is held not just locally, but within the field as a whole, and therefore within the body as a whole. Within a craniosacral biodynamic framework, this process is seen to be a function of the potency of the Breath of Life. As biokinetic forces impinge on the system, potency responds by condensing and becoming inertial to contain and compensate for the forces. The potency of the Breath of Life condenses or coalesces to protect the organism. This can be likened to a quantum-level bioelectric field of action in which the ordering matrix acts as a whole to meet forces that enter its domain. As the unified field of potency responds to the added force, so does the whole tensile fluid-tissue matrix. The fluid-tissue field responds to stressors via densification and contraction. When potency becomes inertial, there is a coiling effect within the field of potency. A vortex of potency literally forms within the matrix as a whole, and the affected tissues contract. This occurs both locally and throughout the field as a whole. Tension or strain patterns within the connective tissue field are generated. As potency becomes inertial in order to contain a stressor, membranes, fascia, ligaments, and tendons all contract in response.

TISSUE MEMORY

If inertial forces cannot be processed at the time of the event, the tissues maintain their contraction. This has been called *tissue memory*. Ho and Knight extend this idea of tissue memory and describe what they call *crystal memory*. Crystal memory is based upon the continuity of the bioelectric field with the fluid-tissue matrix. This is the root of tissue memory. Memory is not just a function of the tissues; it is expressed within the bioelectric-fluid-tissue matrix as a whole. Tissue memory is thus seen to be basically energetic in nature. It is a function of the unified field, not just of the tissues per se.[2]

In craniosacral biodynamic terms, tissue memory is a function of the bioelectric potency of the Breath of Life. The potency maintains the organization of the unified fluid-tissue field. The very nature of the field is to be responsive. As inertial forces enter the field, the potencies naturally track the motion and force of the traumatic impact. Potencies coalesce in a vortex-like manner to contain the biokinetic forces. Fluids and tissues follow this imperative. Fluids become denser under stress, and tissues contract and compress. If these inertial forces are not processed immediately at the time of the experience, then tissue contraction may be retained by the system. Inertial fulcrums are created, and the tissues will continue to organize around them.

Tissue memory is not about the past. It is about unresolved forces that are currently maintaining the disturbance in the present. Patterns of tensile and compressive distress will be retained by the system as a whole and will not resolve until the inertial forces that originate and organize them are processed in present time.

Connective tissue structures are formed within a fluidic ground substance. If inertial potencies are present within the collagen-fluid matrix, the ground substance will be affected by the forming of crystallizations and adhesions and a subsequent reduction in the ability to move and glide freely.

Gel-like substances tend to become denser in the presence of stasis in a process called *thixotrophia*. The gel-like state of the ground substance of connective tissue is maintained its general nature and by the thermodynamics of its immediate area. If inertia and stasis are present, the gel-like ground substance tends to become more solid and sluggish, and less resilient, fluidic, and elastic.

Densification and rigidity can also occur between sheets of connective tissue. The ability of fascial sheets to glide freely is called *fascial glide*. Inertial forces affecting serous fluid can cause the fluid to become denser and even dry up, leading to adhesions between connective tissue sheets. The fascial sheets resist movement instead of gliding easily. Connective tissue adhesions can generate inertial issues throughout the tissue field. Loss of mobility and strain patterns result. The motility and motion of the tissues becomes organized around these fulcrums.

INTRODUCTION TO TRANSVERSE STRUCTURES

In this section we will explore the relationship between the dural membrane system and the connective tissues of the body. Fascia compartmentalizes the body, integrates the motions of various structures, connects structures, and allows structures to express independent motion. Most fascial tissue exists in vertical sheets in the body. These vertically oriented connective tissues meet transverse divisions in the body such as the pelvis, respiratory diaphragm, and thoracic inlet. At these significant horizontal divisions, connective tissues form transverse bands (such as the pelvic floor and respiratory diaphragm) or they attach to transverse structures (such as the clavicles, sternum, and scapulae) (Fig. 13.3). These transverse structures all attach to the pelvis and spine. Inertial issues in their fluid-tissue matrix can therefore be directly fed into vertebral and dural dynamics and generate fixations or adhesions within the vertebral column and dural tube.

We have already encountered the effects of transverse connective tissue relationships. For example, in working with the dural tube we discussed the effects of tension arising from the respiratory diaphragm. Similarly, a transverse diaphragm may have been the location of an inertial fulcrum affecting the vertebrae. Palpation from any vantage point can reveal a fulcrum at a transverse structure, sensed as a connective tissue pull or a distortion through the unified fluid-tissue matrix.

In the approaches described below, we will place our hands in an anterior-posterior relationship to the transverse structure and follow its motility and motion. If the inertial forces are very dense and the related fascial or structural relationship cannot express its motion, you can deepen your contact with the tissues, or work with fluid fluctuation, in order to engage them in a conversation about history, shape, and motion tendencies (Fig. 13.4).

Transverse
structures

Vertically
oriented
fascial planes

13.3 Longitudinal fascia
and transverse structures

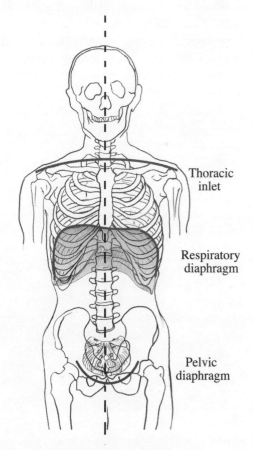

Thoracic
inlet

Respiratory
diaphragm

Pelvic
diaphragm

13.4 The transverse structures
and the vertebral axis

Clinical Application:
The Pelvic Diaphragm

Let's start with the pelvic diaphragm. We are arbitrarily beginning with the pelvis as the inferior pole of the system, but in practice we allow the treatment plan to unfold and work appropriately. The fascial and muscular relationships of the perineal floor are sometimes called the pelvic diaphragm in recognition of their transverse orientation. The pelvic diaphragm is composed of the levator ani (including the pubococcygeus and iliococcygeus muscles), coccygeus muscles, and the fascia covering their internal and external surfaces (Fig. 13.5). The pelvic diaphragm is directly continuous with the other fascial relationships of the pelvis. Familiarity with the anatomy of the pelvis, both male and female, is essential for effective treatment.

Hold the whole of the person in your consciousness. We are a unity of mind, body, and spirit. When you hold the body, you are holding the whole of a person and the whole of their experience. As discussed in Chapter 6, the pelvis can hold very charged personal issues. Issues relating to sexuality, self-worth, value, and abuse may be held in its tissue patterns. As usual, negotiate your contact with the pelvis with respect and clarity. Let the patient know your intentions and why you are making contact there. Give clients the power to say "no" when it is necessary for them to do so.

1. With the patient supine, sit at the side of the table. First place one hand under the sacrum in a transverse position across the patient's sacroiliac joints. Use the hand in the cephalad relationship to the patient's body to do this. When you have established a relationship at the sacrum, place your other hand over the lower abdomen with the edge of your hand just over the pubic symphysis. To find the pubic symphysis in the least invasive way, place your hand on the patient's abdomen and move inferiorly by firmly

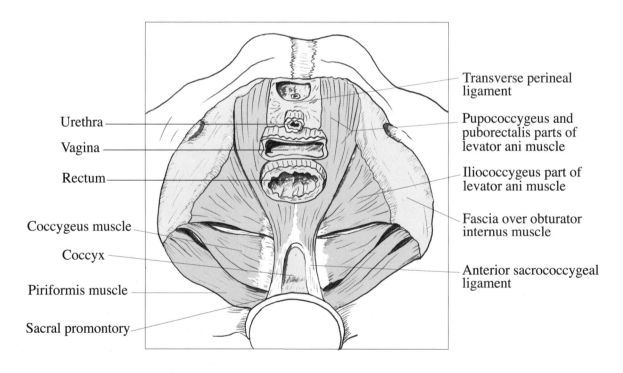

Urethra

Vagina

Rectum

Coccygeus muscle

Coccyx

Piriformis muscle

Sacral promontory

Transverse perineal ligament

Pupococcygeus and puborectalis parts of levator ani muscle

Iliococcygeus part of levator ani muscle

Fascia over obturator internus muscle

Anterior sacrococcygeal ligament

13.5 The pelvic diaphragm

pressing down on the abdominal tissues, finger-width by finger-width, until you are finally just over the pubic symphysis. Let the patient know your intentions before you do this. The pubic symphysis should lie under your hand at the level between your little and ring fingers (Fig. 13.6).

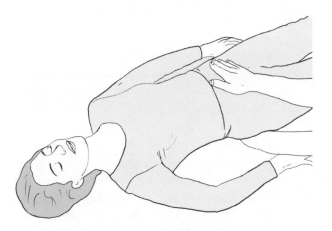

13.6   The pelvic diaphragm hold

2. The hand over the abdomen should be very gently floating on the pubic symphysis and lower abdomen in a firm yet gentle touch. Do not apply any pressure at all; just float on the tissues. The hand under the sacrum should not be grasping it or holding it up in any way. Give the sacrum a lot of space and sense that you are floating on the tissues. Orient to the mid-tide level of action. Remember that the tissues you are holding are part of the fluid-tissue matrix and that you are in relationship to the three fields of potency, fluids, and tissues.

3. In this position, listen to the motility and motion of the tissues that you are palpating. Allow things to clarify. See if you can sense the subtle motions of the pelvic diaphragm. Allow the upper hand to float and follow the movements under it. Include the lower hand and follow sacral and spinal motion also. The fluid-tissue field will express its motion as a whole. Simply listen to

the unfolding story. Follow the patterns that arise using Becker's three-phase healing awareness. Assist a settling into a state of balance, a dynamic equilibrium within all of the tension and force factors present.

4. You may sense a number of phenomena here. Fascia is more elastic than membrane. As the tissues attempt to access a state of balance, there may be a *recoil* effect away from equilibrium. If you sense this, slow down the motion of the fluid-tissue field with a deepening touch. You may find that this requires a deeper engagement of the tissues than we use for the primary respiratory core. Let your physical contact slowly deepen, matching the tension sensed in the tissue field. Try to match the quality of the density or tension you perceive. Your contact becomes a fulcrum for the fluid-tissue matrix and the potency that organizes that field. Do not be heavy-handed here, but bring a quality of a deepening relationship to the tissue field as you clearly meet the densities and tensions.

5. The pelvic diaphragm, as a fluid-tissue field, may not be able to express any motion at all due to the density of the inertial forces. The collagen-fluid matrix that makes up the pelvic diaphragm may be very dense, a qualitative change leading to thickening and crystallization of the ground substance and adhesions within fascial relationships. Density and inertia result. This density is basically energetic in nature. Deepening the contact may create a better relationship with immobilized tissue.

6. Another way to relate to densification in the fluid-tissue field is the use of lateral fluctuation as presented in Volume One. Initiate a lateral fluctuation of potency and fluid between your hands. This may activate the inertial potencies within the fluid-tissue matrix and allow the tissue elements to begin to seek the state of balance. Simply push on the potencies and fluids alternately between your hands in a pendulum-like manner.

7. Listen for expressions of Health within the state of balance. You may sense a drive or permeation of potency into the area. You are waiting for a resolution of the inertial forces and for a soft-ening and expansion within the fluid-tissue field. The pelvic diaphragm may be sensed to soften, settle, and expand.

Clinical Highlight

A woman came to see me with menstrual prob-lems. She also was having difficulty in conceiv-ing a child. In one of her sessions I made contact with her pelvis using the methods described here. Her whole fluid-tissue matrix began to distort around the broad ligament. The fulcrum for the pattern of strain throughout the pelvis seemed to be located within the broad ligament, on the left side near the ovary. As her system settled into state of balance, a memory arose from her adolescence. She had been in a car accident and was not wearing a seat belt. Her pelvis twisted and was smashed against the door. As this mem-ory came up, the shock in her system also was expressed. Strong emotions arose, mainly fear. As I helped to slow the process down, there was a sympathetic discharge from the pelvis through her legs, and shock literally poured out of the fluids and tissues of the pelvis. There was then a resolution of a strong force vector. I experienced it as a welling up of potency and as streaming of energy out of the pelvis, back to the environ-ment. She experienced strong sensations of heat and pulsation. After this settled, the fluid tide strongly expressed itself, her pelvis and pelvic diaphragm expressed a clear motility again, and there was a comprehensive tissue reorganiza-tion and realignment to the midline. Her men-strual problems eased over the next few sessions. She contacted me a few months later to let me know that she had conceived.

Clinical Application: Respiratory Diaphragm

The respiratory diaphragm is a key transverse struc-tural relationship. It is a dome-shaped muscle with large sections of tendon. Its muscular parts can be separated into the sternal, costal, and lumbar parts. The sternal part arises from the dorsum of the xiphoid process, the costal part from the cartilage of the ribs, and the lumbar part from the lumbocostal arches and from the lumbar vertebrae via the crura. The central tendon of the diaphragm is a large and strong aponeu-rosis that is continuous with the pericardium of the heart. The diaphragm thus stretches right across the middle of the trunk of the body from the lower ribs to the lowest thoracic vertebrae (Fig. 13.7). Keep this continuity in mind when approaching the respiratory diaphragm and its patterns.

1. Sitting at the side of the table, place the caudad hand under the spine at the level of T10-L1. Place this hand so that the vertebrae are cupped in the heart of the palm. Your hand is perpen-dicular to the patient's body. After establishing your contact, place your other hand over the lower ribs, sternum, xiphoid process, and upper solar plexus area. You are now in relationship to the respiratory diaphragm and all its related structures (Fig. 13.8).

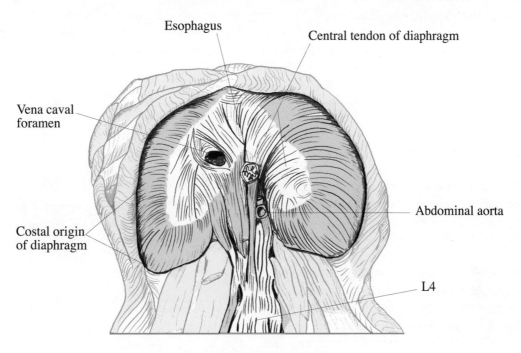

13.7 The respiratory diaphragm

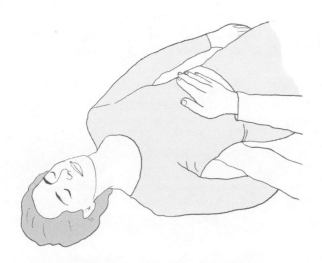

13.8 Respiratory diaphragm hold

2. Allow your hands to float on the tissues that you are palpating. Become aware of the motility and motion of this area within the phases of primary respiration. Be patient and follow the motion of the pattern that clarifies. Work as described above for the pelvic diaphragm, applying the same principles.

237

Clinical Highlight

Many important structures pass though openings in the respiratory diaphragm, including the digestive tract, the arterial and venous blood supply, and the vagus nerve. I once treated a newborn baby who was having severe bouts of colic. She had a seemingly gentle water birth. In listening to her system, I noticed that her cranial base and the osseous structures within the cranium were not holding compressive forces to any great extent. Her vagus nerve did not initially appear to be compromised in any way. As we settled into our relationship, I sensed that her system was organizing around her respiratory diaphragm. As I gently negotiated a contact there, her eyes met mine and she smiled at me. I had the sense that she was telling me, "Yes that's it!" In a short time she communicated some fear, and some tissue shock was processed. Her diaphragm softened and her fluid tide became apparent. Her parents later communicated to me that the colic attacks had ceased. It seems that even though it was a gentle birthing process, she got a little scared along the way, and was holding that fear in her diaphragm. This had compromised the vagus nerve supply as it passes through the diaphragm, leading to her colic symptoms.

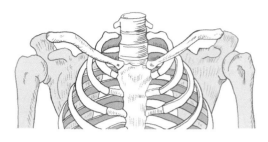

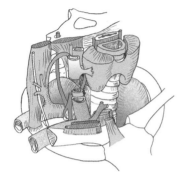

13.9 Thoracic inlet

1. We will use the same approach previously applied to the lower transverse structures. Sitting at the side of the table, place your caudad hand under C7-T3 perpendicular to the patient's body. Once you establish a relationship with the patient's system, place your other hand transversely over the patient's clavicles and upper sternum. Orient to the mid-tide and the motility and motion of the tissues that you are palpating (Fig. 13.10).

Clinical Application: Thoracic Inlet

The thoracic inlet is the opening into the thoracic area created by a continuity of structural relationships. These include the manubrium, clavicle and scapulae, and the inner circle created by the articulations of the first ribs with the manubrium and first thoracic vertebra. Many important structures pass through this area, including the jugular veins and arteries, and the vagus and phrenic nerves (Fig. 13.9).

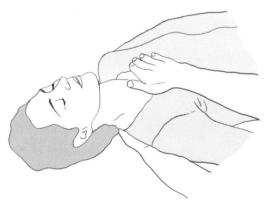

13.10 Thoracic inlet hold

2. Allow your hands to float on the tissues and follow the motion of the pattern that clarifies. Have patience and continue with the same approach described above.

Clinical Highlight

Tension held in the thoracic inlet can generate backpressure against fluid flow in and out of the cranium and can contribute to venous sinus congestion. This can lead to varied symptoms such as headaches, dizziness, and low vitality. Many years ago, I treated a construction worker. He had been off work for some time. His main symptom was dizziness. Neurological tests did not reveal anything to account for the symptoms. I was first interested in his temporal bones and listened for any intraosseous issues or cranial base issues, but compressive forces around the thoracic inlet proved to be the key factor. These manifested as a tense upper chest, compressed upper thoracic vertebrae, and much lateral fluctuation of fluid within the area. A clear backpressure within the fluid tide could be sensed as fluid echoing and lateral fluctuation within the vertebral and dural axis. The thoracic inlet was the first area to be highlighted as the Inherent Treatment Plan engaged. The potency began to drive towards these relationships as I listened to his system. As I supported the treatment plan, I attended to the thoracic inlet and related vertebral fulcrums. We later discovered that this was coupled with an occipito-mastoid issue and related venous sinus congestion. Over a three-month period, his dizziness cleared up and he was able to return to work. The key was the initial highlighting of inertial forces around and within the relationships of the thoracic inlet.

VERTICAL CONTINUITY OF MAJOR FASCIAL TRACTS

Next we turn our attention to the vertical arrangements of fascia. I will discuss the major connective tissue tracts from the top down, as all of these relationships should ideally function as though they are hanging from the cranial base. Incredible as it may sound, the major fascial relationships can be tracked superiorly to the cranial base and are literally hanging from it.

Let's first look at the cervical area. The connective tissue tracts that descend from the cranial base and mandible can be thought of as a series of tubes that are continuous with the connective tissues below. The anterior tract begins with the pretracheal and buccopharyngeal fascia. The pretracheal fascia descends from the mandible and hyoid areas to cover the anterior aspect of the trachea. The buccopharyngeal fascia descends from the cranial base and pterygoid processes of the sphenoid bone to enclose the trachea and esophagus and it is continuous with the pretracheal fascia anteriorly. This tube descends inferiorly to merge with the pericardium of the heart.

Posteriorly, the sheaths of fascia surrounding the internal carotid artery, internal jugular vein and vagus nerve are called the *carotid sheaths* and are connected medially by a sheet of fascia called the *alar fascia*. The alar fascia merges anteriorly and inferiorly with the buccopharyngeal fascia and the pericardium. The carotid sheaths are loosely continuous with the most posterior tube of fascia, the prevertebral fascia. The prevertebral fascia forms a tube around the cervical vertebrae and the deep cervical muscles. Inferiorly it is continuous with the longitudinal ligaments of the vertebral column (Fig. 13.11 a and b).[3]

These tubes of the cervical area are continuous with the fascial relationships below. This is extremely important. The anterior tube is continuous with the pericardium and diaphragm below. The carotid sheaths also merge with the pericardium and are also connected to the prevertebral fascia. The alar fascia merges with the buccopharyngeal fascia and pericardium. The

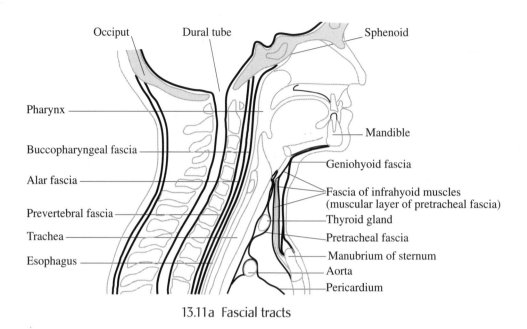

13.11a Fascial tracts

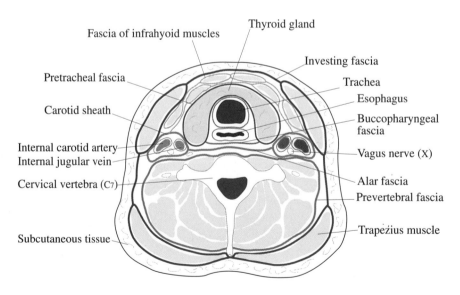

13.11b Fascial tubes

prevertebral fascia is continuous with the connective tissue of the vertebral column all the way inferior to the sacrum. There is an important space between the alar fascia and the prevertebral fascia called the retropharyngeal space. This space allows ease of glide between the cervical tubes. It is continuous all the way down to the thoracic area and, in some cases, all the way to the respiratory diaphragm.

All these sheets of fascia are an integral unit. The pretracheal, buccopharyngeal, and alar fascias and the carotid sheaths all merge with the pericardium and diaphragm below, and the carotid sheaths are continuous with the prevertebral fascia and therefore with the connective tissues of the vertebral column (Fig. 13.12).

Following the major tracts inferiorly, we find more continuity below the diaphragm. One important vertical tract to emphasize is the continuity from the diaphragm to the falciform ligament of the liver and then to the round ligament and the umbilical ligament, and on down to the pubic arch. Thus, we have a continuous connective tract from the cranial base anteriorly down to the pubic arch, and posteriorly down to the sacrum.

The connective tissues of the visceral and organ systems show a similar continuity. Fascia covering the organs and muscles of the body can also become inertial, with adhesions between facial layers and tracts. The viscera have double layers of fascia, lubricated in their gliding action by serous fluid, so all the principles described for fascial tracts also apply to viscera and muscular systems.

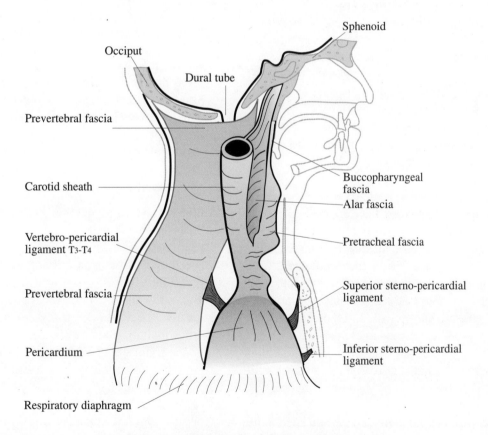

13.12 Cervical fascia and their continuity

Clinical Application:
Sensing for Fascial Drag

This section explores the relationships of fascial and connective tissue patterns and their organizing fulcrums. We will sense the fascial tracts and learn to become aware of inertial fulcrums and related tissue issues such as adhesions and loss of mobility. We will also be sensing the ability of fascial sheets to glide in relationship to each other and learning to palpate fascial restrictions. This is similar to the approach we used with the dural tube (see Chapter 4), when we used traction to sense the resistance from the occiput or sacrum. Inertial fulcrums may generate sites of compression, adhesion, and congestion, manifesting as joint compressions, adhesions between fascial sheets, eccentric motion patterns, or adhesions between fascial tissue and other structures such as organs.

Traction is a useful initial learning process, providing a way to recognize and relate to specific fulcrums that organize the whole system. Traction can be used to initiate a conversation with the forces that organize not just the inertial pattern, but also the whole fluid-tissue matrix. Once you have a relationship to the connective tissue field as a whole, a more intuitive approach of listening can then be used. With patience, the whole fluid-tissue field will communicate its history and priorities to you.

Here we introduce a subtle traction into fascial relationships. This intention has the quality of a conversation with the fluid-tissue field about the ease of its dynamics. As you sense the quality of fascial glide, you may also sense specific fulcrums and sites of crystallization. We will induce/suggest a subtle intention of traction in various places in the body, first noticing the ease of fascial glide locally and then noticing the flow of traction through the larger fluid-tissue matrix. For learning purposes, we will start at the feet and work up the body, but in practice you can work with any body area rather than using a set sequence.

1. Orient to the biosphere and mid-tide. Hold the whole of the person and the field around them within your perceptual field. Place your hands on the dorsal (anterior) side of the patient's feet. Perceive/sense that you are holding a unified fluid-tissue matrix. You may sense that the field you are holding is fluidic, yet it is also a tensile field. That is, it expresses a tensile motion within the cycles of primary respiration. First sense the general quality of the fluid tide and then add the tissues to this awareness. You may sense the connective tissue field expressing a tensile motility and motion. Then subtly suggest a caudad traction within this field. Suggest/intend traction rather than using any heavy physical pressure. Hold the whole of the field in your awareness as you do this. You are not just tractioning the local connective tissues, but the whole of the fluid-tissue field all at once.

2. As you suggest an inferior traction, see if the fascial relationships glide freely. Sense if there is a feeling of ease of glide within your subtle traction. Try to sense into the deeper layers of fascia. You may be able to sense through the pelvis, up to the respiratory diaphragm and beyond. Slowly and gently sense superiorly up the body without narrowing your perceptual field. Notice any resistance to the intention of glide. The whole tissue field may respond to your conversation. As you sense a boundary, see if you can determine its location in the body.

3. Slowly move your attention up the body, section by section between joint relationships and transverse structures. You want to sense and locate specific sites of inertia within fascial dynamics. Doing this section by section, you can locate and map out sites of connective tissue and fascial inertia. It is a useful learning process. Critical areas include places of fascial connection to bones and transverse structures such as knees, hips, sacroiliac joints, pelvic and respiratory diaphragms, ribs, shoulders, thoracic inlet, and cranial base. All the joints are of interest here because the fascial planes are continuous with the connective tissues of the joints and their joint capsules. When there is inertia within a joint rela-

tionship, you may sense a fascial drag that has its fulcrum within the joint. You can become very precise in sensing the exact location of the fulcrum within the joint relationship (Fig. 13.13).

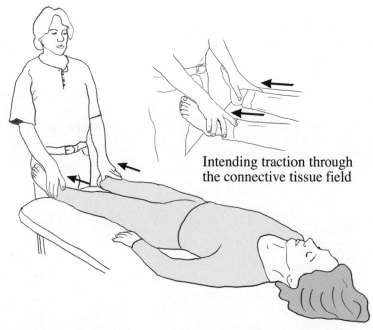

Intending traction through the connective tissue field

13.13 Traction and the connective tissue field

ALTERNATIVE LISTENING APPROACHES

The skill of traction is a very useful entry into the organization of the tissue system, but it is by no means the ultimate way to work with connective tissue. As you become familiar with this process, you will find that you can hold a wide field of awareness and sense the body as a whole without the idea of tracking attention through the fascial field. By holding a wide perceptual field and truly having a sense of holding a unified fluid-tissue matrix, the information naturally emerges. With patience, the treatment plan engages from within and the treatment decision is made by the Breath of Life, not by our clinical investigations. The fluid-tissue matrix will distort as a whole around the fulcrum. In other words, the biodynamic potency distinguishes which issue is addressed, and this includes fascial and connective tissue fulcrums. Given

time, the potency begins to show a pattern of organization, and something engages from within. The tissue field distorts around the priority issue at hand.

For instance, I may be holding a person's feet within a wide perceptual field. I sense the fluid tide and include the tissues within my field of awareness. I orient to the mid-tide and motility and motion within the phases of primary respiration. With patience, a form begins to emerge. Perhaps I sense a drive of potency towards a fulcrum. Then the whole fluid-tissue field may literally distort around a particular fulcrum. Listening from the feet, I may sense a drive of potency towards the right hip joint. I may then sense a literal distortion within the whole fluid-tissue field organized around that particular fulcrum within the hip. I did not have to introduce traction into the field in order to know this. Indeed, that may get in the way of the treatment plan.

243

Clinical Application: Inertial Issues within Fascial Relationships

Here we will be intending a traction to the site of the inertia encountered within fascial relationships. We will then relate to the fulcrums present with our familiar clinical skills. For the purposes of this exercise, we will again start the session from the feet and work cephalad up the body.

1. Intend/suggest a cephalad traction into the fascial tracts. Try to sense into the deeper layers of fascia. This intention has the quality of a conversation. It is not meant to make any demands; it is a joint inquiry into the conditions at hand. Listen to the response of the fluid-tissue matrix to your inquiry. As you engage the fluid-tissue field, you may sense a limit to your intention of traction. Do not override this boundary with any force whatsoever. Try to sense the location of it within the body. Your intention of traction allows you to directly engage an inertial fulcrum in a conversation about both history and Health.

2. Maintain your intention of traction to the boundary generated by the inertial fulcrum. This directly engages a particular pattern within the whole fluid-tissue field. Does this unified field of action begin to organize in some way around this fulcrum? Help access the state of balance and employ Becker's three-phase awareness here.

3. Listen for expressions of Health. You may sense various expressions of potency and fluid fluctuation. You may sense heat, pulsation and a streaming of energy as the biokinetic forces resolve. As biokinetic forces are resolved, you may sense an expansion within the fluid-tissue matrix. The fascia may now be able to glide freely past the original site of inertia.

4. Continue your work, moving through each segment of the body. From the thighs place your hands on the lower abdomen and repeat the inquiry. Then place them above the diaphragm on the ribs, then on the shoulders. Each time

sense for ease of fascial glide and for any inertial issues present. Sit at the head of the table and place your hands under the shoulders and traction cephalad so you are now tractioning the posterior aspect of the body. Proceed as above.

The above exercise can give a fairly complete picture of the patient's fascial patterning. You can perceive joint and vertebral restrictions and even sense into the organ systems and perceive adhesions and congestion within visceral relationships. Another useful exercise is to work in pairs on a third person. One person listens to the expressions of primary respiration at the occiput, while the other works through the fascial relationships of the body. The practitioner at the cranium may be able to sense the fulcrums explored by the other practitioner as well as their related cranial patterns.

ALTERNATIVE APPROACHES

Other conversation skills can be used with fascial issues. These may include listening locally for the state of balance and lateral fluctuation, directing potency and fluids, and local stillpoint processes. Of course these are the same basic skills we use with any inertial fulcrum.

Working Locally

As you discover a particular site of inertia within the fascial field, you can move directly to that site and hold it in any appropriate way. As you hold the site, listen for the dynamics generated by the inertial fulcrum. Assist in the attainment of the state of balance and listen for Becker's three-phase healing process. If the connective tissue area does not express any motion dynamic, you can gently deepen your contact to initiate a conversation with the fluids, tissues, and inertial forces present. This is not an introduction of compression into the relationship; it has the quality of a subtly deepening physical contact and letting your palpating hands settle into the fluid-tissue field. Once the fluid tissue field seems to be seeking a neutral, facilitate the state of balance if necessary.

Disengagement

Compressive issues may often be sensed in a joint relationship such as the hip joint, leading to a sense of limited motion or motility. The potencies, fluids, and tissues within the joint area may seem to be locked up. You can use the principle of disengagement to start a conversation about space and possibility here. There are a number of ways to initiate this conversation. Using the hip joint as an example, you might hold it with one hand under the hip and the other over the inguinal area above the joint. As you listen, get a sense of where the compressive forces lead you. For instance, you may be pulled into a particular area of the joint or notice a tissue pull into a related area.

Subtly engage the tissues in a conversation about space by drawing your hands in opposite directions, gently intending a spreading across the joint through the fluid-tissue field. You are initiating a conversation about space, and once this is accessed, listen for the action of potency within the system. Help the potency-fluid-tissue matrix access a state of balance if appropriate, and listen for expressions of Health. You may sense a resolution of inertial forces, the release of shock affects, and a softening and expansion of the field. Listen for the realignment to natural fulcrums and the midline.

Lateral Fluctuation

You can also apply your understanding of lateral fluctuation to the relationship being explored. Using the hip joint again as our example, hold the hip as described above. As you listen to its dynamics, you may not be able to sense much motility or motion. The area may be perceived as dense and inertial.

An initiation of lateral fluctuation may help the inertial potencies express themselves beyond the conditions present. You can start fluctuations by "bouncing" potency and fluids from one hand to the other back and forth until the system takes up the intention. As potency begins to express, follow the process as usual (see Volume One, Chapter 18).

Direction of Fluids

You can also use the direction of fluid process to enhance the expression of potency within the area. Let's say that you perceive an inertial fulcrum within the left sacroiliac joint. You may sense the tissue field organizing around this area, fluid fluctuations around it, a tissue pull into it, or a boundary to your intention of traction. Place one hand under the person, posterior to the sacroiliac joint. This can be in the form of a V-spread on either side of the joint, or just use the fingers or palm of the hand more generally. Place the palm of your other hand over the inguinal area and over that sacroiliac joint to direct fluid and potency towards the sacroiliac joint.

To direct potency and fluid, sense the fluids between your hands and generate a subtle backpressure toward the sacroiliac joint. As with all direction of fluid processes, you are stimulating the expression of potency in the area. You are working with the potency within the fluids as a whole. You are not directing a current of energy or fluid to the area. Notice the nuances of the tide as you do this. Are there any echoes from dense and inertial joint areas? Are there lateral fluctuations around the inertial fulcrum within the joint? Wait for a sense of pulsation, enhanced potency and for softening and expansion of the joint relationship.

All of these skills can be used in relationship to inertial fulcrums anywhere in the human system. They are used as conversations appropriate to the communications given to you. Once you have these skills in your hands, you will find that they smoothly merge and interrelate. For instance, you may be holding the sacroiliac joint as described above, and you may deepen your contact with the joint to initiate a conversation with its dynamics. You may then help access the state of balance. The state of balance may not be able to be attained, or the area may be very dense. You may then initiate lateral fluctuations in the area. You might even direct fluids to the specific site of inertia within the joint relationship. The essence of the work is to deeply listen to the system with understanding and empathy. It is amazing and humbling to watch how the system heals itself. Healing is found within the conditions present and our role is to deeply appreciate and encourage this potential.

WORKING WITH JOINTS

All of the above skills can be applied in relationship to any joint in the body, but knowing the specific anatomy of each joint is essential for effective treatment. Use whatever methods are necessary to gain deep knowledge of each site, including studying textbooks and videos, cadaver studies, tracing or drawing each joint from a number of positions, or constructing models from clay. Include all ligaments and joint capsules in your drawings or constructions. It is important to have visual images of the relevant anatomy in your hands. Once you know your anatomy, let it recede into the background as you listen and relate to the living anatomy as it speaks to you.

Essentially, working with joints is about re-establishing space. It is about inquiring into the nature of space and of the organizing forces involved in the conditions present. Every joint needs space, no matter what its nature. Space allows motion and intelligent organization in every joint action. The space within a joint relationship enables mobility and also an inner motility. An inner motility is generated within bones and tissues in the inhalation surge, as described in Volume One. Space is generated within every aspect of the joints during this expansive phase including both internal (intraosseous) and external (interosseous) relationships.

As you listen to the motility and motion of a joint within the phases of primary respiration, orient to the inhalation phase and notice the quality of space that manifests. If no inertial forces are present, the space generated will seem expansive and the inhalation motion of the joint will feel easy and open. If inertial issues are present, you may sense resistance, eccentric motions, density and fluid fluctuation, to name just a few possibilities. When inertial issues are present, proceed as normal. The first step is always to listen, orient to motility and motion, and follow the unfolding process. As you listen and respond to the

priorities of the system, any of the skills outlined above may come into play.

PERIPHERAL JOINTS AND AUTOMATIC SHIFTING FULCRUMS

Like any tissue form in the body, the motility of peripheral joints orient to midline automatic shifting fulcrums. L5 is the midline fulcrum for the lower limbs, while the upper limbs orient to C7. These are embryologically derived: The limb buds extend from these fulcrums in the embryo, and C7 and L5 remain the suspended automatic shifting fulcrums of the limbs throughout life. When first palpating the joint, see if there is a clear relationship to these fulcrums and to the midline (Fig. 13.14).

Clinical Application: Peripheral Joints and Suspended Automatic Shifting Fulcrums

In this application we will assume an inertial fulcrum at the knee, but the same general approach can be applied to any peripheral joint. We will first relate to the knee as described above and then contact both the knee and its ideal fulcrum at L5.

1. Hold the knee in both hands. As always, the first priority is to establish a relationship and listen. Orient to the biosphere and mid-tide. Listen to the expression of potency and motion within the system and within the specific joint. You may sense its motility and motion within the mid-tide. Listen for ease of motion, expression of motility, and for the generation of space within the inhalation surge. Note the sense of potency and fluid fluctuation within the joint and related tissues.

2. Follow any inertial pattern that clarifies. Orient to the fulcrum that organizes the pattern of motion present. The first intention might be to help access the state of balance. Again remember Becker's three-phase awareness and wait for an expression of potencies and for the processing of inertial forces. Wait for a sense of expansion within joint relationships and for a

realignment to the midline and to automatically shifting fulcrums.

3. Other conversations such as lateral fluctuation, direction of fluids, and disengagement processes

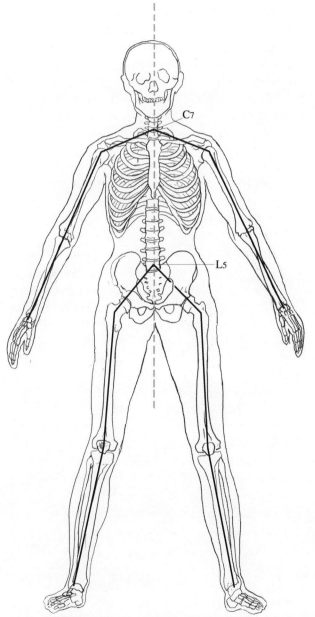

13.14 The midline of arms and legs orient to automatic shifting fulcrums located at C7 and L5

might come into play as you meet the inertial situation. As the conversation between you and the unified potency-fluid-tissue field develops, you can use any of the skills described above. For instance, you may sense a very inertial joint with fluid congestion and tissue adhesions. The potency-fluid-tissue matrix may not easily attain a state of balance. You may then want to bring in other clinical conversations. You might initiate or enhance lateral fluctuations of fluid and potency to help in the expression of inertial potencies within the organizing fulcrum. In this case, you might initiate a lateral fluctuation between your hands as they hold the knee. You might direct fluid towards the site of the fulcrum, or use an intention of disengagement to gently place a subtle traction.

4. When there is a sense of expansion and reorganization within the knee, you can then relate the joint to its natural fulcrum in the midline, orienting the knee to its natural automatically shifting fulcrum. With the patient in a supine position, hold L5 in the palm of one hand, and contact the knee joint with the other, holding posterior to its popliteal area at the posterior of the joint.

5. Listen for the motility of the joint relative to L5 and the midline. You may sense a rising and widening in relationship to the midline in inhalation. Any pattern of motion may then clarify. Follow these motions and, if appropriate, encourage a state of balance within the L5-limb dynamic. Help slow the motion down at both poles until the system settles into a stillness within a state of balance. Listen for expressions of Health here. As inhalation is expressed, you may notice a surge coming through the fluids. The joint then expresses a clearer relationship to its fulcrum at L5 and to the midline generally (Fig. 13.15).

The same process can be used for any peripheral joint. For example, if you are holding an elbow, relate it to its fulcrum at C7.

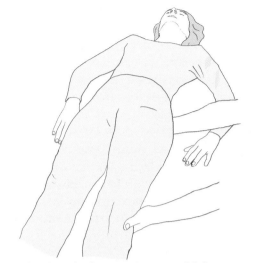

13.15 Orienting the knee to its natural fulcrum at L5

Clinical Highlight

An elderly woman diagnosed as having a calcified and fused right ankle joint was referred to me. Her orthopedic consultant wanted to fuse the ankle with the hope that the pain would be reduced and the joint stabilized. The woman was afraid of having this surgery and was very motivated to explore alternatives. She had to travel a long distance and the journey was difficult. On palpation, there was still some mobility present and her system had a fair expression of potency. She was a very resilient person and a fighter. She had stress patterns that manifested as worry, anxiety states, and sleeplessness.

I saw her over a six-month period. During this time we worked with her ankle locally for many sessions and related it back to its natural fulcrum at L5. Many sessions were also about following the Inherent Treatment Plan as it arose. We worked mainly via states of balance and lateral fluctuation. Sometimes we both entered what I would describe as the Dynamic Stillness within a state of darkness, or timelessness. I can remember one session where both she and I came back to a present awareness together and realized that something special had happened. Her overall stress symptoms softened after that session.

Pelvic issues soon clarified and her right hip joint was highlighted as a critical site of inertia. Her pelvis was very inertial; it was as though her ankle had supported her all these years and finally given way. Many sessions were focused on her hip and its very compressed forces. Vertebral and cranial base issues also arose, as did some issues that went all the way back to birth. In each session I always checked in with her ankle and finished with some specific work in relationship to it. She needed to be held at the ankle each session, or she would feel anxious and not well met. Although each session was not necessarily oriented to the ankle, it was really important to "touch base" with it. It allowed her to feel contacted at her perceived issue.

Session work was slow, but I saw gradual progress. Although the major inertial forces organizing the tissue changes in her ankle were remote, the ankle showed deep changes in tissue form and function. In one session, we again went through the mysterious gateway while palpating her ankle, and something dramatic seemed to occur. There was Stillness, a sense of rhythmic balanced interchange, a reorientation to the midline, and a settling and lengthening throughout her system. She terminated sessions soon after that and I received a simple thank you note with a comment that her situation had changed and she could not come any more. I assumed that she had become discouraged or had decided to opt for the operation.

A year later a young women came to see me. She said she was a friend of the woman's daughter. A few months earlier the elderly women's daughter had returned from a year's trip abroad and had found her mother dusting kitchen shelves balanced on her ankle. Her ankle issue had resolved through our sessions and I had never known it!

UNWINDING AND MACRO-MOTIONS

Working with connective tissues as described in this section may elicit movements of whole body areas. Parts of a patient's body can express larger motions during this kind of session work. I call these macro-motions. An arm may begin to move in a certain way, or a leg begins to express some motion, or a patient's head may move or rotate rhythmically. Perhaps as you palpate a knee, hip, or shoulder joint as explored above, the patient's limb begins to move in some way. These motions are sometimes called unwinding motions. *Unwinding* has the connotation that something is releasing or being processed. However, when tissues and tissue structures move, they are not necessarily releasing or resolving anything. Macro- or micro-motions, whether they arise spontaneously or by practitioner initiation, are patterns of organization around fulcrums.

Macro-motions are commonly expressions of traumatic experience and are manifestations of trauma schemas. They are the shape of an experience, not the organizing factor itself. In essence, tissues do not really unwind; they show a pattern of motion and organization around a fulcrum. The fulcrum organizes the motion. This kind of motion is thus a factor of unresolved forces within the patient's system. To understand the motion, you must access the fulcrum and the forces within it that generate the motion.

Furthermore, during Stage Three of the Becker three-phase healing process, tissue motions commonly arise. These are also not "unwinding" motions. When inertial forces and fulcrums resolve, tissues are freed to seek their natural fulcrums, and a period of reorganization and realignment to suspended automatically shifting fulcrums often occurs. These motions must be given space so that a new organization can be accessed and expressed. If you treat these motions as unwinding of tissues or as new tensile strain patterns and engage them in any way, you may get in the way of the completion of a healing process.

Macro-motions can be a manifestation of a frozen need to protect. When a motion like this is expressed, it may be a sign that a frozen fight or flight intention is beginning to surface. For instance, a patient's arm may begin to move and an intention to guard, to strike out, or to protect, may begin to surface. Or the patient's head may begin to rotate rhythmically, attempting to express the orienting response. It may move into a particular position expressing an unresolved experience such as birth trauma. Almost any kind of motion can arise with almost any kind of origin. These motions are often expressions of frozen stress responses and are expressions of unresolved trauma. Chapter 22 in Volume One contains a discussion of skills related to frozen intentions in limbs. These skills largely have to do with accessing the intention, slowing the process down, and helping the patient to physically prepare to do whatever is being expressed before they actually slowly do it. The preparation phase mobilizes the muscle and joints and resets the nervous system to help complete the intention present. The idea is to mobilize the system in a resourced manner to complete the frozen fight or flight intention. Rather than continually repeating the need to protect through the cycling of the sympathetic nervous system, the energies of the intention can actually be completed.

If macro-motions arise, the intention is to access the forces at work that are generating the form of organization and the motions being expressed. One way to approach macro-motions is to follow the form of the motion and to sense its organizing fulcrum. As the form clarifies, gently slow the motion down until a state of balance around the inertial fulcrum is accessed. The principles are the same as in all of our work. Stillness is accessed, and this enables the engagement of potencies.

Traditional ways to initiate macro-motions include countering gravity as you hold a limb, or placing compression into a joint or tissue structure to initiate motion. For example, you might be holding a patient's arm and sense motion arising. You might then subtly lift the arm in such a way as to counter the force of gravity. This can be a delicate process of balancing the motion, the weight of the arm, and the intention to support the arm. This process can allow a motion to arise as a pattern of organization around whatever fulcrum is being accessed. As this motion arises, the art is then to help the arm access a state of balance, a stillness, as an integral part of the whole tensile tissue field. I find that I do not ever need to initiate these kinds of motions. If they arise, I simply listen and help slow the motion down without getting in the way of it, until a state of balance is attained. The important thing here, as always, is to access a stillness in which the forces at work that generate the motion clarify and resolve.

1. Mae-Wan Ho, Ph.D., and David P. Knight, Ph.D., "Liquid Crystalline Meridians," Institute of Science in Society, *American Journal of Complementary Medicine.* Also, Mae-Wan Ho, *The Rainbow and the Worm: The Physics of Organisms* (World Scientific Publishing Co., 1998).

2. Ibid.

3. For an excellent discussion of the cervical area and its related fascial and muscular relationships and their interrelated spaces see *Craniosacral Therapy Vol. II,* John Upledger, D.O., (Eastland Press, 1987).

14

Infants and Birth Trauma

Birth is one of our most formative experiences, a universal rite of passage that can generate significant lifelong physical, emotional and mental effects. Craniosacral biodynamics offers profoundly effective support for resolving the issues of the birth experience in children and adults. Working with babies and adults who are processing birth experiences is one of the most significant and gratifying applications available to practitioners, because of birth's central role in psycho-emotional, structural and energetic patterning.

In this chapter we will:

- *Introduce basic birthing concepts.*
- *Talk about the basic therapeutic skills needed in birth work.*
- *Describe shock and traumatization in infants.*
- *Introduce the Birth Schema.*
- *Talk about important terminology.*
- *Introduce the stages of birth and related concepts.*

INTRODUCTION

As we enter this area, let's first acknowledge that babies are conscious and aware little beings. Conventional medicine's longstanding view that babies have little awareness or intelligence is a gross misconception leading to enormous damage, even today. Hospital personnel and parents routinely handle babies insensitively and administer medical procedures as if the child has no awareness and is not affected. However the research evidence is overwhelming that babies are extremely aware, even as fetuses in the womb. They perceive threats, register pain, and even comprehend verbal and nonverbal messages with astonishing sensitivity, in some cases even greater than an adult's.[1]

Similarly, current medical beliefs underestimate babies' emotional needs for bonding and loving trust. Recent studies have clearly established the enormous survival value of bonding with mom and avoiding major threats and pain in the earliest days and months. Yet even today babies' medical interventions are often delivered as if the baby's bonding needs are not a priority, and nurseries lack essential human contact arrangements. The medical community's resistance to well-researched facts in this area is one of the mysteries of our modern culture. Suffice it to say, if you are a pregnant mom or know any pregnant moms, and you encounter a health professional who says that (or behaves as if) babies have no feelings, don't experience or remember pain, don't really need full and immediate skin-contact bonding, and/or do not comprehend the psycho-emotional content of their surroundings, find a provider with a different belief-system.

The damage done to babies and the hidden societal costs of all this are enormous. I suspect that a high percentage of baby and adult health issues can be traced to natural and unnatural events surrounding pre- and perinatal experience. These effects live on long after the circumstances of birth are forgotten, and surface in numerous autonomic nervous system dysfunctions, as well as structural issues, later in life.

There is good news as well. Timely treatment can definitely reverse the effects of a difficult birth. Preventative care with craniosacral biodynamics and related methods is clearly effective in resolving these issues. One of the best descriptions of the value of this kind of support surrounds the work of Robert Fulford, D.O., presented in chapter two of *Spontaneous Healing* by Andrew Weil, M.D.[2] This inspiring account beautifully shows how simple treatment at the time of birth allows the system to settle into its new environment and avoid a wide range of childhood problems such as ear infections, colic and other common issues.

As a final preliminary comment, be aware that working with babies often invokes issues for the practitioner. This is true for many other therapeutic situations, but it is especially relevant when treating babies. The problem is that our own unresolved birth issues may arise. I always recommend that practitioners work with their own birth issues in order to understand the birth process more clearly, and to be more able to hold a neutral ground for patients in treatment sessions. This means a commitment to taking on our own unresolved prenatal and birth issues and the related forces and psycho-emotional structures still at work within our systems. This can be done with cranial sessions, psychotherapy, or other therapeutic methods. I have done personal work around my own prenatal and birth trauma over the years and have even sensed and worked with my earliest felt-sense experience of conception and implantation. This exploration has been critical in understanding and opening up my personality structure. It has also greatly enhanced my ability to empathize with infants and to hold a steady neutral ground with their sometimes very intense processes.

LIFE TAKES SHAPE

It is the nature of life to take shape. Life takes shape around experience. As we respond and react to our experience, our body-mind takes on the shape of that experience. We are conscious, living beings, and it is the natural tendency of consciousness to generate form and shape. As we meet our world and have experiences, we tend to create shapes in response or reaction to these experiences. These responses are psychological, emotional, and physical. So as we have experiences, we make decisions about them, and shape ourselves in response to them. The potency of the Breath of Life centers the forces of all of this within our body-mind. As always, when working with birth related issues, the intention is to process the forces involved and liberate the inertial potencies centering the conditions.

Neonates and birthing infants are conscious, sentient beings who make decisions about their experience and take shapes accordingly. Over the last thirty years much evidence has accumulated to show that neonates and infants are aware of their environments and register and respond to their sensory experiences. In this vein, I would like to quote Raymond Castellino, D.C., from his paper, "Somatotropic Facilitation of Prenatal and Birth Trauma:"[3]

Evidence is mounting that prenates are sentient, conscious, feeling beings who have much to express to those who receive them into their arms at birth. David Chamberlain, Ph.D., has amply pointed out to us that, at seven weeks, prenates [the baby in the womb] have been observed to be sensitive to touch and at fourteen weeks prenates have been observed to move away from light sources even though their eyelids are still closed. At fourteen weeks prenates have clearly responded to sound. Thomas Verney cites cases which more than suggests that language development begins in the womb... David Chamberlain cites other video ultrasound studies where prenates appear to be expressing affection and emotions such as joy, gladness, fear, anger and sadness. Prenatal twins have been observed gently caressing each other. In another case a prenate has been observed making a fist and actually hitting the shaft of an amniocentesis needle invading his womb space.[4]

A wealth of empirical evidence over the last three decades from the field of prenatal and birth psychology points to the sentience of prenates and newborns. Over a thirty-year career, William Emerson Ph.D., a pioneer in the field, has gathered voluminous evidence in his regression work with clients and with direct work with infants that points to this conclusion with certainty. I have had the privilege to work and collaborate with Emerson and Castellino, and I can confirm their observations. In my own work with infants, it is clear to me that they respond directly to the quality of presence of the practitioner and understand what is said and communicated to them. Emerson writes about the prenate in a similar manner:

> The prenate (i.e., the unborn baby) is vulnerable in a number of ways that are generally unrecognized and unarticulated. Most people think or assume that prenates are unaware, and seldom attribute to them the status of being human. I recall a recent train trip, where an expectant mother sat in a smoking car filled with boisterous and noisy people. I asked her whether she had any concern for her unborn baby, and whether she thought the smoke or the noise would be bothersome to her unborn child. Her reply was, "Well of course not, my dear. They are not very intelligent or awake yet." Nothing could be further from the truth.... Theory and research from the last twenty years indicates that prenatal experiences can be remembered, and have lifelong impact ...[5]

There is no longer any doubt that newborns must be related to as sentient, aware beings who deserve the best of our attention, respect, and understanding. Communicate with babies as if they know the language, because somehow they are able to derive the intended meaning. Similarly, communicate in a style appropriate for a small person, using a soft, gentle, slow voice that respects their extraordinary sensitiv-ity. Avoid the practice of talking about babies in their presence as if they are unable to understand, respecting how we would naturally feel uncomfortable if someone did this to us.

Experiencing babies as sentient, aware beings is a great paradigm shift with the capacity to revolutionize our pregnancy, birthing, and child care practices. This is the foundation of using craniosacral biodynamics with babies, without which any therapeutic techniques are grossly limited. Really take this in deeply and notice the effects, and make it the central basis of your work with babies.

EMPATHY AND NEGOTIATION OF BOUNDARIES

The baby's acceptance of a practitioner is of critical importance, so special attention is given to negotiating a relationship. The newborn has not come to the session of its own accord, but rather it has been brought by its parents or primary caretakers. We have to gain the baby's permission for the session work. Introduce yourself, explain what is happening and describe your intention. Infants can understand all this, in their own way. In addition to verbal statements, use the quality of presence, the slowness of approach, a gentle touch and the clarity of intention to engage the baby's trust and participation. The infant must sense our integrity, full attention, and communication skills. Sincere enjoyment of being with babies is also a great support for creating a workable relationship.

Negotiation of boundaries with an infant can be quite different from creating a relationship with an adult. The world of infants is totally unified. They perceive and sense everything all at once. Experience is whole and is sensed to arise in present time. All input has equal weight and intense input, such as a contact made too quickly, or your loud voice, can be overwhelming. It is important to respect this when approaching infants. Furthermore, their world is undifferentiated from their mom's world. They are truly a unified field of consciousness. Their physical and psycho-emotional world is not separate from mom's or the primary caregiver's presence. So approaching the baby means approaching the mom, and vice versa. If trust is well-established in the whole field, gradually the baby recognizes the practitioner as part of the whole system.

THERAPEUTIC SKILLS

Working with newborns and infants requires special practitioner listening skills. We seek an openness and receptivity through all of our sensory doors, simultaneously. We communicate and listen through touch and through all of the senses, as if compensating for the language difference. Put yourself in the baby's place and imagine how sensory input must be a total integrated experience, relatively undifferentiated, and not yet biased in favor of words and interpretations. We use the same basic skills within all craniosacral biodynamics, but they are used with particular delicacy and insight when working with newborns. How we work communicates how we receive the infant and how we respond to what is received. Castellino writes,

> The practitioner perceives visually, aurally, and kinesthetically. The practitioner sees, listens and feels. The way the practitioner uses his or her attention during treatment sessions has profound effects on the course of treatment. It is the practitioner's responsibility to pay attention to and learn how the application of their attention affects the course of treatment.[6]

The first therapeutic practice is to sink into stillness and to simply listen in empathy with clear intention and attention. As you stay in relationship to infants, they will begin to show you their prenatal and birth history in macro- and micro-movement patterns. They will communicate via sound, facial expression, and body motion. The action of potency, the related fluid fluctuations and membranous-connective tissue patterns relay their stories. Initially, just listen and appreciate this story using the mid-tide and Long Tide as the appropriate levels for listening. Let the sessions unfold with pacing and a therapeutic process that is noninvasive and appropriate to the infant's emerging process.

A second general skill relates to pacing. Working with babies we discover their great sensitivity. In their intrauterine watery life sounds were muffled, and environmental changes were buffered from sudden changes. In the outside world an airy pacing prevails. Sounds are louder and environmental changes arise quickly. Babies therefore appreciate a slow pace consistent with their former world. The practitioner can establish such a pace through soft low voice tones, slow movements, and gradual "slow-motion" actions. This style of contact is valuable for infants and also is helpful with adults when infant processes are encountered.

The sensorial basis of the infant's reality leads us to a third skill focus area. Psychologically, the baby's ego and psychological defenses are not formed until later in early childhood. Infants experience everything through their bodies and bodily sensations. There is no clear differentiation between self, body, and environment. In prenatal and birth psychology the nature of the prenate and newborn ego system has been called a *body ego*.[7] The baby's experience is mediated entirely through its body senses. Therefore the craniosacral biodynamic skills of listening through actual palpatory contact can be extremely valuable, meeting babies within their own natural medium of physical contact. With adults, we palpate a wide range of physical/emotional/mental phenomena, but with babies the picture is in some ways simpler because it is more body-centered.

INFANT RESOURCES

It is important to appreciate the resources of the baby. Session work must be carried out in a resourced environment, within the resources available to the infant. Safety is by far the top priority, the preeminent resource for babies. Skills of contact and negotiation can establish safety for the infant. Over time, the infant may begin to experience your presence and touch as a resource. The infant has recently experienced a dramatic change of environment from inside to outside, and the journey is usually strenuous at best. Their survival equipment, the autonomic nervous system, has been at the least engaged, and more commonly fully taxed. Even the mom, the initial focus of a baby's instinctual survival strategy, may be anaesthetized, feeling endangered herself or exhausted. The combination of factors can make a deep impression that lasts for extended periods of time. The practitioner can provide a much-needed counterbalancing experience of steady safety and confidence for the baby and the family.

Session work without a firm basis in relational safety can be retraumatizing. Infants can reexperience their unresolved prenatal and birth issues as if the events are happening all over again. Because of this, as the practitioner begins to work with unresolved prenatal or birth forces, the baby may start to become overwhelmed. The signals of overwhelm are generally quite visible, giving the practitioner plenty of opportunity to guide the unfolding process to a favorable completion. These signs are outlined below. The practitioner sees the signs of activation and helps the infant stay in present time. This can be done as long as the relationship is secure and positive; if the baby experiences the practitioner as invasive or disrespectful, the whole process is jeopardized.

In addition to the primary resources of contact with mom (and dad, if bonding and protectiveness has been established) and quality of attention and relationship with the practitioner, babies may have other resources that can be cultivated in the session environment. The baby may prefer to lie on one side more than the other, like to move in a certain direction, or enjoy contact in a certain location. These kinds of preferences are commonly part of the *birth schema*.[8] There may be a certain way of being held or approached which resources them, including certain sounds, songs, textures of cloth, or other factors. The intention is to follow babies' processes, to support their healing and to respond appropriately to their individual trauma patterns and birth schema.

TRAUMA AND STRESS RESPONSES

Parts of the birth process can be perceived to be traumatic by the infant even in the best circumstances.

The forces of the birthing process can be extreme, and the nature of the experience can be overwhelming. Therefore, working with babies often means working with trauma and states of autonomic shock (see Chapters 21 and 22 in Volume One) including dissociation, or *splitting*.[9]

Working with babies at this level is a tremendous service to the baby and the family, as these states can be perpetuated and cause significant problems for a long time if they are not resolved. Practitioners will need all the skills we have discussed and high levels of competence in trauma resolution strategies to really meet the needs of babies. Under ideal conditions, the autonomic system can reset with the support of mom's loving contact and a safe, peaceful environment. Unfortunately, conditions are not always ideal, and additional assistance can have tremendous benefits.

The autonomic nervous system can strongly affect a baby's birth experience. Practitioners need to be able to recognize the various signs of autonomic activation and respond appropriately. The large topic of autonomic function is covered elsewhere, but a brief overview here will set the stage for understanding craniosacral biodynamic treatment methods.

The autonomic nervous system is part of our repertoire of survival mechanisms, constantly operating beneath our conscious awareness and control. Autonomic functions are hard-wired into our core physiology. If we feel threatened, the intelligence of the system immediately invokes a series of responses to address the problem, initiating a cascade of neuroendocrine-immune chemical changes that we experience as physical and emotional shifts. Normally the system shifts back to a baseline state after the danger is passed, but if the threat is overwhelming, the system can become fixated at a particular phase of the autonomic cycle, constantly attempting to fulfill its natural sequence. These autonomic issues can be at the root of many health problems.

The autonomic nervous system evolved over the entire history of life forms, and three distinct stages have been identified. Conventional anatomy and physiology recognizes only two of these three stages, the sympathetic and parasympathetic nervous systems, but recent work by Stephen Porges, Ph.D., has articulated a third branch, the social autonomic system. This new finding is extremely important in understanding human stress responses and deserves mainstream adoption. We will discuss this concept in much more detail in Chapter 18.

The social engagement system is the newest and most sophisticated autonomic function, characterized in babies by instinctual maternal bonding strategies. Babies know how to recognize mom both visually and aurally, how to find mom's breast, elicit her affection (via oxytocin and endorphin inducement) and how to irresistibly acquire mom's attention.

If the social engagement strategies do not work, babies will turn to their older autonomic layer, the sympathetic nervous system, best known as the locus of "fight or flight" capabilities. It is common to hear angry cries coupled with physical motions when a baby's needs are not being met. Babies can express anger and fear, but their real effective usage of this layer is minimal, since they are physically incapable of either fight or flight. However the neurochemistry of fight/flight (cortisol, adrenaline, norepinephrin, and related neurotransmitters) is still activated even if physical action is not possible, and a protective contraction of the muscles and connective tissues inevitably arises.

Assuming failure of the sympathetic to solve the problem, the system has one card left to play, the parasympathetic response. This is the oldest layer of the system, derived from simple relatively immobile organisms. The parasympathetic response is to "play possum" or go immobile, in hopes that the danger will pass on its own. In infants, dissociation, freezing responses, and withdrawal are primary examples of this response. A traumatized baby may thus sleep a lot, be very quiet and slow in orientation. They may, however, be sensed to make poor contact, have bonding or attachment issues, or to be very "far away" or listless.

The autonomic system is designed to deal with ordinary novelties and threats, and generally functions quite well to keep us alive and operational. However extreme circumstances can "overwhelm" the capacity of the autonomic system. Overwhelm is the distinctive point at which "novelty and stress" becomes "trauma." When the system is overwhelmed and has inadequate resources to cope with the event, the system does not give up, but rather keeps trying to fulfill its intended functions. It continues to cycle, often at the precise point of overwhelm. The resulting neurochemical responses are the ground from which sprouts the whole spectrum of post-traumatic stress disorder symptoms.

Generally, babies' autonomic nervous system experience is underestimated or unrecognized in modern health care. I am convinced that simple awareness of autonomic effects of various birthing and infant-care events would have a huge benefit for our world.

AUTONOMIC STRATEGIES FOR BABIES

Let's go through these stages in more detail. The social engagement system is baby's best bet for any perceived survival issue. Unfortunately, this level is frequently defeated by routine birthing procedures, and much more so by events arising from major medical interventions. Babies need and expect protection from pain and nurturance from their mothers. But if mom is anesthetized, her capacity for meeting the baby is at least compromised, and baby's capacity for meeting mom can be equally reduced because the anesthesia is fed to the baby through the umbilical cord. If the baby is immediately removed from the mom for cleaning and examination, the expected bonding encounter is interrupted. If painful pressures, suctions, surgeries, or shots are given without explanation, the expectation of protection is at least undermined. All of these may be experienced as a betrayal of the bonding process at the time of birth. When this occurs, the social nervous system, and its orientation to safety, contact, and nurturance, may be overwhelmed. Once non-protection and non-connection are experienced at a social autonomic level, the baby may respond to novelty and stress by immediately bypassing the social engagement processes and going straight to sympathetic nervous system activation. I suspect that this is a root source of our current

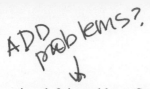
ADD problems?

epidemic of attention deficit problems. Scandinavian research has similarly linked the use of anesthesia in birthing with the modern epidemic of drug use.

The sympathetic system in babies lacks muscular coordination and strength to implement its programmed response mechanism. The neurochemistry is present, but there is little chance for actual fulfillment. Sympathetic nervous system problems in babies commonly present as hypertonic or tense tissues, sleeplessness, extended inconsolable crying, and similar excited states. The infant's cries may seem anxious and angry.

Emotions are an important feature of the sympathetic response, in that fight/flight responses have direct correlates in anger and fear, in the extreme, rage and terror. Babies are just as subject to the neurochemistry of sympathetic activation as adults, and we can actually palpate these emotions in a raw form in traumatized infants.

The parasympathetic state is the default strategy of last resort for the baby. Unable to make contact, unable to move, the baby deals with perceived threat (absence of mom, physical pain) by going into a dissociative state. This can present as non-contact, hypotonic tissues, excessive sleeping, inability to move the head, and similar placid states. Ironically, these babies may be identified as "good" babies, and indeed the neurochemistry of parasympathetic response (serotonin, dopamine, endorphins) is generally pleasurable in the short term. However, in its extreme, a fixated parasympathetic state is dangerous because metabolic function slows down to the point where the heart/lung's supply of oxygen-rich blood to the brain is too low. I wonder if parasympathetic shock may be a factor in SIDS.

Parasympathetic-shock children are not commonly recognized as having problems until later in life. They may appear as quiet babies who sleep a lot and give no trouble, and if they do not like your contact they are likely to just turn away instead of crying. But later they may have learning difficulties, and in adult life may have issues such as chronic fatigue, endogenous depression (atypical depression), and states of low energy and low motivation. These are people who

tend to collapse under stress and can sleep for weeks on end in response to stressful or threatening life experiences.

The remarkable endurance of nervous system patterns has been well-established by Emerson, Castellino, Chamberlain, and others. The trauma schema may become ingrained and habitually held within the system and become a habitual way of responding to threat. Under stress, the child or adult begins to live in *trauma time*,[10] and the ability to respond to stress is greatly diminished over the long term. Researchers have proposed that an autonomic set point or adapted default strategy can be instilled semi-permanently so that the individual habitually goes to sympathetic or parasympathetic strategies instead of having their full autonomic repertoire available. My experience is that the inherent equipment for a full spectrum of autonomic responses is never lost. The system can be reset back to the original intention. Craniosacral biodynamics is superbly effective for this purpose because the work is at a blueprint level.[11]

PHYSICAL TRAUMA

Birth process is a very physical experience. Strong physical forces are present even in the most ideal natural scenario. In a vaginal birth, strong forces are encountered as the baby moves though the birth canal. In medical emergency situations, these can be greatly compounded. Contractions of the uterus are intense and forces will be introduced into the baby's body as it meets the inner surfaces of the womb. mom's sacrum and pubic bone are powerful contact points. All of these forces are intensified if the baby becomes temporarily stuck in the birth canal. Even in optimum conditions, passage is likely to involve uncomfortable, physiologically straining positions. Upon exit, drastic changes of environment are encountered, including different air pressure and temperature. The baby ideally resolves these forces naturally via mom's welcoming contact and nurturance.

However the more common experience involves a host of other physical challenges. Labor may be induced, disrupting the natural neurochemical pre-requisites for natural self-regulation. Anesthesia may be used, generating dissociative experiences at the very time when authentic contact is most needed. Physical means of extraction such as forceps may be used, painfully squeezing the cranium. If vacuum extraction is used, the fluids and contents of the brain are literally sucked cephalad. Cesarean births pose a whole cluster of different issues, which vary depending on whether the infant was engaged in the birth canal or not. The list of physically stressful or painful possibilities goes on and on, including the customary examination, air passage suction, inoculations, and, just a bit later, circumcision for the boys. All of these physical experiences may generate protective tissue contractions that can endure for a lifetime, especially if bonding and attachment is sub-optimum.

From a craniosacral biodynamic viewpoint, it is really the field of potency that contracts and becomes inertial in order to center the various forces and disturbances within the system. The forces of the birthing experience are centered and contained in ways that are appropriate to the resources of the infant. Potency condenses to center and accommodates the shock within the system and protective patterns are retained as the trauma becomes bound in the system.[12]

RECOGNIZING TRAUMATIZATION AND SHOCK AFFECTS

Recognition of trauma's telltale signs in babies is an essential skill for effective treatment. *Shock affect* means any physical, physiological, emotional, or psychological aftereffect of autonomic nervous system overwhelm. These affects are often clearly observable. The following description of important shock affect characteristics in infants is gleaned from the work of Castellino[13] and Emerson with additions from my own experience. Sadly, we have become so used to seeing traumatized babies that some of these affects are thought to be normal.

Recognition is just the first step in treatment. We will go on to employ all our skills to support healing. Working with babies is obviously different from work-ing with adults, but the underlying intentions are the same. We slow the process down when we encounter a trauma vortex, work to establish disengagement and space in compressed situations, and work with fluids and potency to help resolve underlying issues. These need a certain delicacy and insight when working with infants, but they are all skills that we have already learned. We use voice contact and sensitive listening, or specific methods such as EV4s at the sacrum for dissociative states, all in ways that are consistent with a craniosacral biodynamic approach.

Motion Affects

Discontinuous patterns of motion are an early indicator of a traumatized infant. The traumatized infant's motion patterns may seem jerky and have clear breaks in body motion continuity. The infant may tend to move more easily toward one side as opposed to the other. She may lose orientation when moving towards the midline. For example, the infant may tend to stay on her left side. As mom moves to the right, she may express jerky motions or trembling as she approaches the midline. She may express jerking and/or shaking motions of the extremities and be unable to physically orient herself. Traumatized infants will thus not be able to coordinate their physical responses to the environment or to a caretaker's movements. At the other end of the spectrum, in parasympathetic shock, infants are overly quiet and placid. Their muscle tone may be hypotonic, and they may be developmentally slow in motor skills.

Traumatized infants also have difficulty holding their heads up. This shock affect is also so common that it is thought to be normal. An untraumatized infant can partially hold its head up and can turn its head from side-to-side to orient itself to its environment at will, without breaks in motion continuity. I have seen untraumatized infants lift and turn their head to orient to my voice, mom's presence, and other sound.

These kinds of shock affects are so common that it has become assumed that it is normal for an infant to express discontinuity of physical movement and jerky, disoriented motions. However, untraumatized infants will not express such discontinuous motion dynamics. I have had the pleasure to attend to a number of infants who had relatively untraumatized births. In all cases their motions were smooth, they could make eye contact, they could orient to their environment, and they did not express startle reflexes inappropriately.

Motion affects often have coupled tissue affects, such as compression on the birth lie side, vertebral and pelvic distortions, and various cranial molding issues. As the child grows older, if the forces present remain unresolved, these can become formalized as intraosseous distortions, unsymmetrical structures, or other tissue patterns.

Reading these breaks in continuity has great clinical importance. Become sensitive to them and be able to see and feel babies' birth traumas as you watch their motions and see breaks in the continuity of their movement patterns. These motions and patterns are communications. They tell the story of the birth and its unresolved issues and are a call for attention and help.

Hyper- and Hypotonicity and Skin Color and Tone

Infants with shock affects may exhibit hypertonicity or hypotonicity, or a blend of the two. For instance, there may be a general hypertonicity present with specific areas of hypotonicity. Alternatively, hyper- or hypotonicity of tissues may be localized to areas which met the forces of birth. Hypertonicity is an expression of the sympathetic nervous system's protective tissue tension held in relationship to the forces and pressures of the birth process, while hypotonicity is an expression of the collapse into parasympathetic shock.

In hypo- states, tissues lose their tone and resiliency. There may also be a lack of skin color, a paleness, or a mottled look to the infant's skin. Coloration can also be mixed (red for sympathetic, pale for parasympathetic), and occasionally the coloration can seem to flash back and forth.

Hyper- or hypo- toned tissue within the occipito-atlanteal junction and occipital triad generally is a

common manifestation of this affect.[14] The occipito-atlanteal junction is under extreme compressive force during the birth process. Potencies will condense within the O/A area and occipital triad in response to the birthing forces. The tissues of the O/A junction respond to the birthing forces by contracting to protect the infant from traumatic compressive forces. If the birth process is excessively prolonged, a hypertonic defensive contraction can become locked into the O/A junction and the occipital triad as a compressive strain pattern. This is often coupled with intraosseous occipital distortions. If the system went into shock, the tissues may alternatively collapse under the continual compressive forces and a hypotonic, hypermobile state may result. Castellino cites the study of Schneier and Burns[15] as a basis for stating that hypotonicity at the O/A junction has been clinically implicated in sudden infant death syndrome. I have personally noticed this hypotonic affect in many infants.

With an infant's system you are basically in relationship to a fluid-tissue field of potency. The intention is always to re-establish the relationship of the fluid-tissue field to potency and the ordering matrix. In hypertonic states, it may be beneficial to work with CV4s, stillpoints, direction of fluids, and states of balance. The offering of space via the principle of disengagement may also be very helpful here. In hypotonic states, direction of fluid, lateral fluctuation, and EV4s may be very helpful. The intention is to re-establish the relationship of hypotonic tissues to the fluid tide and its healing potency. Of course, the ability to be still and listen to the deeper forces at work is the foundation of treatment, as usual. I basically work with infants through stillness and the offering of space.

Sensory and Attention Affects

Traumatized infants' eyes may seem glossy and dissociated, as though they are not fully present. Untraumatized infants' eyes are clear and fully present. The eyes of infants who have experienced shock trauma may not converge normally, but may cross or split as they move their head. This is both an expression of dissociation and of physical birth trauma involving the sphenoid bone, the frontal bone, the superior orbital fissure, the cavernous sinus, and the cranial base generally. Similarly, the infant may not be able to orient to the environment. There may be total or partial inability to orient to visual, auditory, and tactile stimuli. This is again an expression of the dissociative process in traumatization.

Attention affects are another trauma indicator. An infant may seem unable to be fully alert during waking states, unable to hold an object within her attention for even the briefest moment, or she may shy away from any eye contact at all. Infants may have difficulty holding an object within their visual field, or maintaining contact with an object. Infants may also have difficulty in voluntarily holding or shifting their attention from person to person. They may have difficulty in negotiating a shift of attention from their inner world to the outside world or vice versa. They may seem "spaced out" much of the time. These are signs of dissociative processes. These are all difficulties in the areas of alertness and attention and are all signs of traumatization and of the presence of either hyper- or hypoarousal states.

Sensitivity to Contact and Touch

Traumatized infants are highly sensitive to boundary issues and are easily retraumatized by touch or contact. Babies relate to the world much more directly through the body than adults do. Their world is literally mediated through their body and its senses, not through their mind and thought processes. They may be very sensitive to near or direct touch, especially if contact is made inadvertently on trauma sites and force vector pathways. Unconscious contact with these sites can be experienced as overwhelming by the infant and can touch off a shock response.

Castellino notes another important touch or contact affect. He writes that traumatized infants may have "total or partial inability to match gentle pressure from direct touch with extremities, head, or trunk of the body."[16] In other words, traumatized infants

cannot appropriately respond to your touch. They may recoil, become agitated, or express discontinuous motions when touched. Touch may invoke their trauma schema, and they may become lost in their shock response.

Many times I find that I have to first make contact with traumatized infants via their energy field. It is sometimes easier for the infant to initially negotiate contact with an *off the body touch*. Emerson calls this *far touch*. Far touch can be surprisingly effective in revealing the nature of the force vectors present, areas of traumatic impact, and even cranial patterns. Some infants will begin to process their shock affects even more with this kind of touch than with physical contact. For these babies, actual physical tissue contact may become appropriate gradually, over a period of sessions.

Crying Affects

Many times parents will bring their baby in to see me because of issues around the infant's crying. The baby may cry almost constantly, or cry all night, or seem to become lost in their crying. These affects are commonly due to traumatization. Untraumatized infants cry according to their needs, and their crying varies according to what is being communicated. Traumatized infants cry inappropriately. Their crying seems to be not about present needs, but about the present experience of past trauma. Their bodies may hurt, they may experience the present in terms of their birth trauma, and it may even feel like the trauma is still happening, or that it may again happen at any moment. It is important to remember that in all of this, they are trying to communicate how it is, and it is important to learn to listen to their story. They may express high-pitched piercing crying, crying that is alternately weak or shallow, and crying that is frequent, perhaps almost constant and without apparent reason. Within a cranial context, cranial base and compressive issues can actually hurt. But we are not just treating physical patterns and problems. Babies are fully conscious beings, and their cries are attempts to communicate their suffering.

Traumatized infants may cry inconsolably and may get lost in their emotions. In this state they cannot make visual, auditory, or tactile contact and cannot orient to their present environment. They are not in present time, but are in trauma time. It is common in sessions with infants to have periods where these crying processes occur. If the infant gets lost in their trauma schema, it is important to bring them back to present time and to resource them in mom's presence, and in your present and conscious contact. One simple way of doing this that can be successful in the short term, is to lift the infant and to consciously, physically, and verbally bring them back into physical contact with mom.

Other Autonomic and Reflexive Affects

An infant expressing shock traumatization may display seemingly bizarre autonomic affects during sessions when birth trauma is re-experienced. The infant may have rapid involuntary changes in autonomic responses, such as rapid variations in pulse rate, respiratory rate, skin color, and pupil size. These are all autonomic functions still cycling from the stress response.

Inappropriate expression of the Moro reflex (the startle response) can also indicate trauma. Traumatized babies may seem to continually express this reflex when stimulated. Alternatively, they may also express the reflex while sleeping. This is so common that it is often considered to be normal, but untraumatized infants only express this reflex when it is appropriate.

An infant may react to your presence with dissociative fear responses. This is very common. They may go quiet and freeze. This is not the sign of an accommodating and resourced infant. The intentions of the practitioner can be too overwhelming for their systems. They can experience the practitioner's presence as a new invasion or new stress upon their system. It seems to happen more when the practitioner gets into a "doing" mode without really listening and negotiating the contact. The infant becomes overwhelmed by the practitioner's presence, goes into parasympathetic affect states, dissociates, and becomes seemingly accommodating. The practitioner may interpret

this passive state as positive and apply more techniques. The structural issues may be helped, but the trauma is driven deeper and the child may even be driven into deeper hypo-states. They may sleep better after sessions, but this is the sleep of parasympathetic affect, not of resolved trauma, and the child may be actually set up for future problems. Do not confuse the hypo-state with a quiet, resourced, and present baby.

Sleeping, digestive, and eliminative problems may also be present in traumatized babies. Respiratory affects are another common sign of trauma. These may include difficulty breathing, fitful breathing, mouth breathing, and other expressions of respiratory dysfunction. These affects may be due to the cycling of sympathetic energies within the brain stem and its effects on the autonomic nuclei of the central nervous system. They may also be generated by various cranial issues. Cranial patterns may generate pressures that impinge on major cranial nerves. For instance, compression of the occipital base, intra-osseous distortions of the occiput, temporal, or sphenoid bones, medial compression of the temporal bones, O/A compression, and almost any other kind of cranial base pattern can compress the jugular foramen and vagus nerve, leading to digestive, respiratory, and sleeping problems. Issues involving the glossopharyngeal nerve can precede difficulties with the sucking reflex and feeding, while spinal accessory nerve problems can affect the orienting response.

Clinical Highlight

A number of years ago, I worked with a newborn infant who expressed the startle response with any contact and had continual spasticity in her upper and lower limbs. She could not orient and inappropriately expressed fear responses and displayed almost continual shaking or trembling. Orthodox medical investigation did not uncover neurological damage or pathology. This seemed to be a situation in which her system was continually trying to resolve its shock, but did not have the resources to complete the process. She was caught in a hyperarousal stress response. The trauma-bound energy within her central nervous system could not successfully be processed, and this affected the cerebellum and midbrain structures that relate to muscular coordination and tissue tonicity. This was all coupled with a fear response.

It took a number of months of slow and careful work for her to resolve a large part of her trauma and to orient to her world appropriately. What seemed most important was the slowness of my approach to her, the establishment of a resourced space with infant, myself, and mom, and the very gradual negotiation of physical contact. The negotiation of contact was most critical so that the cycling energies within her system were not driven deeper by a fear response to my presence. She needed to be empowered to say yes or no. Stillpoints, stillness generally, and EV4s were all useful starting points. Over a period of six months, this infant resolved a great deal of her sympathetic cycling, her spasticity softened, and her development sped up. She was able to bond with her mother better and she oriented more easily to her environment.

I have treated many infants who expressed hypertonic spasticity throughout their bodies and especially in their limbs. This is a sign of frozen fight or flight stress responses. It needs to be slowly and carefully resolved. Again, this is a direct effect of the traumatic energies cycling within the system. Resource these infants within their relationship to mom and work to gradually liberate the potency within the system.

THE BIRTH SCHEMA

The phrase *birth schema* covers a lot of territory. It encompasses the whole matrix of interwoven effects of the birthing process, including all physical, physiological and psycho-emotional effects. It is the totality of processes held in the system due to the birth process. Physical components may involve patterns, restrictions, fixations, and specific motions. Each person's birth schema is unique and personal and relates directly to responses and reactions during the birth process.

To appreciate the full scope of a birth schema, we need to expand our horizons beyond the actual birth event. Subtle factors at the very first moments of incarnation including conception and implantation may be registered in the total condition. The parents' relationship may be a factor, or events during pregnancy such as a physical injury, illness, or major family events. The baby is an energetic-emotional-physical composite expression of all these factors. The following is a summary of some important aspects of the birth schema.

BIRTH SCHEMA COMPONENTS[17]

- Psychological correlates and trauma memory.
- Shock traumatization.
- Force vector patterns and related inertial fulcrums.
- Ignition issues.
- Patterns of energy, fluids, and potency.
- Birth lie position.
- Conjunct sites (sites of impact).
- Conjunct pathway.
- Cranial and whole body inertial patterns and micro movement patterns.
- Macro (gross) movement patterns and body position, tissue tone, and patterns of tension, contraction, and flaccidity.

Psychological Correlates[18]

Psychological correlates are the attitudes and expectations that we hold, derived from family, culture and other sources. These can set the stage for the person's sense of self and how they perceive their world. The experience of the prenatal and birth period sets a tonal quality for our perception of ourselves, our world, and other people. Life statements such as "the world is good" or "the world is bad," or "I always get what I need," or "life is a struggle" can derive from our earliest experiences. Some psychological correlate categories are the following.

Mistaken Assumptions

These are beliefs about self or the world based on the limited perspective of the infant in the womb and in the birthing process. These may be things such as, "I never get what I need," or "the world is a bad place and I want to escape it." These assumptions can infuse their way into our sense of the world and into all of our relationships.

Life Statements

These are deeply held beliefs about the world and our sense of self within the world based on our experience and reactions to experience in the prenatal and birth period. Life statements like, "I always get hurt in intimate relationships," or "the closer I get to someone, the more threatened I get," or "the closer I get to someone, the more space I need," can obstruct true intimacy. Such statements may be derived from the pain of the birth process, relating to the very intimate relationship with mom.

Survival Strategies/Character Strategies and Psychic/Psychological Strategies

The first period of life can color our early childhood experience as the foundations of character formation and psychological defense systems are developing. These affect how we later negotiate our way through

life. Psychodynamic strategies are based upon the foundation of our earliest experience. Prenatal and birthing experience must not be neglected when doing work within a psychological or psychotherapeutic context.

Emotional Patterns

Prenatal and birth experience can set the foundations for later emotional life. The emotional affects of prenatal and birthing experience can underpin our later feelings about ourselves and our world. How we negotiated the birth experience can set the stage for how we later express or repress emotions. We may live our life through the sensations of these emotional affects. Thus, some people live their lives in constant states of anxiety, fear, and anger. Alternatively, these strong emotions may be perceived to be overwhelming and life threatening and some people will organize their personality system, and their life choices, in ways which protect against experiencing them. All of these processes may have had their roots in the prenatal and birth experience.

Boundary Issues

The birth process is the first real physical experience that brings us clearly into relationship with physical boundaries and potentially traumatic experience. How we negotiate this experience as an infant sets the stage for our perceptions of personal boundaries and an integrated sense of self with clear and functioning boundaries. I have worked with clients[19] diagnosed as "borderline personality" whose poor sense of boundary and self-construct was traced back to traumatic birth processes and subsequent poor bonding with mom.

Orienting Issues

Loss of boundary, and the cycling of shock trauma within the system, can lead to difficulties in orienting. Orienting is the part of the sympathetic response sequence in which we scan our surroundings and identify the threat. A person may lose the ability to orient to stressful situations or processes, or even to life itself. People with orientation issues may set up their lives so that they live in a narrow band of experience which is easier or safer to manage. Unique or novel situations may be experienced as threatening. Alternatively, orientation issues may arise mainly when under stress. The person may lose the ability to respond to situations which are stressful or novel and will develop personality systems that avoid conflict or the need to assert themselves. They may have great difficulty in asserting their needs.

Intimacy Issues

The prenatal and birthing experience is one of the most intimate experiences of our lives. The intense intimacy of bonding with mom is perceived as critical to survival. How this is experienced sets the stage for later issues around intimacy. How do we enter relationship? Do we expect to have our needs met? Is there trust? Do we protect ourselves from intimacy? How do we do this? Do we find close and intimate contact painful or joyful? When a relationship gets "too close," do we withdraw and run away? These questions and related issues all can arise out of our earliest experience. For many people the most painful emotional and psychological life issues revolve around the safety and trustworthiness of intimate relationships.

Life Goals and Tendencies

Our sense of self in the world and our life goals and direction can be supported or impeded by our response and reactions to prenatal and birth experience. I have met many people who, whenever they attempted a new direction in life, were stopped by feelings of impending doom or suffocation. Alternatively, I have met people who could not stick with the intensity or struggle of reaching their goals. All of these kinds of issues can reflect our birthing experience.

TRAUMA AND EMOTIONAL MEMORY

The psychological correlates discussed above are commonly coupled with emotional memories of traumatic origin. *Trauma Memory* refers to emotionally charged implicit memories derived from traumatic experience. These are often coupled with autonomic cycling and tissue patterns. It is important to understand that the infant's defensive and emotional responses to stress are fully operational during the birthing process. If the infant is overwhelmed, these unresolved memories and stress responses can continue to cycle in their systems if not resolved during or soon after the experience.

Implicit emotional memories are generated by processing in the amygdala which accesses the importance of an experience and gives it emotional tone, and the hippocampus, which relates the present experience to the past, leading to short-term associative processes. This eventually leads to long-term indexing and storage of the experience elsewhere in the cortex. Though the anatomy is still forming, I believe that this system is fully functional in the infant. But in the presence of trauma, the homeostasis of the system can be disturbed. If the amygdala assesses an experience as an overwhelming threat, neurochemical changes occur that may continue to cycle in the system. Memory becomes less reliable, the system may become hypersensitive to sensory input, and responses may no longer relate to present-time life experience. Traumatized babies and children may then experience anxiety, hyperactivity, depression, hyper- or hypo- sensitivity and/or dissociation, all unrelated to apparent current events. It is not uncommon during sessions for babies and adults to re-experience these early trauma memories as the forces are activated and resolved.

CONJUNCT SITES AND PATHWAYS

During the birth process, the infant makes firm physical contact with mom's pelvis. The *conjunct site* is the site, or part of the infant's cranium or body, that makes contact with the maternal pelvis. High levels of force can be applied at these sites. Some babies show significant bruises from these sites when they first appear. The conjunct site patterns in the baby's body generally show these points of impact, often in great detail. The position of the baby in the womb and in the birth canal, the shape of the mother's pelvis, and the nature of the delivery (such as a mobile vs. a restrained mom) all contribute to the conjunct site content.

There are obviously many conjunct sites during the birth process. Specific parts of the baby will contact specific parts of mom's pelvis. Some contacts are of particular significance in cranial molding and distortion patterns. mom's sacrum and pubic bones are especially potent sources for conjunct sites.

Conjunct pathways are the pathways of conjunct sites, or parts of the body that are in contact with mother's pelvic structures as the infant passes through the birth canal. There are typical conjunct pathways for the different stages of birth and for the different pelvic shapes.

If the infant experienced trauma at a conjunct site, it then is also a trauma site. Force vectors will become associated with it, and, if the infant is later touched at or near the site, a trauma response may arise. This may include a startle response or an expression of shock affect such as dissociation or strong emotion. If the infant was stuck there, and was overwhelmed by the experience, then hypersensitivity and reactivity is more likely. The site may be hypersensitive and become associated with trauma.

FORCE VECTORS AND VECTOR PATTERNS

The forces encountered as the baby meets conjunct sites in the birth canal will introduce force vectors and vector patterns into their system. We have discussed force vectors earlier in Chapter 8. Force vectors can be important parts of the total birth schema, as specific physical events during birth are registered in the tissues. Force vectors have outside origins, so in the birth context we expect to find their origins in the baby's being pushed against a hard pelvic bone, being pulled out with forceps or vacuum extraction, or experiencing similar external stressors. Working with force vectors in babies is similar to how we treat adults; however, all the special cautions described above are also brought into play.

Castellino writes about force vectors:

> If the baby's ability to integrate the experience psychically, emotionally or physically is compromised, these vector patterns are especially amplified in the baby's memory systems. The vector forces actually transmit the trauma through the baby's structures. In the cranium the vector patterns will cause cranial lesion patterns which are birth-stage specific.[20]

Thus, the vector forces introduced within the birth process literally transmit the traumatic experience throughout the body structures. These vector patterns are amplified within the baby's memory systems. These memories are mainly emotional and physical in nature. Remember that the infant experiences the world through the body and its sensations. There will thus be psychological and emotional processes of traumatic origin coupled to the force vector and structural issue. The whole of this is sometimes called a *force vector pattern*. A force vector pattern may seem to have a particular directionality to its expression, reflecting the actual lines of force and echoes of the original impact.

Force vector patterns can be sensed as both physical tissue patterns and as energy patterns within and around the cranium and baby's body. These vectors give rise to, and are consistent with, cranial molding patterns, inertial fulcrums within the cranium, and with whole-body strain and compressive patterns. They are also consistent with the trauma sites and movement pathways of the birth process as the infant passes through the birth canal. Babies will exhibit movement patterns that relate to the force vectors that are held in their systems. Thus, fragmented and discontinuous motion patterns are a direct expression of the birthing process and of the force vector patterns still held in an infant's body. Unresolved force vectors will commonly become coupled with fight or flight emotions such as fear and anger, and/or with parasympathetic freezing and dissociative states. They will also generate tissue patterns that can be held throughout life if not resolved in some way.

TISSUE MEMORY AND TISSUE PATTERNING

Tissue memory refers to the connective tissue patterns held within the body as a result of past experience, especially traumatic experience. Tissue memory is not just about past experience. It is about how the system is now organized to manage the unresolved forces still present. Connective tissue responds to the forces of birth by contracting. If these forces remain unresolved, the resulting contracted state can be held indefinitely.

Tissue memory, and related connective tissue patterns, are often coupled with emotional memory. The original stress elicited a sympathetic nervous system response with an emotional component (fight and flight being coupled with anger and fear, respectively). The emotional affect becomes coupled to the tissue pattern and structural issue. Thus, if you are working on a structural issue, you must listen to the whole of the story. It is not separate from the entirety of the infant's experience.

For example, an infant may have experienced strong compressive forces during birth which were accompanied by fear and contraction in their system. As an adult, the same person may respond to stress at work or in a close relationship in the same way that they responded to birth. Thus, under stress, the person may re-experience their shock trauma, may react emotionally and psychologically inappropriately, and may express physical symptoms such as headaches or digestive problems. This is because the energy and the forces of the original experience are still held in their neuroendocrine, fluid, and tissue systems, and they are physically expressed as protective tissue contractions and compression in their body.

The concept of tissue memory obviously includes cranial and body patterning. These patterns may include various types of cranial base patterns, compressive fulcrums, intraosseous distortions, overriding of cranial structures, membranous strains, dural torsion and vertebral compressions, connective tissues torsioning and tension, and others. These inertial patterns will become frozen within the tissues of the body and will tend to become expressed as tension and strain within its defensive processes. Under stress, the system will tend to defend itself by contracting in relationship to already existing strain patterns. Thus, the response to new stress can reinforce the existing trauma schema. This can set the stage for both infant and adult pathologies.

FLUID SHOCK

The trauma of the birth process can generate what is known as *fluid shock*. Fluid shock is commonly coupled with tissue memory and related cranial and body patterning. Fluid shock occurs when there is systemic shock held in the system. Potency acts systemically to center the shock affects present. In birth process systemic shock is especially centered within the cerebrospinal fluid. The infant's fluid core may seem to be inertial and the fluid tide may be difficult to perceive. I have palpated newborns' craniums which were dense and deeply inertial with a loss of resiliency and motility due to this type of systemic shock. Some babies I have seen have had such extreme tissue compression and fluid congestion present, that their heads felt like small cannon balls. This is especially the case in cesarean births. It is sad and sobering to see this in such young infants. I have even palpated chronic shock states within cerebrospinal fluid that were traced back to conception itself. Perinatal psychologists call this *conception trauma*. The shock seems to be stored as a traumatic memory within the cerebrospinal fluid itself.

Furthermore, venous sinus drainage may be compromised due to the strain placed on the reciprocal tension membrane system by the birthing forces. This can also lead to inertial cerebrospinal fluid, resultant fluid stasis and lowered vitality, and to lethargic and hypotonic babies. Coupled with shock trauma, fluid congestion can be a significant source of devitalization. The system may be unable to constitutionally resource itself, and thus potency cannot be fully expressed. Practitioners can relate to these affects by appreciating the interdependence of membrane, bony, and fluid systems.

I have also noted traumatically induced fluid congestion and shock affects due to vacuum extraction (ventouse). The vacuum force placed upon the cranium is an abnormal force that the system is not naturally designed to meet. The Aqueduct of Sylvius (the cerebral aqueduct) can be lifted cephalad during the vacuum extraction procedure. Due to the induced shock affects, unresolved force vectors, and membranous strain and cranial molding patterns, the aqueduct may not return to its natural anatomical position. This can generate important repercussions, especially in later life. The dynamics of potency and fluid can be compromised as potencies will become inertial within the cerebrospinal fluid in order to center the forces and shock experienced. The person may have back-pressure against the normal circulation of CSF to the fourth ventricle, as well as compromised fluid fluctuation in the third ventricle. The result is lowered potency and vitality. Direction of potency and fluid towards the Aqueduct from above can be a useful starting point when you meet this condition in an infant or adult.

IGNITION ISSUES

Ignition is a dual process whereby the intentions of the Breath of Life manifest in form. There is a primal ignition at conception in which the blueprint of the human system is laid down as an organizing factor within the conceptus. It occurs as the Long Tide manifests its ordering winds, and a stable ordering matrix is laid down. Space is enfolded as organizing fulcrums and midlines are expressed. Within this process, the ordering matrix of a human being ignites within the fluids of the embryo as an ordering force for the generation of form. This transmutation process can be perceived throughout life. The embryological blueprint of a human being is continually maintained, from the moment of conception until the day we die.

A second ignition within the cerebrospinal fluid occurs at birth. When the umbilical cord stops pulsing and the first breath is taken, a powerful inhalation of potency arises within the fluid midline. This is expressed as an ascension of potency in the cerebrospinal fluid and as an ignition of potency in the third ventricle of the brain (Fig. 14.1). It is an expression of our empowerment to incarnate as a human being. If there is traumatization during the birth process, this ignition process may not be fully expressed. Umbilical trauma and too-early cutting of the cord will affect this ignition process. In Sutherland's terms, the "bird" may not take flight. The ventricle system may not fully ignite with the potency of the Breath of Life, and the cerebrospinal fluid may not fully potentize with its intention.

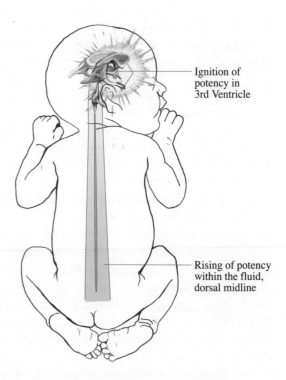

14.1 Ignition of potency after birth

Ignition issues are very common, and they often derive from use of anesthesia. I have found many adults with chronic fatigue and exhaustion whose etiology traces back to anesthesia. I do not totally condemn the use of anesthesia; obviously it has great value in certain situations. My point is that it should be used cautiously, effects on the autonomic nervous system should be recognized, and follow-up care should be expected in order to resolve the resulting ignition issues or other effects.

BIRTH LIE POSITION

In our description of the birthing process, we will be using terminology that is different from orthodox obstetrics. In orthodox obstetric terminology, the *lie position* relates to the general position of the infant in the womb. The traditional lies are longitudinal, in which the long axis of the infant is parallel to the long axis of the mother, and transverse, in which the long axis of the infant is perpendicular to the long axis of the mother (Fig. 14.2).

Our use of the term *birth lie* derives from the work of Emerson. In this model, the birth lie of the infant relates to the aspect of the infant which is conjunct, or in relationship, with the mother's spine and sacrum. Hence, a *left birth lie* means that the left side of the infant's cranium is in contact with the mother's spine and lumbosacral promontory (see Fig. 15.1). Alternatively, a *right birth lie* means that the infant's right side is conjunct with the maternal spine and sacrum. When I discuss specific birth dynamics in the following chapters, I will also use the term *non-birth lie side* to denote the side opposite the birth lie side. The non-birth lie side commonly conjuncts with the anterior aspects of the mother's pelvic structures, especially the pubic symphysis and the pubic arch.

The birth lie position is the starting point for the baby's journey through the birth canal. Determining the birth lie side helps us visualize the birth process and follow the baby's birth patterns with greater clarity and empathy. Visualizing the birth lie also gives a clear reference point for perceiving the rest of the baby's birth pattern and motions.

THE TRUE PELVIS AND THE PELVIC INLET AND OUTLET

The pelvis is divided into two basic areas, the false pelvis and the true pelvis. The false pelvis lies above the pelvic brim. The true pelvis lies below the pelvic brim and is the bony canal through which the infant

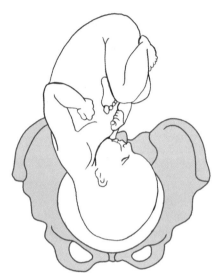

Longitudinal lie

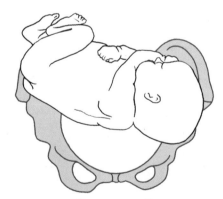

Transverse lie

14.2 The longitudinal and transverse birth positions according to conventional obstetrics

must pass. The true pelvis is composed of the pelvic inlet, the pelvic cavity, and the pelvic outlet. The pelvic inlet is bounded anteriorly by the pubic symphysis and arch, laterally by the iliopectineal lines on the innominate bones, and posteriorly by the sacral ala and promontory. It is basically a plane between the sacral promontory and the pubic symphysis. The pelvic outlet is bounded anteriorly by the arcuate pubic ligament and the inferior aspect of the pubic arch, laterally by the ischial tuberosities and sacrotuberous ligaments and posteriorly by the tip of the coccyx. It is basically the plane between the most inferior coccyx bone and the inferior aspect of the pubic arch. The mid-pelvis is the space between these two (Fig. 14.3).

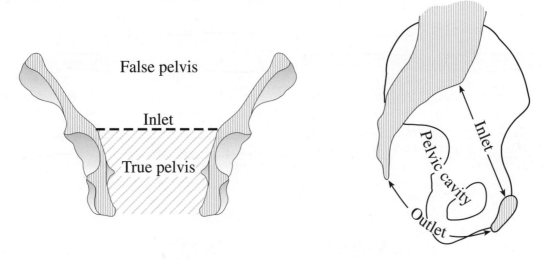

14.3 True Pelvic and pelvic inlet and outlet

PELVIC SHAPES

Each birthing mother will have her own unique pelvic shape and structure, and these are also part of the birth schema. Different pelvic shapes can have strong influences upon the birthing process. The pelvic shape categories were determined and named in the 1930s by medical researchers Caldwell, Moloy, and D'Esopo. They x-rayed and studied the pelvic shapes of over 500 women in the era before x-rays were considered to be dangerous. They discovered four basic pelvic shapes which they called Gynecoid, Android, Anthropoid, and Platypelloid.

The *gynecoid pelvis* is apple or oval shaped. Its transverse diameter is a little longer than its anterior-posterior diameter. Its widest transverse dimension is located approximately one-third of the distance from the sacrum. It is the most common type. According to Oxorn,[21] it is present in fifty percent of Caucasian women.[22] Some other authorities quote fifty-five percent. The *android pelvic* shape is sometimes called *heart-shaped*. It is triangular in shape, has a narrow pubic arch, and its transverse dimension is slightly wider than its anterior-posterior dimension. Its widest transverse dimension is closer to the sacrum than in the gynecoid pelvis. The *anthropoid pelvis* is oval or olive shaped. Its anterior-posterior dimension is longer than its transverse dimension. Its widest transverse dimension is almost halfway between the sacrum and the pubic arch. It is the most common type in African and Asian women. Finally, the *platypelloid pelvis* is plate-like, very flat transversely—a long transverse oval. It is long in its transverse dimension and short in its anterior-posterior dimension. It is the least common pelvic shape and is the most difficult for birthing. Each pelvic shape will be outlined in greater detail when we explore the various types of typical birth patterns in our next two chapters (Fig. 14.4).

SYNCLITIC AND ASYNCLITIC POSITIONS

Just before labor begins, the infant's cranium and body may be in a number of positions relative to the mother's pelvic inlet. These positions relate to the angle in which, in a head-first birth, the infant's cranium enters the inlet of the pelvis. This is called the *angle of descent*. The angle of descent is defined by a flat transverse plane through the infant's head at the level of the sphenoid bone and the relationship of that plane to the mother's pelvic inlet. This transverse plane is called the *occipito-frontal plane*. The transverse diameter across the infant's cranium is called

the *biparietal diameter* (Fig. 14.5). The positions are named according to the angle this plane makes with the mother's pelvic inlet. These angles of descent have clear repercussions for the types of inertial patterns seen in infant and adult craniums. We will explore these in our next two chapters.

If the infant's occipito-frontal plane descends parallel to the plane of the maternal pelvic inlet, the entry is called *synclitic*. Synclitic births generally occur when the pelvis is spacious and there is plenty of room to descend. In synclitic births, the mother's uterus is basically perpendicular to her pelvic inlet, the infant's occipito-frontal plane is parallel with the mother's pelvic inlet, and its sagittal suture lies midway between the sacral promontory and the pubic symphysis.

If the infant's cranium descends into the inlet at an angle it is called *asynclitic*. There are two types of asynclitic births, anterior and posterior. In most women,

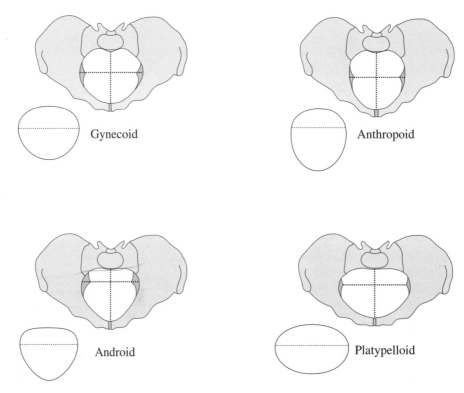

Gynecoid

Anthropoid

Android

Platypelloid

14.4 Pelvic shapes

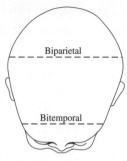

14.5 The biparietal and bitemporal diameter

the pregnant uterus is held in a relatively upright position by the abdominal wall, parallel to the mother's spine and it is in a posterior position relative to the plane of the pelvic inlet. This generally prevents the uterus from lying in a plane perpendicular to the inlet. As the infant descends in this position, the posterior parietal bone is lower than the anterior parietal bone, and the sagittal suture is closer to the pubic symphysis than it is to the sacral promontory. Thus, the posterior parietal bone descends first. The occipito-frontal plane is at an oblique angle to the pelvic inlet. This

position is called *posterior asynclitic*. This is the most common position of descent.

In synclitic positions, the infant's parietal eminences enter the pelvic inlet at the same time. In asynclitic presentations, the parietal eminences enter one at a time, making the diameter smaller and less subject to pressure. There is thus a mechanical advantage in posterior asynclitic entries, with a narrower diameter presented to the pelvic inlet than that found with a synclitic position.

If the mother's abdominal muscles are lax (as is common in overweight women), the uterus and baby may fall anteriorly and the bulk of the baby's body is then held more anteriorly in the abdomen. In this position, the angle of descent is different from that of a synclitic or posterior asynclitic descent. The angle of descent is again oblique, but, unlike in posterior asynclitism, the anterior parietal bone descends first and is lower than the posterior parietal bone. The anterior parietal bone is conjunct with the pubic symphysis, and the sagittal suture lies closer to the sacral promontory than to the pubic symphysis. The descent is then called *anterior asynclitic* (Fig. 14.6).

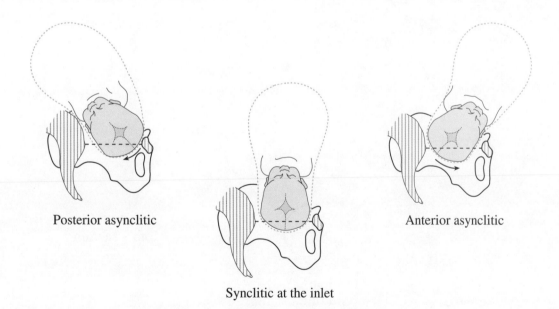

Posterior asynclitic

Synclitic at the inlet

Anterior asynclitic

14.6 Asynclitic and synclitic position

TRADITIONAL TERMINOLOGY FOR POSITION

In traditional obstetrical terminology, position is the relationship of a particular part of the baby, called the *denominator,* to the mother's pelvis. The terminology is used to describe the presenting position of the baby. The most common denominator is the occiput. Others are the *frontum* (forehead) for brow presentations and the *mentum* (chin) for face presentations. There are three sets of abbreviations used to describe the position of the baby as it presents to the obstetrician or midwife. These are:

- *The denominator:* O = occiput, M = chin, Fr = forehead (frontal bone)

- *Contact or conjunct site with the mother's pelvis:* The side of the mother's pelvis that the denominator is in contact with; L (left) indicates the left side of the mother's pelvis, R (right) indicates the

right side of the mother's pelvis, and no letter indicates that the dominator is directly anterior or posterior.

- *The position of the denominator relative to the mother's pelvis:* "A" (anterior) indicates that the denominator is in an anterior position in the pelvis; "P" (posterior) indicates that the denominator is in a posterior position in the pelvis, and "T" (transverse) indicates that the denominator is in relationship to the side of the mother's pelvis, and the cranium is thus transversely oriented in the pelvis.

Thus, *LOA* indicates that the occiput is conjunct with the left anterior side of the mother's pelvis. In other words, the baby's occiput is pointing to the left anterior side of mother's pelvis. *OA* would indicate that the baby's occiput is directly pointing anterior and is conjunct with the pubic arch (Fig. 14.7).

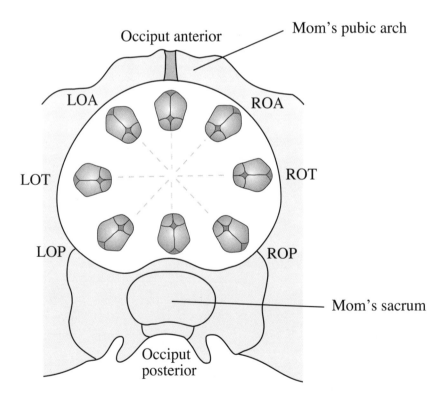

14.7 Traditional terms for positions of the occiput: for example "ROA" means right-occiput-anterior

STATION

The word *station* denotes the relationship of the presenting part of the infant to an imaginary line drawn between the ischial tuberosities of the mother's pelvis. This line is a reference point that helps obstetricians and midwives to talk about the depth of descent that the infant has accomplished at any time. The imaginary line across the ischial tuberosities is called *station zero,* or 0. Above the spines the next station is minus 1 (one centimeter above 0), and this continues to minus 5, which is an imaginary line across the pelvic inlet. Below the spines, the station is plus one, two, three and so on, until at plus five the infant is crowning at the pelvic outlet (Fig. 14.8).

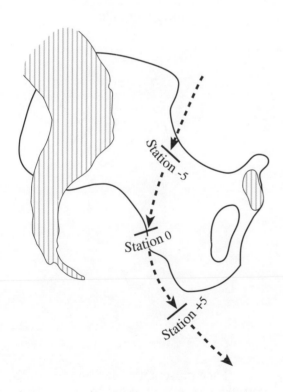

14.8 The "station" of the
presenting part of the baby

INLET ATTITUDES

Inlet attitudes refer to the attitude or entry position of the infant's head at the beginning of labor. It indicates the position of the head as the infant enters the maternal pelvic inlet. The attitude of the infant as it enters the pelvic inlet can obviously have major implications for its experience of Stage One and for the subsequent stages of birth (Fig. 14.9). The basic attitudes are:

The *military attitude,* or *median presentation*: The infant's head is aligned with its spinal axis. It is neither in flexion or extension. The vertex of its cranium is centered within the inlet.

Bregma presentation: The infant's bregma presents to the maternal inlet.

Brow presentation: The infant's brow presents to the maternal inlet.

Face presentation: The infant's face presents to the maternal inlet.

STAGES OF THE BIRTH PROCESS

Different birthing dynamics occur in each region of the pelvis, as described by the *stages of birth.* Mainstream obstetrics uses a three-stage birth process description; however, I prefer the four-stage categorization developed by Sills and Emerson and further elucidated by Castellino. It relates much more directly to the actual motions within the birthing process and to the experience of the infant. Emerson has also developed typical psychological correlates relating to each birth stage and to each pelvic type.

In the common obstetrical view, there are three stages of labor. The First Stage begins at the onset of labor and ends at the complete dilation of the cervix. The Second Stage begins at the complete dilation of the cervix and continues to the birth of the baby. Finally, the Third Stage begins at the birth of the baby and continues to the delivery of the placenta. Both Emerson and I have concluded that these stages do not give a clear description of the baby's journey and do not reflect the baby's own experience and the tasks

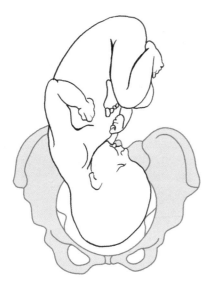

Flexion of the head

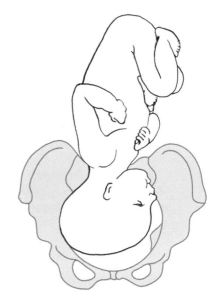

Military attitude

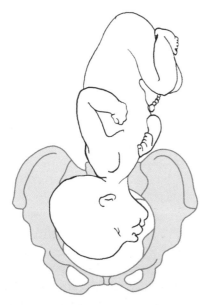

Brow presentation leading to
partial extension of the head and neck

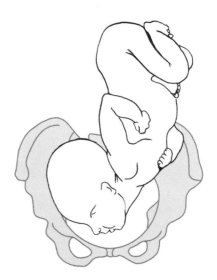

Face presentation leading to
complete extension of the head and neck

14.9 Inlet attitudes

that must be negotiated for successful birth and bonding. Having four stages seems to enable a more accurate description. In the four-stage system, Stage One relates to the dynamics of the pelvic inlet, Stage Two relates to experiences of the mid-pelvis, Stage Three relates to the dynamics of motion around and through the pelvic outlet, and Stage Four relates to actual birth of the head and body, to umbilical issues, and to the entire process of bonding and attachment. We will introduce these stages below and describe the process in much more detail in our next chapter. Having an accurate image of these relationships helps in visualizing the infant's journey though them (Fig. 14.10).

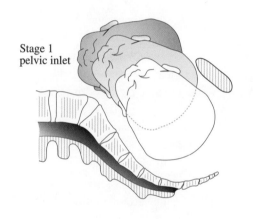

Stage 1
pelvic inlet

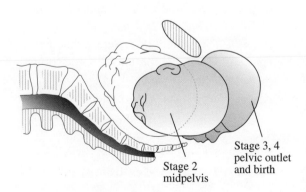

Stage 2
midpelvis

Stage 3, 4
pelvic outlet
and birth

14.10 Stages of birth

Stage One—Inlet Dynamics

Following the beginning of contractions, the infant descends into the pelvic inlet. This stage is therefore also called *Stage One, inlet dynamics*. The baby's head experiences the first of a series of compressive forces as the uterus pushes against the resisting pelvic tissues. In a gynecoid pelvis, it is generally a transverse or oblique descent, and this position will vary with each different pelvic shape. Stage One has two basic phases. Phase one is the descent into the pelvic inlet, and phase two occurs when the infant laterally flexes over the sacral promontory. Stage One ends when the cervix is fully dilated and the infant enters the mid-pelvis as its head begins to rotate towards the maternal sacrum. In Stage One the lie side cranium is in strong contact with the maternal lumbosacral promontory. If the infant gets stuck here, the conjunct site can become a strong source for generating inertial fulcrums, cranial patterns, and overwhelming experiences.

Stage Two—Mid-Pelvis Dynamics

Stage Two occurs mainly within the mid-pelvis. In Stage Two, the cervix is fully dilated and the infant's cranium commonly rotates toward the maternal sacrum. Stage Two ends when the infant is facing the sacrum. Different pelvic shapes and sizes will greatly influence the nature of this descent. In some cases there may be little or no rotation, such as in a posterior birth or platypelloid pelvis.

Stage Three—Outlet Dynamics

Here the infant must negotiate its way through the pelvic outlet. In this phase, the infant's cranium is typically oriented in an anterior-posterior position relative to the mother's pelvis. This stage also has two phases. In phase one, in a typical birth, the infant's cranium is in lateral flexion, and its nose is towards its shoulder. As the infant descends, its cranium must first go into a flexion position to negotiate its movement around the pubic arch. In the second phase the baby's head moves into an extension position in order to continue its descent through the arch. Medical interventions such as forceps delivery commonly occur here.

Stage Four—Restitution, Head and Body Birth

This is the last birth stage and includes a number of processes. Restitution occurs when the baby's head is born and realigns with its shoulder position. The body is then born. Once the baby is born, its umbilicus must stop pulsating, the placenta must be born, and self-attachment and bonding to the mother occurs. Self-attachment denotes the baby's own intention to connect with mom and attach to her breast. The untraumatized baby will actually push itself up its mother's body to reach the breast and will naturally attach itself to her breast. This takes time and nurturing both for baby and mom and does not usually occur in hurried modern hospital births, a great loss for us all. Some authorities consider this process important in the bonding process and in the empowerment of the infant to get what it needs. Medical interventions commonly occur here, interrupting the natural process of bonding in favor of examining and cleaning the baby. Stage Four also includes the month of life outside of the womb, a period in which loving contact and bonding can naturally heal much of the shock or trauma experienced during the birth process. In our next chapter, we will look at these stages in some detail in relationship to different maternal pelvic shapes.

1. For a detailed discussion of infant intelligence and awareness see David Chamberlain, *The Mind of Your Newborn Baby* (North Atlantic Books, 1998).
2. Andrew Weil, *Spontaneous Healing: How to Discover and Enhance Your Body's Natural Ability to Maintain and Heal Itself* (Balentine Books, 1996), Chapter Two.
3. Castellino pioneers new approaches to prenatal and birth trauma resolution in newborns and young infants. He has also developed a process workshop format for adult processing of prenatal and birth trauma in a small group setting.
4. Raymond Castellino, D.C., "Somatotropic Facilitation of Prenatal and Birth Trauma," draft of class notes and text for forthcoming book.
5. From *The Vulnerable Prenate,* a paper by William Emerson, Ph.D., an edited and elaborated version of the same-titled paper presented at the 1995 San Francisco APPPAH Congress, published in the *Pre- and Perinatal Psychology Journal* 10(3), Spring 1996.
6. Ibid.
7. *Body ego* is a term coined by Emerson.
8. The term *birth schema* refers to the internalization of the birth experience by the infant. This may include such things as the nature of traumatization held within the baby's system, related motion patterning, tissue patterns, and psycho-emotional reflections.
9. *Splitting* is a psychological term denoting the felt-experience of dissociation. The psyche literally splits from the soma. Psychological splitting can be very subtle with some aspects of the self-sense split off from other aspects; the most extreme is the classic *split personality.*
10. The person responds as though the trauma is still happening within the present.
11. See Bruce Perry, MD, Ph.D., Ronnie Pollard, MD, "Homeostasis, Stress, Trauma, and Adaptation, A neurodevelopmental View of Childhood Trauma," *Child and Adolescent Psychiatric Clinics of North America* 7(1), January 1998. Note: rather than epinephrine, norepenephrine, CRF, and cortisol as in fight or flight responses.
12. Again, see Perry and Pollard, note 11. See also Chapters 21 and 22 in Volume One, and Vreny, *The Secret Life of the Unborn Child* (Summit Books, 1981).
13. Raymond Castellino, "How Babies Heal," paper, 1995.
14. The occipital triad relates to the interwoven

dynamics of the occiput, atlas, and axis. See chapter 7 of this volume.

15. Schneier and Burns, "Atlanto-occipital Hypermobility in Sudden Infant Death Syndrome," *Chiropractic: the Journal of Chiropractic Research and Clinical Investigation* 1991 July, 7(2):33–14.

16. Op. cit., Castellino, "Somatotrophic Facilitation."

17. After Castellino and Emerson.

18. After Emerson.

19. This has to do with my work as an accredited psychotherapist. The borderline personality system is complex and can be extremely challenging to the practitioner. These people have very poor boundaries, are very diffuse in their sense of self, see the world in terms of black or white and are very prone to transference. You may be either their savior or the cause of all of their problems. They can also be very projective and threatening. They may be a thousand miles away, but you sense their presence in the room. You may seem threatened by their projections or made to feel like you are the greatest thing that has ever happened to them. Beware, their view of you can shift dramatically to the other pole. You must respect their reality, but must also be very grounded in your own reality. Please refer clients like these to competent therapists who have experience with the borderline strategy.

20. See note 1.

21. Harry Oxorn, *Oxorn-Foote Human Labor and Birth,* 5th ed. (McGraw-Hill, 1986).

22. Ibid.

15

Basic Birth Dynamics

Using our overview of the birthing process, this chapter will present the specific forces at work in each birth stage. A detailed knowledge of birthing gives practitioners a deeper capacity for empathy and more accurate comprehension of factors affecting their patients, leading to more precise facilitation and more efficient clinical results.

This chapter's discussion makes use of terminology previously introduced to describe cranial patterns, including flexion/extension, side-bending rotation, torsion, lateral or vertical shear, and compression. In this chapter we will describe how the stages of birth can generate these patterns. The birthing process also generates patterns of compression, traction, torsion, and shear throughout the body. Whenever cranial base patterns are mentioned, we are always talking about membranous articular strain patterns. Think of the cranium of the infant as a fluid-membranous being, rather than as a bony structure. These patterns are most likely to arise if the infant becomes stuck in any position and if its system has become overwhelmed by the experience.

To help understand the birthing process, I highly recommend a good textbook on birth and labor, such as *Human Labor and Birth* by Harry Oxorn.[1] These chapters are not meant to be a full course on working with infants, but rather to serve as an introduction to the subject. To work with infants, the best training is to apprentice with an experienced practi-

tioner. I also recommend courses on pediatric cranial work and birthing dynamics.[2]

In this chapter we will:

- *Explore the most common birth process, which is a left birth lie through a gynecoid pelvic type.*
- *Go into each stage of birth in detail in relationship to its conjunct pathway and conjunct sites.*
- *Note the major strain patterns that may arise in each stage.*
- *Summarize typical birth motions through other kinds of pelvic shapes.*

TYPICAL BIRTH PROCESS

As introduced in our last chapter, we will begin our exploration of a typical birth process in terms of four stages. These are not the traditional obstetrical stages, but are derived from an appreciation of the baby's physical and emotional experience during the birthing process. In this exploration we define the stages of birth in terms of the tasks the infant must complete in order to be born. During the birth process the infant experiences positional and movement changes as well as great variations in sensations of pressure, compression, torsion, and shear. All of these factors are expressed within every level of the system. The inertial potencies generated by the experience affect potency, fluids, and tissues as a unified field. Bone, membrane, CNS tissue, and fluids are all affected by, and express, the forces at work. The total response is not just structural or physical, but includes the full spectrum, from tissue and fluid effects, to emotional processes, to autonomic shock states, including both sympathetic and parasympathetic responses.

The infant begins the birth process in a variety of positions when true labor starts (when maternal contractions are regular and about twenty to thirty minutes apart). Many babies start in a posterior position and then rotate to one side or the other. The most common pelvic type in Caucasians is the gynecoid pelvis, and the most common beginning position is baby lying with her left side conjunct to mother's spine. The left side of the baby's head and body contacts the mother's lumbosacral promontory and spine. Some variation of this starting position is seen in fifty to fifty-five percent of births[3] (Fig. 15.1). We call this the *left birth lie* position.[4]

The common positions of entry into the pelvic inlet include *left occiput anterior, left occiput posterior,* and *left occiput transverse.* The following explanation is based on a common starting position, the left occiput

transverse engagement (LOT). In this position, the infant's cranium is in a transverse relationship to the maternal pelvis; the sagittal suture of the infant is in

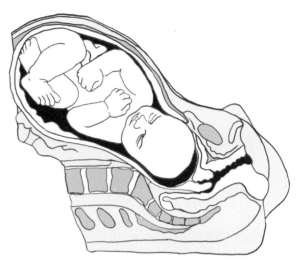

15.1 Left birth lie position: baby's left side is conjunct with mother's spine

the transverse diameter of the pelvis. Oblique starting positions are also common, as are posterior positions. Other common left birth lie positions include left occiput anterior (LOA) and left occiput posterior (LOP), each yielding an oblique orientation (Fig. 15.2).

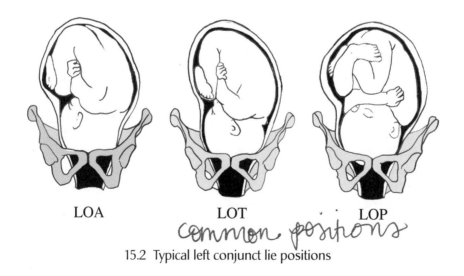

LOA   LOT   LOP

common positions

15.2 Typical left conjunct lie positions

In the following sections, we will describe the dynamics of a birth through a *gynecoid pelvic inlet*. As described in our last chapter, the gynecoid pelvic inlet is an oval-round shape. Its transverse diameter is a little longer than its anterior-posterior diameter. It is sometimes called an apple-shaped pelvis. Its inlet shape is oval to round, and its widest transverse dimension is located approximately one-third of the distance from the sacrum (Fig. 15.3).

Many variations in positions and forms of movement are possible. These describe typical birthing motions. All of the different cranial base patterns described in Chapter 8 can be generated during birth process.

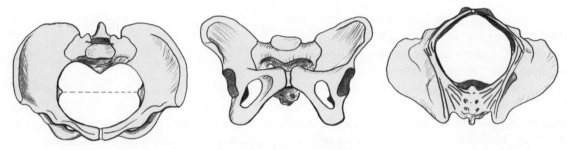

15.3 Gynecoid pelvic shape

STAGE ONE: PELVIC INLET DYNAMICS

Stage One begins when contractions begin. In the LOT position, the infant's left side is lying against mother's spine with the left side of the head conjunct (in contact with) with the maternal lumbosacral prominence. The infant's first task is to negotiate its way past the pubic arch so that it can enter the pelvic inlet. The posterior asynclitic entry position is the most common, with the baby's left parietal bone lower than the right and leading the way into the pelvis (see Fig. 14.6).[5] The infant generally starts the birthing process with her head partially flexed toward her body. The infant's occipito-frontal diameter is the common presenting diameter. As the pressures of descent build, the head is forced into increased flexion, the neck is more fully flexed and the suboccipito-bregma diameter becomes the presenting diameter (Fig. 15.4 and 15.1).

In Stage One's early phase, the infant's head meets the mother's pubic bone with the posterior parietal bone leading the way. The pubic arch is the first strong resistance. Either the sagittal area of the cranium, or

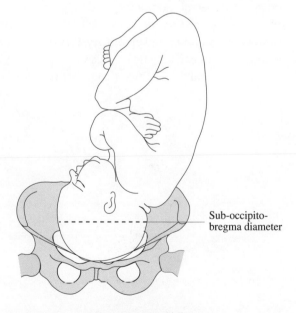

Sub-occipito-bregma diameter

15.4 Outset of labor

the superior aspect of the right parietal bone, may contact the pubic symphysis (Fig. 15.5).

If the sagittal suture is conjunct with the maternal pubic symphysis, force vectors may be introduced in a caudad direction. The non-birth lie parietal bone (right parietal bone) may be subjected to strong pressures in both caudal and oblique directions via its contact with the pubic arch. Caudal vector patterns may affect the cranial base generally and generate compressive cranial base fulcrums; oblique vectors may affect the opposite (birth lie) occipito-mastoid and O/A areas. Compressive fulcrums may be introduced into these areas. This may give rise to cranial base and SBJ compressions and general compressive vectors through the longitudinal axis of the body. If the right parietal bone initially is conjunct with the maternal pubic bone, then oblique force vectors may be introduced into the cranium (see Fig. 15.5).

In the later phase of Stage One, the infant must change direction to pass under the pubic bone, rotating over the maternal sacral promontory (Fig. 15.6). Both sacrum and pubis exert a dragging effect on the cranium as the baby passes. The baby's body rotates anteriorly, along with the mother's uterus. As this occurs, the infant's left parietal bone is conjunct with the maternal sacral promontory and may experience strong transverse pressures. As the baby's cranium rotates over the sacral promontory, this transverse pressure moves caudad and creates pressure against the left temporal bone. Thus, a conjunct pathway is

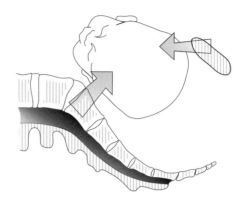

15.6 Middle stage one

generated from the superior aspect of the left parietal bone caudad to the left temporal bone, forcing them into internal rotation with corresponding membranous patterns. The baby may be in this stage for some time; the longer a pressured contact is held, the more likely that the system will gather potency at the site to contain and manage the disturbance, leading to lasting force vector patterns and other effects such as a right side-bending cranial base pattern (a convexity bulge) being generated on the non-birth lie side.

At the end of Stage One, the infant is in a synclitic position and is fully engaged in the birth canal. If the infant is in this position for some time, strong transverse forces can be fed into the cranium, leading to medial compressive issues, temporal bone intraosseous compression, and exhalation-extension patterns (Fig. 15.7).

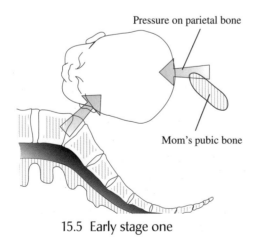

15.5 Early stage one

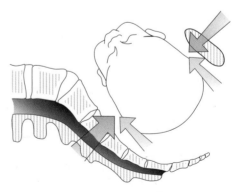

15.7 Late stage one dragging and compressive forces

STAGE ONE: CRANIAL BASE PATTERNS

Lateral forces may be placed on the greater wing of the sphenoid on the birth lie side, and a lateral shear of the cranial base may be generated here. As the compressive forces are fed in via the conjunct site at the sacral promontory, a right lateral shear distortion may result. As the infant experiences dragging forces along this conjunct pathway, the left greater wing of the sphenoid may be dragged inferiorly on the birth lie side, generating a right torsion pattern (a superior greater wing on the non-birth lie side). The medially compressive forces introduced via the sacral promontory may also give rise to medial compression of the cranial base on the birth lie side. A medially compressed left temporal bone may be generated (see Fig. 15.7).

Stage One General Inertial Issues

- Extension patterns may be introduced into the dynamics of the cranium.

- Axial compressive issues are introduced into the body, especially on the birth lie side.

- Various cranial base patterns may be generated, usually on the non-birth lie side.

- Medial compressive issues may be generated, especially on the birth lie side.

STAGE ONE: INTRAOSSEOUS DISTORTIONS OF THE SPHENOID

Intraosseous compressions within the temporal and sphenoid bones may also arise in Stage One. The sphenoid bone is in three separate parts, the body and its lesser wing, and the two greater wing and pterygoid sections (Fig. 15.8). Under birth stress, these parts can become distorted or displaced in relation to each other. In one instance, the greater wings can become relatively fixed by medial compression while the cranium is experiencing downward forces. This can generate a shearing of the greater wing complexes relative

to the body or cause the body to shear inferiorly relative to the greater wings. This will be sensed as a strong shearing force in the infant's cranium and will also persist in adults. Vertical shear can be found on just one side, if one greater wing complex is dragged inferiorly while the other is held fixed against the maternal sacrum or pubic arch.

Vertical shear in the sphenoid can produce dramatic effects in the facial area. The sphenoid wings pull the maxillae up via the pterygoid processes, while the sphenoid body pushes the vomer down. This situation can affect the vomer (leading to a compression or S-shape) and cause restricted glide and range of motion between the pterygoid processes and the palatines. Facial effects of shearing can also be one-sided, corresponding the unilateral vertical shear of one greater wing only.

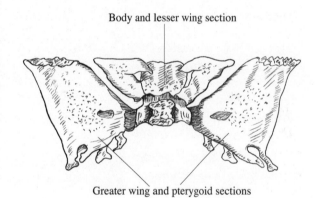

Body and lesser wing section

Greater wing and pterygoid sections

15.8 The sphenoid bone
is in three sections at birth

It is also possible to have a vertical shear of the wing sections relative to the body in the opposite direction, with the body pushed up and both or one of the wings pulled down. This occurs when the inferior dragging forces on the greater wings are stronger than the inferior compressive forces transferred to the body of the sphenoid. The greater wing sections are dragged inferiorly and the body is left in a superior position, creating a strong tension in the hard palate (Fig. 15.9).

283

MEDIAL COMPRESSION OF THE SPHENOID

The greater wing sections may also become medially compressed into the body of the sphenoid. Negotiating the motion around the sacral promontory can place great pressure on the birth lie side, in this case the left side. This intraosseous compression can be a factor in intransigent side-bending and torsion patterns, generating great sensitivity to touch contact at the greater wings. Some people cannot initially be contacted at the greater wings due to these strong intraosseous compressions. The vault hold may bring up a sensation of intense crowding and pressure. Contact needs to be carefully negotiated by the practitioner. In late Stage One, bilateral compression of the wing sections into the body of the sphenoid can arise (see Fig. 15.9).

Stage One Intraosseous Distortions of the Sphenoid Bone

- Shearing patterns between the greater wings and the body of the sphenoid (various forms of lateral and vertical shearing).

- Torsion patterns between the greater wings and the body of the sphenoid.

- Compression between the parts of the sphenoid.

INTRAOSSEOUS DISTORTIONS OF THE TEMPORAL BONE

The temporal bone is originally composed of three parts, the petrous and squamous parts, and the tympanic ring. These can become compressed together during Stage One, and later this may be the origin of persistent medial cranial base compression. Initially such compression patterns may seem to be interosseous, arising from fulcrums at the sutures. But insightful palpation may reveal that the organizing fulcrum is located within the temporal bone itself. No matter how much attention is given to the cranial base as a whole, the pattern will not be amenable to resolution unless the nature of the intraosseous forces within the bone are appreciated

OTHER EFFECTS OF STAGE ONE PRESSURE

The TMJ may be affected by dragging and compressive forces. The TMJ and its ligaments on the birth lie side may become compressed and hypertonic. The TMJ and its ligaments on the opposite side may become tractioned and hypotonic in compensation.

In the late phase of Stage One, the infant's head is now in a *synclitic* position (head parallel to the pelvic inlet) relative to the pelvic inlet. If the infant becomes stuck here, strong lateral forces arise from both the sacrum and pubic arch yielding bilateral medial compression of the cranial base. This can generate extension (transverse narrowing) patterns (see Fig. 15.7). Intraosseous distortions of the sphenoid and temporal bones may be generated and either or both parietal bones may be flattened, puckered, or forced to overlap at the sagittal suture.

While this is occurring, the mother's pelvis must widen to receive the infant's head. This motion is called *counternutation*. The pelvis widens at the pelvic inlet and narrows at the ischial tuberosities. The sacrum moves into flexion and the ilea rotate externally (Fig. 15.10). The infant has now descended into the pelvic inlet and is in a synclitic position (parietal bones level with each other). The infant will now begin its rotational descent within the mother's mid-pelvis, the beginning of Stage Two.

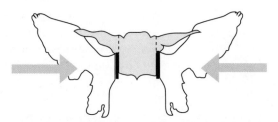

Medial compressive forces

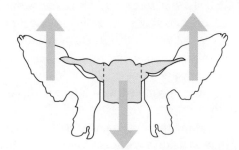

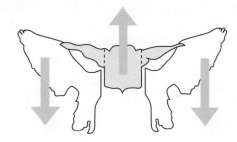

Vertical shearing of the body relative to the greater wing / pterygoid parts

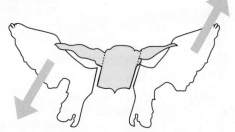

Lateral shearing of greater wing / pterygoid parts relative to the body

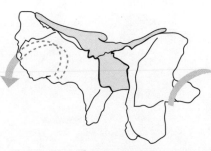

Torsioning of greater wing / pterygoid parts relative to the body (common in stage two)

15.9 Common intraosseous distortions of the sphenoid bone

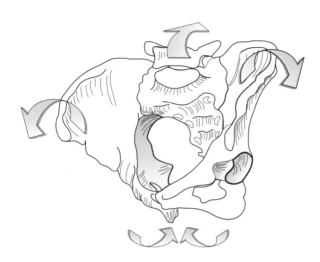

15.10 Inlet dynamics: counternutation
of mother's pelvis

BODY RELATIONSHIPS

Spinal and Structural Repercussions

Infants experience strong compressive forces along their longitudinal axis throughout the birth process, leading to possible vertebral issues. Axial compression through the vertebral column is a common clinical finding in both children and adults, and birthing forces are a common origin. Specific vertebral fixations result, but commonly the axial force must be addressed as a whole for full resolution to occur. See Chapter 5, "Vertebral Dynamics," for clinical approaches to these issues.

In Stage One, these forces are especially felt on the birth lie side (Fig. 15.11). The infant may contract muscles and connective tissues on that side, setting up a pattern that can continue indefinitely. In our current example this would show up as a left-sided body contraction, a chronic pattern of tissue tension, and/or a habitual posture of self-protection from stress. This may produce patterns of scoliosis and asymmetric compression in the spine and structural system, yield-ing patterns of side-bending in vertebral relationships and a possible narrowing of the discs on the birth lie side. A low shoulder, a generally contracted left side, and posteriorly rotated hip bone on the birth lie side will give the appearance of a "C" curve on that side of the body. If the sacrum is posterior and inferior on the birth lie side as described below, then a full "S" curve may arise. A general pattern of contraction on the left side of the body may also be seen (Fig. 15.12).

Compressive forces often generate fulcrums within places of transition, such as areas of change in the spinal curve. Inertial forces may also lodge within specific areas of transition such as the atlanteal-occipital junction, the cervical/thoracic junction and the lumbosacral junction. Compressive forces impinge on the occipito-atlanteal-axial area leading to compression patterns coupled with intraosseous distortions of the occiput.

In the infant these structural patterns may be sensed only as tendencies, not as full-blown structural issues. The sensitive hands of the cranial practitioner can perceive these tendencies and the forces involved and detect related patterns of distress in the fluids and tissues of the system. It may take years of habit-

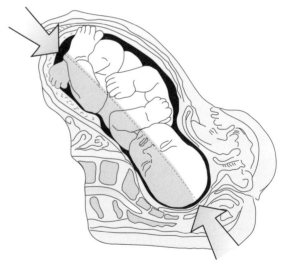

15.11 Stage one axial compression especially affects the birth lie side

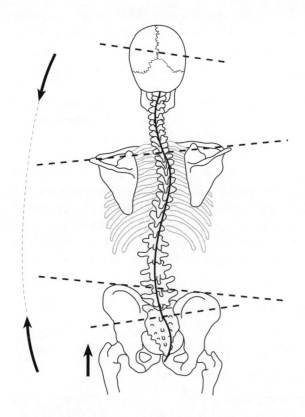

15.12 Adult structural distortion based on stage one experiences, left birth lie

Dural Repercussions

The compressive forces generated by the birth experience can also affect the dural membranes. The dural tube may seem denser along its entire length due to the presence of these forces. Commonly, forces come to rest within specific areas of the dural tube, and these may be coupled with local vertebral issues.

Central Nervous System

The central nervous system also experiences extreme compressive forces during the birth process. If these forces become entrapped within neural tissue, potency will condense to center the forces involved and the motility of the central nervous system can be affected. The ventricle system also has to organize around the unresolved compressive forces introduced. In a left birth lie, the infant experiences more extreme forces on its left side. In this case, the left ventricle may be slightly contracted when compared to the right. A right side-bending pattern in the cranial base may be coupled with the narrowed ventricle. This will have ongoing repercussions for both infant and adult.

Pelvic Repercussions

Stage One forces especially impact the pelvis on the birth lie side, particularly at the hip and sacroiliac joints. In a left birth lie, compressive pressures build on the left side of the body, and the left innominate bone is forced to rotate posteriorly. This drags the sacrum on that side in a posterior and inferior direction. The patterns that are generated may include a posteriorly rotated innominate bone on the birth lie side and a torsioned sacrum. The sacrum tends to be held inferior and posterior on the birth lie side—the left side in the example here. Both hip bone and sacrum may express inertial patterns that fulcrum around left-sided cephalad-caudad force vectors. Posterior rotations of the hip bone and a posterior-inferior sacrum on the left side of the body are reported to be most common by osteopaths and chiropractors, probably because a

ual maintenance of these forces before they are expressed in clear structural forms. I have treated many infants who retained these birthing forces in their spinal relationships. The sacroiliac pain or migraine headache of the thirty-year-old may have had its beginnings in the experience of birth.

Infants often habitually pull up the leg of the birth lie side in a contracted manner. In this case it would tend to be seen on the left side. As the birth continues, these left-sided compressions are reinforced by the ongoing nature of the birth contractions. Babies who are born from a posterior presentation, and who remained posterior during the whole birth process, tend to pull both legs up and tend to suddenly pull their head posteriorly if they are startled.

majority of people start the birth process in a left birth lie position (Fig. 15.13).

Psychological Considerations

As birth contractions build, the infant begins to descend towards the cervix that is not yet dilated. This is sometimes called the "no exit" phase of the birth process, as the infant meets strong resistance from the undilated cervix. This can bring up feelings of confusion, loss, and even abandonment as the infant enters and moves through the birth canal. Some infants seem to have a clear sense that they are going to an outside world, but for others it can be a confusing and even terrifying experience as if they are entering a dark tunnel with no apparent end in sight.[6]

The infant may experience loss of contact with mom and this alone may be disorienting and scary. Infants live in "present time" and usually have no sense of past or future. Strong forces and overwhelming pressures at any time in the birth process may have the sense of being endless. Furthermore, when these experiences are stimulated within clinical sessions, it may seem to the infant that the trauma is occurring again. It is extremely important to resource the infant in mom's presence and for the practitioner to gradually become a resourcing presence for them. The various stages of birth process can re-stimulate earlier prenatal trauma or stress. Stage One can re-stimulate conception issues as the infant is again in transition from one world to another.

Left-sided compressive forces make the innominate bone rotate posterior. The sacral base on the same side is then forced to rotate posteriorly and inferiorly creating sacral torsion.

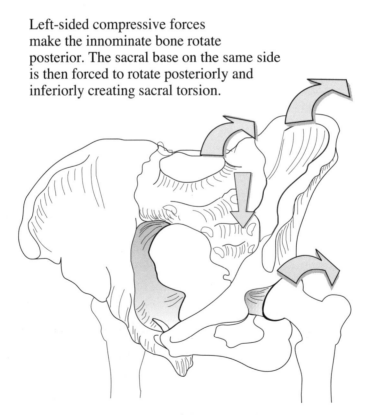

15.13 Pelvic repercussions

Summary of Stage One Pelvic Inlet Dynamics

Summary of Motion (Fig. 15.14)	Cranial and Whole–Body Impacts
Early Stage One Infant descends in posterior asynclitism, pressures against the left parietal-temporal and sagittal areas (Fig. 15.5).	• Diagonal and oblique force vectors on cranium. • O/A compression on birth lie side. • Occipito-mastoid compression of birth lie side. • Ongoing caudad compression yielding compressive patterns in the cranium and spine.
Middle Stage One Infant's cranium meets pubic arch, cranium rotates around lumbosacral promontory in lateral flexion (Fig. 15.6).	• Medial compression of the left temporal bone and cranial base. • Intraosseous distortions of the sphenoid and temporal bones. • Right side-bending. • Right lateral shear. • Right torsion. • TMJ compression on birth lie side. • Intraosseous distortions of sphenoid and temporal bones.
Late Stage One Infant is in synclitic position and has descended into the pelvic inlet in a transverse position (Fig. 15.7).	• Extension patterns. • Medial compression of the cranial base. • In all stages: possible over-riding of sutural relationships— sagittal suture is especially vulnerable— flattening or puckering of parietal bones.
Body Patterns (Figs. 15.11, 15.12, 15.13)	• Compressions in the body on birth lie side. • Dural and spinal compressions. • Posterior innominate bone and inferior sacrum on birth lie side. • Short leg on birth lie side.

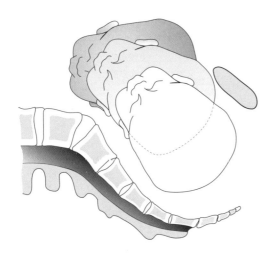

15.14 Summary of motions in stage one descent

In early Stage One the mother's pelvis counternutated. The pelvic inlet opened. During the later phases of Stage One, the pelvic floor and outlet must begin to open, and nutation, which is the opposite of counternutation, occurs. In nutation, mom's ischial tuberosities spread apart, the sacrum moves into extension, and the two ilea move into internal rotation. The result is that, as the infant continues its descent in the birth canal, the pelvic floor opens to allow the infant easier passage (see Fig. 15.24).

STAGE TWO: MID–PELVIS DYNAMICS

Stage Two begins the transition from an inside world of the womb to the outside world. It begins when the infant moves through the pelvic inlet and begins to negotiate passage through the mid-pelvis. The pelvic inlet in the gynecoid pelvis is basically an apple-shaped oval with a transverse dimension slightly longer than its anterior-posterior dimension (see Fig. 15.3). The pelvic outlet, however, is an oval that is wider in the opposite dimension (anterior-posterior) (Fig. 15.15). In order to more easily enter the pelvic outlet, the infant's head must turn in the birth canal so that its longitudinal dimension enters the outlet anterior-posterior. To do this, the infant will generally rotate its head posteriorly toward the maternal sacrum as it

continues its descent through the birth canal. Rotation is mainly of the head, not the body, with strong cranial contact on the mother's sacrum and pubic arch. The whole process is facilitated by the shape of the birth canal and the downward force of uterine contraction working together to generate a firm corkscrew-like motion. Because of the rotation that commonly occurs in this stage, it sometimes called *rotational descent.* By the end of Stage Two, the infant's head is facing the maternal sacrum (Fig. 15. 16, 22).

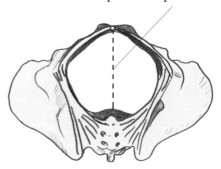

A-P axis is the widest part of the pelvic outlet

15.15 Pelvic outlet in a gynecoid–shaped pelvis

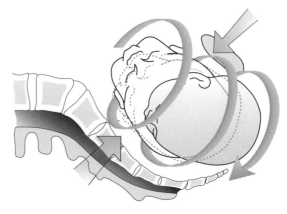

15.16 The corkscrew–like motion through the mid-pelvis

OVERVIEW OF ROTATIONAL MOTION AND RELATED FORCES IN STAGE TWO

Torsion

During Stage Two, torsion is generated within the infant's tissues, especially within the reciprocal tension membrane, the cervical spine and related connective tissues, and through the vertebral axis and dural tube generally.

Dragging Pressure

A dragging force is generated by the contact with the sacrum and pubic bone on the infant's cranium (Fig. 15.17). The mother's sacrum becomes a common *moving fulcrum* for conjunct sites and force vectors. Pressure begins at the baby's parietal-temporal area on the birth lie side and moves inferiorly along the greater wing of the sphenoid, zygoma, and maxilla, and then the TMJ area. This generates a rotational torsioning force against all of these structures. Meanwhile a similar pressure is exerted by the contact with the pubic bone on the back side of the baby's head, at the parietal and occipital bones on the side opposite the birth lie. The dragging pressure here moves inferiorly and toward the occiput.

Force Vectors

If the infant becomes stuck in any position during rotational descent, any area contacting the sacrum or pubic arch at that point can become a fixed fulcrum, with force vectors introduced. Lateral and diagonal vectors in both infant and adult craniums can be present due to Stage Two rotational descent pressures, and can register in all layers of the system.

Sphenoid Pattern

The left greater wing of the sphenoid may be dragged inferiorly on the birth lie side, giving rise to a torsion pattern on the side opposite the birth lie side. In this case, a right torsion pattern will result as the left greater wing is dragged inferiorly. The left side of the head will also experience strong lateral forces that may yield a right side-bending pattern, or reinforce an existing one that began during Stage One. These forces may also reinforce an existing lateral shear pattern, or may induce one. In this case, since the forces are directed from left to right across the infant's cranium, a right lateral shear will result. Intraosseous distortions of the sphenoid bone may also be reinforced or generated here (see Fig. 15.9).

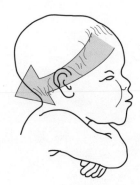

Conjunct pathway with pubic bone (left side lie)

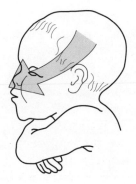

Conjunct pathway with sacrum (left side lie)

15.17   Dragging forces in stage two

Sphenoid-Maxillary Patterns

Another pattern that can be generated in Stage Two is sphenoid-maxillary torsion. As the infant's head corkscrews past the sacrum, the fulcrum of contact shifts from the left side of the head to the left side of the face. As this occurs, the head is also descending, and a dragging force is experienced from the greater wing of the sphenoid inferior across the zygoma and maxilla on the left. This can be visualized as a moving fulcrum of contact from the greater wing anteriorly and inferiorly across the left side of the face. If the forces are great enough, the maxillary complex may be forced into a torsioned relationship with the sphenoid bone. This is a true torsion pattern where

the sphenoid-maxillary complex is forced to rotate around an anterior-posterior axis (Fig. 15.18). This can also generate compression within the TMJ on the high maxilla side. It is common to see maxillary torsion in relationship to TMJ compression. This pattern is common in both infant and adult and can have important clinical repercussions (See Chapter 11, "The Hard Palate," for clinical approaches to maxillary torsion).

By the end of stages one and two, forces have been fed into the cranium that can create a "C" curve on one side of the infant's head. This is generated by a combination of the concavity of a side-bending pattern with sphenoid-maxillary torsion on the side opposite the concavity, plus TMJ compression on the same side. It is usually seen on the birth lie side.

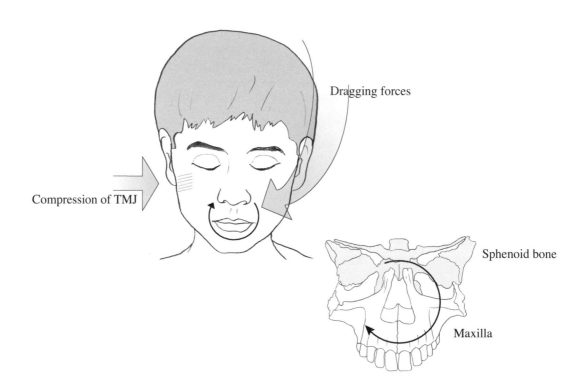

Dragging forces

Compression of TMJ

Sphenoid bone

Maxilla

15.18   Sphenoid–maxillary torsion

Stage Two General Inertial Issues

- Rotational patterns throughout the cranium and body; rotational issues within the membranous-osseous system.

- Generation or reinforcement of cranial base patterns expressed on the non-birth lie side.

- Torsional issues that involve the sphenoid-maxillary complex leading to a true torsion of the maxilla and vomer relative to the sphenoid bone.

- Compressive issues in TMJ dynamics.

INTRAOSSEOUS DISTORTIONS OF THE OCCIPUT

The baby's occiput is in four distinct parts: the two condylar parts, the basilar part, and the squamous part (Fig. 15.19). In Stage Two, the occiput's contact with the maternal pubic arch can generate strong moving pressure across the back of the infant's head. These forces can impact the parts of the occiput and affect their later coalescence into a single bone. The squamous portion is being rotated while the other occipital parts are relatively fixed by the downward descent forces. In a left birth lie, the occipital squama may be rotated clockwise (when viewing it from the rear) and its right side is forced inferiorly into compression with the right condylar part. Meanwhile the left side of the occipital squama is forced away from the left condylar part. The infant would end up with compression between the right side of the squama and the right condylar part and a spreading, or wedging apart, of the left side of the squama and left condylar part (Fig. 15.20). The spread side may generate more pain later in life than the compressed side. The forces of the birth process are literally introduced into the tissues of the occiput. These biokinetic forces, if not resolved, will maintain compressive and torsioned tissue patterns within the inner relationships of the occiput. These intraosseous issues may, in turn, generate autonomic activation, cranial nerve entrapment neuropathy, and various cranial base patterns.

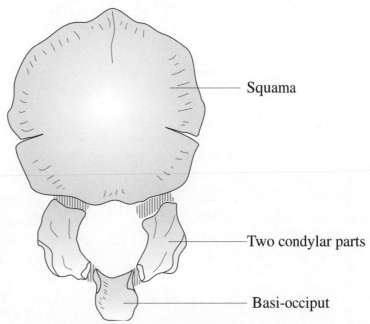

Squama

Two condylar parts

Basi-occiput

15.19 The occiput is in four parts at birth

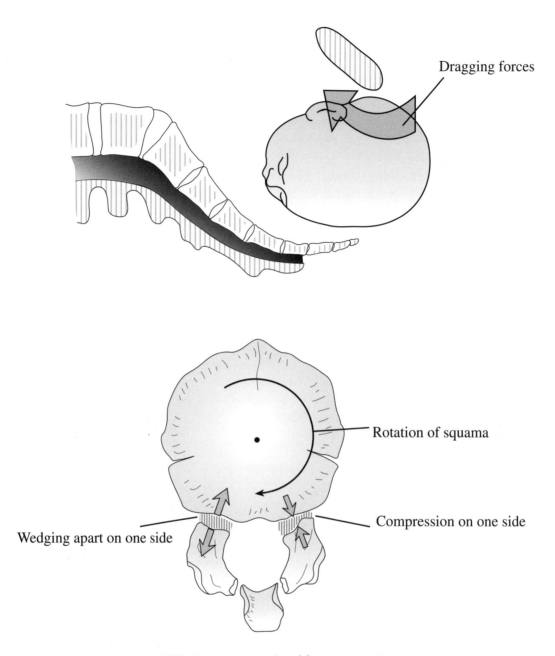

Dragging forces

Rotation of squama

Compression on one side

Wedging apart on one side

15.20 Stage two rotational forces on occiput

Stage Two Intraosseous Distortions of the Occiput

- Rotation of the occipital squama relative to the condylar parts.
- Compression between the squama and condylar part on the non-birth lie side.
- Wedging apart of the squama and the condylar part on the birth lie side.
- Torsioning of the squama, condylar parts and basi-occiput around the foramen magnum.

INTRAOSSEOUS DISTORTIONS OF THE SPHENOID

In Stage Two the infant may also experience forces that generate tensions between the three parts of the sphenoid. The baby may have to pause or may become stuck at any part of the corkscrew descent process, and the forces may press the wings of the sphenoid in opposite directions, generating a torsion effect between the wings and the body. This may also create strain patterns in the reciprocal tension membrane (torsion and shear in the tentorium and falx), the cranial base, and the cerebral hemispheres.

If the infant's head is stuck in a position that generates medial pressures and force vectors from one side of the cranium toward the body of the sphenoid, then the greater wing can become medially compressed into its body as described above. Almost any variation of intraosseous distortion can occur between the greater wing sections and the body of the sphenoid, creating torsioned relationships, vertically or laterally sheared patterns or wedging of the structures in every direction (see Fig. 15.9).

Intraosseous forces in the tissue of the sphenoid bone can give rise to many different cranial base patterns. These are often first interpreted as cranial base issues, but they will more resistant to change than normal if the inertial forces and fulcrums within the sphenoid are not appreciated. The same applies for the other components of the cranial base (the temporal and occiput); intraosseous issues may underlie the apparent cranial base pattern, and need attention before the interosseous and other factors can be resolved.

Intraosseous issues have both physiological and structural repercussions. Intraosseous distortions of the occiput can cause discomfort and contribute to compression of the vagus nerve at its exit through the jugular foramen. These pressures can also affect the spinal accessory nerve and the glossopharyngeal nerve. Symptoms of these effects include digestive disorders, colic, respiratory difficulty, and sucking problems. These problems can persist and manifest in children and adults as a long list of problems, such as respiratory and/or digestive issues, migraine headaches, autonomic dysfunction, learning disorders and even depressive states. I have seen such wide-ranging effects clinically in both infants and adults.

INTRAOSSEOUS DISTORTIONS OF THE TEMPORAL BONE

The temporal bone is subject to the same pressures as its neighbors and can also acquire intraosseous distortions in Stage Two. These may be new at this stage, or they may be a continuation of the medial pressures described in Stage One. But Stage Two places special rotational pressure on the inner relationships of the petrous portion. The intraosseous forces present, and the resulting compression/torsion pattern within temporal bone, can generate symptoms for a long time. Intraosseous distortions of the temporal bone can manifest later as "glue ear," ear infections, tinnitus, and learning disorders (Fig. 15.21).

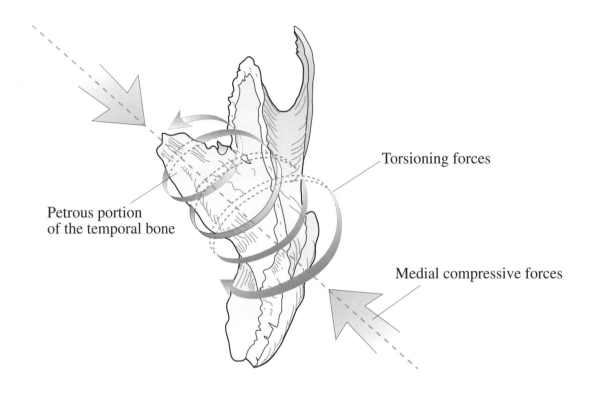

15.21 Compressive and torsioning forces placed upon the temporal bone

Stage Two Intraosseous Distortions of the Temporal Bone

- Medial compression within the petrous portion of the temporal bone.
- Compression and torsion issues within the petrous portion.
- Inertial patterns between the petrous portion and the squama of the temporal bone.

BODY PATTERNS IN STAGE TWO

Forces at work in Stage Two can also affect the whole body, similar to the patterns described in Stage One. The strong downward pressure continues to compress the vertebral axis, particularly the cervical area. Meanwhile the rotational component adds to the picture. The head turns while the body is relatively fixed, yielding torsion patterns in general and torsion of the spine, dural tube, and pelvis in particular. Dural torsion may become coupled with vertebral torsion, pelvic compensations, cranial base patterns, and rotational patterns throughout the body. Stage Two torsion can also contribute to adhesions of the dural tube to the inner walls of the spinal column and to a torsioning of the denticulate ligaments within the dural canal. The respiratory diaphragm can also reflect the torsion pattern by tensing, leading to a host of secondary symptoms including shallow breath, tight chest, and general inflexibility. I have seen this as a common finding when working with infants and adults alike.

<table>
<tr><td colspan="2" align="center">

Summary of Stage Two Mid-Pelvic Dynamics

</td></tr>
<tr><td>

Summary of motion (Figs. 15.16, 15.22)

Cranial Patterns

Infant's head is engaged in the pelvic inlet and must rotate toward the sacrum to enter the anterior-posterior diameter of the pelvic outlet (see Figs. 15.16, 15.17, 15.18, 15.20).

</td><td>

Cranial and whole-body impacts

- Cranial torsion patterns on the side opposite the birth lie side.
- Right side-bending.
- Right torsion.
- Right lateral shear.
- Intraosseous distortions of the temporal bone, occiput and sphenoid.
- Torsion patterns across the foramen magnum and condylar parts, sphenoid-maxillary torsion, and TMJ compression.

</td></tr>
<tr><td>

Body Patterns

Torsional and rotational forces are placed on the infant's body.

</td><td>

- Dural rotations.
- Cervical compressions, rotations and side-bending.
- Pelvic torsions and shear.
- Vertebral rotations.
- Respiratory diaphragm torsions.
- Whole body torsions.

</td></tr>
</table>

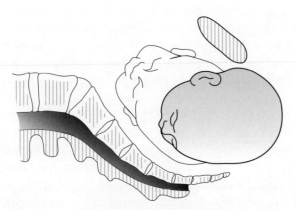

15.22 Stage two motions

STAGE THREE: PELVIC OUTLET DYNAMICS

At the end of Stage Two, the infant's head has rotated toward its left shoulder and her face is pressed against the maternal sacrum, chin pushed toward the neck. The cervical area is compressed and torsioned though the body does not generally rotate very much. The baby is now in a position to descend through the pelvic outlet. Infants must negotiate their way around a ninety-degree angle at the pubic symphysis while their face is being dragged across the maternal sacrum and coccyx. Stage Three has two basic phases. In early Stage Three, the infant's head is in anatomical flexion. In late Stage Three, the infant's head moves into extension as it descends around the pubic arch (Fig. 15.23).

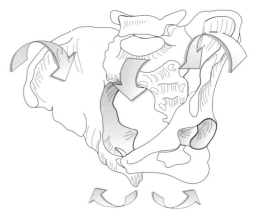

15.24 Nutation of the maternal pelvis

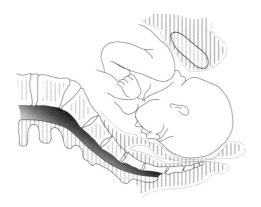

Early stage three: infant's head is in flexion towards the sacrum

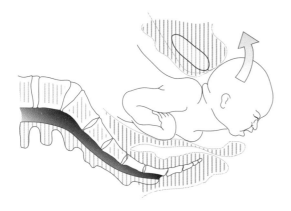

Late stage three: infant's head descends into extension to move around the pubic arch

15.23 Basic movements in stage three

Meanwhile the mother's pelvis is shifting into nutation at this time with the iliac crests moving closer together and the ischial tuberosities moving wider apart. This helps the infant in its Stage Three descent as the pelvic outlet widens and opens to its motions (Fig. 15.24).

EARLY STAGE THREE: FLEXION PHASE

In early Stage Three, the infant's head is in anatomical lateral flexion. Her head is oriented in an anterior-posterior position in mom's pelvis, with her frontal bone conjunct with the mother's sacrum and the occiput conjunct with the mother's pubic bone. The compressive forces and pressures are mainly anterior-posterior in orientation. The conjunct pressures of the mother's sacrum on the frontal area tend to drag the greater wings of the sphenoid into a flexion position and may also force the frontal area to bulge out. Meanwhile the pressure on the occiput from the pubic arch tends to hold the occiput in extension. The sphenoid will be forced into relative flexion, while the occiput is in relative extension, a position counter to their natural dynamics (Fig. 15.25). This is the source of the superior vertical shear pattern as described in Chapter 8. This will occur if the infant was stuck in this position for a period of time and if the forces involved could not be processed at the time or immediately thereafter. In this case the baby has a distinctive bulge at the frontal area.

During the whole of Stage Three, anterior-posterior pressures can also feed compression into the sphenobasilar junction and the occipital base. Thus, cranial base compressions can arise here. The falx can also go into a protective contraction, and the SBJ tends to be held in a flexion pattern.

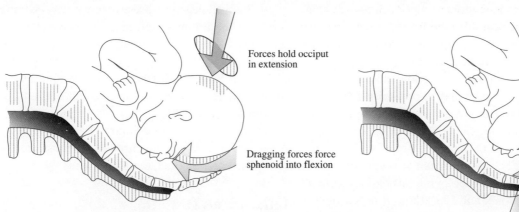

Forces hold occiput
in extension

Dragging forces force
sphenoid into flexion

15.25 The generation of superior vertical shear

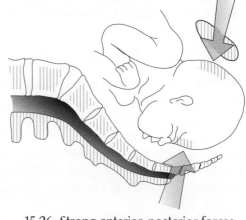

15.26 Strong anterior–posterior forces
in stage three

As early Stage Three continues, the conjunct point against the occiput moves toward the foramen magnum and creates a moving fulcrum from the upper occipital squama toward the foramen magnum. The occipital base can become extremely compressed because of these pressures. If the infant becomes stuck at any point, the moving fulcrum of the pubic symphysis on the occiput can become a fixed fulcrum, introducing a force vector affecting the occipital base, the cervical area generally, the O/A junction, and the Occiput/C1/C2 relationship. The forces involved can also impact the dynamics of C7 and T1 and the upper thoracic vertebrae (Fig. 15.26).

LATE STAGE THREE: EXTENSION PHASE

As the infant's head moves around the mother's pubic bone, the conjunct site becomes the occiput and foramen magnum. This signals the arrival of late Stage Three and anatomical extension (lengthening and narrowing). This can be a reversal of the paradoxical pressure experienced in early Stage Three, as the sphenoid bone is now held in relative extension while the occiput is held in relative flexion because of the pressure against the pubic bone. This can give rise to an inferior vertical shear pattern. This situation is indicated by the distinctive ski slope look at the frontal area at birth (Fig. 15.27).

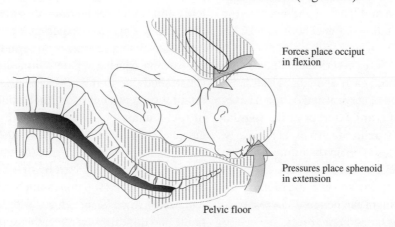

Forces place occiput
in flexion

Pressures place sphenoid
in extension

Pelvic floor

15.27 The generation of inferior vertical shear

Meanwhile the anterior-posterior pressures continue, with the frontal bone flattened against the sacrum and coccyx. Compressive force is applied directly to the two parts of the frontal bone, but also impacts the sphenobasilar junction and the occipital base. The infant's vomer may be pressed into the body of the sphenoid. This is a relatively common inertial issue: thumb-sucking can be a natural self-corrective attempt to alleviate the discomfort of sphenoid-vomer compression. These forces can also generate contraction and compression in the falx and tentorium, the ethmoid bone, and the ethmoid notch of the frontal bone.

The mandible, sphenoid-maxillary relationships and TMJ are also affected by the birthing forces of Stage Three. The pressure of the face against the sacrum and pelvic floor can travel through the mandible into the TMJ, affecting one or both sides. The same pressure on the face can push the maxillae firmly into the palatines and the pterygoid processes of the sphenoid bone.

BODY PATTERNS

During Stage Three compressive forces are introduced commonly into the O/A junction, occipital triad, cervical area generally, upper thoracic area, and lumbosacral junction. The C/D junction (C7 and T1), and T2-T3 are particularly vulnerable to compressive forces at this time. These forces can later generate vertebral compression and fixation and become the basis for possible facilitation of spinal nerves and CNS function.

The downward pressures described in Stages One and Two continue in both early and late phases here, so the earlier discussion of cervical and occipital issues (i.e., impingement of cranial nerves at the jugular foramina) is equally true in Stage Three. Similarly, the dural tube issues described in the prior stages are equally possible here. The dura may lose elasticity and thicken, thin, or dry out, and become taut. Again, the respiratory diaphragm can be tensed in response to the compressive and torsioning forces.

In any birth stage, compressive forces may be transferred to the infant's sacrum, sacroiliac joints, and lumbosacral junction. Intraosseous distortions of the sacrum are common. If the sacrum is fixed in its articulations or holds intraosseous forces, the motility of the central nervous system can be compromised. The sacrum will not be able to express its natural rising in the inhalation phase of primary respiration, and a dragging force may be generated and transferred to the spinal cord via the lamina terminalis.

Intraosseous Distortions of the Occiput

Stage Three can deeply affect the occiput due to a phenomenon known as *telescoping* in which the occipital squama is so firmly pushed against the condylar parts that it wedges them apart and moves them anterior. They in turn press against the basilar part and the body of the sphenoid, and all of these structures telescope together in compression. Telescoping is another type of intraosseous distortion of the occiput. The axis can also become involved due to the ligamentous continuity between the occiput, C1, and C2, becoming wedged between the condylar parts of the occiput. Telescoping may produce a range of symptoms, from simple discomfort to cranial nerve entrapment and autonomic issues as described in our previous chapter. Resultant issues may include sucking problems, respiratory problems, digestive problems, and even later learning disorders.

The infant may also experience a "shelving" of the occipital squama relative to the condylar parts. Here the squama, which is separate from the condylar parts, is flattened due to the pressures encountered as the infant moves around its mother's pubic arch. A part of the squama becomes flattened and an angular indented shape is created instead of the normal smooth curve. At the level of inion and the transverse sinuses, as the squama is stabilized by these structures, a literal folding of the squama at inion may result. Strain patterns will then be introduced within the dural membrane and this can even affect the central nervous system (Fig. 15.28).

Stage Three Intraosseous Distortions of the Occiput and Cranial Base

- Telescoping and wedging together of the axis, atlas, occipital squama, occipital condyles, basi-occiput, SBJ and body of the sphenoid bone

- Forming of an internal shelf on the occipital squama.

Intraosseous Distortions of the Sphenoid

In early Stage Three, a superior vertical shear pattern may be generated within the sphenoid bone itself. If compression is present between the body of the sphenoid and the occiput, the sphenoid's body will follow the occiput. In this case, while the greater wings of the sphenoid may be forced into a flexion position by

the pressures from the frontal bone, the body can be forced into a relative extension position by the occiput. This is more likely to happen if there is a telescoping of structures as described above. The infant may then be left with a superior vertical shear pattern whose fulcrum is within the sphenoid itself.

Likewise, in late Stage Three an inferior vertical shear pattern within the sphenoid bone may be generated. In this case, while the greater wing portions are forced into an extension position by the pressures from the frontal bone, the body of the sphenoid is forced into a flexion position by the occiput. An inferior vertical shear pattern is generated with its fulcrum within the sphenoid itself.

Alternatively, almost any kind of intraosseous pattern within the sphenoid bone may be generated. The most common kinds are shearing patterns between the sphenoid's greater wing sections and its body. The greater wing sections may shear superiorly or inferiorly relative to its body, dependent on the inertial forces present (see Fig. 15.9).

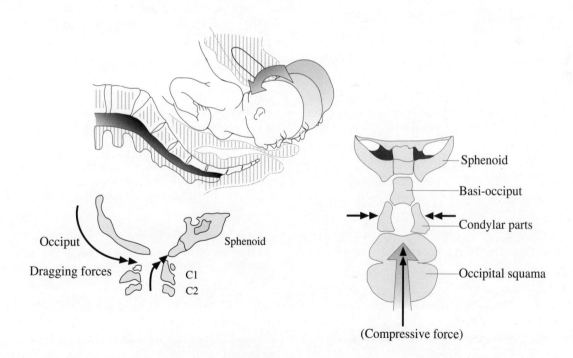

15.28 Intraosseous telescoping of occipital base structures

Summary of Stage Three Pelvic Outlet Dynamics

Summary of motion (Fig. 15.23)	Cranial and whole–body impacts
Cranial Patterns, Early Flexion Phase A-P descent in the flexion position; face is conjunct with the sacrum; occiput is conjunct with the pubic symphysis. (Figs. 15.23, 15.25, 15.26)	• Superior vertical shear, flexion patterns. • Compression at the SBJ. • Compression at the occipital base and through the falx. • A-P compression in cranium. • Ethmoid compression in ethmoid notch of the frontal and in glabella area. • Vomer-sphenoid compression. • Vomer-maxillary compression.
Cranial Patterns, Late Extension Phase A-P descent in extension, cranium rotates around the pubic arch (Fig. 15.27).	• Inferior vertical shear. • Flexion or extension patterns. • Compression at cranial and occipital base. • A-P compression through falx. • Intraosseous distortion of occiput that telescopes the squama, condylar parts, basilar part, body of sphenoid and C1 and cervical structures. • O/A and O/C1/C2 compressions. • TMJ compression. • Flattening of frontal bone. • Shelving of frontal bone. • Shelving of occipital squama. • Compression of ethmoid into the ethmoid notch and sphenoid. • Compression of the vomer into the body of the sphenoid.
Body Patterns, Both Phases	• Continued compression through the body yields occipito-atlas and axis compression, and cervical and upper thoracic (C7, T1, T2, T3) compression. • Sacroiliac and lumbosacral compression and torsion of the sacrum within the ilea. • Compression in respiratory diaphragm, dural tube, and ribs.

STAGE FOUR: HEAD BIRTH, RESTITUTION, BODY BIRTH, AND BONDING

The baby's head is born at the end of Stage Three, signaling the beginning of Stage Four. Relieved of pressure, the infant's cranium springs open in an expansive process. Ideally any birthing forces present are resolved and the infant's cranial structures remold and orient to the midline and Sutherland's fulcrum. However, during head birth intracranial pressures are dramatically lessened, and the sudden change may elicit a protective response in fluids and tissues. The sudden change in pressure can even invoke a shock response, and this may later generate dural tension and fluid congestion. This can further affect the motility of the central nervous system and the fluid drive of primary respiration, and it can impact the ignition process (introduced in Chapter 3 and explored in more detail below).

The process of *restitution* occurs next. In restitution, the infant's head rotates and realigns with the rest of the body. If the midwife or doctor forces restitution, a strain can be fed into the cervical area or can reinforce compression and strain patterns already held in the cervical vertebra. Dural torsion can also be exacerbated (Fig. 15.29).

Birthing the body involves several events. First, the anterior shoulder must be born. In our current left-side case, the right shoulder is anterior and is conjunct with the mother's pubic symphysis. The infant's

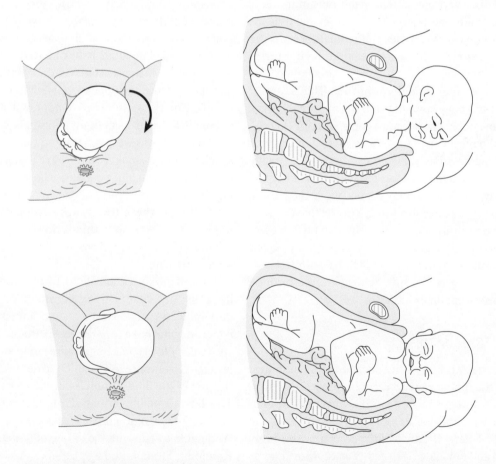

15.29 Restitution: the head rotates to the natural position relative to the shoulder

shoulder may become stuck at the pubis, and the forces involved can generate a low shoulder on the side opposite to the birth lie side. Midwives and doctors often try to help here by pulling the baby's head posteriorly, to help the infant's shoulder clear the pubis. The forces applied can yield shoulder strains, sprains and even cervical damage, usually on the side opposite the birth lie side. Clavicle fractures can also occur. Other interventions here can also be problematic. Strong contact attempting to help the movement may generate forces leading to an internal rotation of the shoulder. Lifting via the armpit can generate rotator cuff strain. Other strain patterns that can arise due to intervention at this point include rib head strains and shoulder muscle damage. Castellino has noted an adult condition that he terms "pseudo cervical disc syndrome."[7] The symptoms mimic cervical disc syndrome, but on investigation the discs are not pathological. When these individuals process the original traumatic forces generated during birth, marked improvements in symptoms are gained.

Next, the other shoulder is birthed. The posterior shoulder has been conjunct with the maternal coccyx and perineal floor; now it must come anterior (in relation to the mother). Patterns may arise that are similar to those described above, but here they are usually less intense, and they are located on the birth lie side.

Finally, the infant's body comes out. If the baby is pulled out with excessive force, a protective contraction can occur throughout the body, and further compression, rotation, and torsion patterns may be fed into the infant's system. A compressive pattern yielding a "C" curve on the side opposite to the birth lie side is also sometimes induced.

Umbilical Issues

Now the baby is born, still attached by the umbilical cord. If the umbilical cord is cut before it stops pulsing, it may be experienced as very shocking. The connection with mother is suddenly ended, and the pulsing of her blood within the cord is suddenly stopped and not allowed to gently cease. Most importantly, when the cord is suddenly cut, the baby's system is not given an opportunity to adjust to its new relationship with its mother.

When the umbilicus stops pulsing and the first breath is taken, there is a natural ignition of potency within the cerebrospinal fluid. This manifests as a strong ascending expression of potency within the fluid midline. This key event is centered in the third ventricle. The Breath of Life infuses the fluids of the newly-born living system with intelligence as the baby becomes a more independent being in its new world. If this ignition is only partial, low vitality and lethargy may result in later life. Vitality issues may even arise in early childhood. Issues of low ignition are commonly generated by birth trauma and fluid shock affect. Anesthesia in the infant's system is also a common origin of partial ignition, evidenced by a dampened fluid tide with sub-optimum drive. Respiratory issues such as breathing difficulties and asthma have been noted by practitioners in relation to this type of trauma, as have digestive and eliminative issues. I have treated a number of adult colitis cases that had their origin in umbilical shock. Once the shock resolved, the system was relieved of the colitis. See Chapter 3 for a more detailed clinical discussion of ignition issues.

If the cord was wrapped around the infant's neck, specific patterns may result. I have experienced this kind of trauma in adult patients who experience feelings of suffocation, umbilical tension, and solar plexus activation as these forces are accessed. Here it is important to help slow things down and to make a relationship to the umbilicus and the forces and shock affects present.

Umbilical shock can lead to umbilical affects, including low vitality, tissue contraction, poor sense of empowerment, low esteem, and lumbar vertebral issues, to name but a few. The tissue around the umbilicus (solar plexus and diaphragm) may contract in a protective response. As mentioned above, low potentization of the fluid system is another possible result. This has two major origins. One relates to interference with the ignition process as previously discussed. Another has to do with the nature of umbilical energy. Randolph Stone noted a spiral-like pulsation which naturally arises from the umbilicus upon birth. This is easily palpated within the space above the umbilicus. When the cord is cut too soon, it as though the infant has had to draw this umbilical energy inward in order to survive. This sense of umbilical *implosion* can be very palpable in session work. Later on, a sense of low motivation or powerlessness in life may result.

If umbilical shock arises during a session, you may see the infant or adult spasm around the umbilicus and solar plexus area. Autonomic and emotional responses such as hyperarousal and fear may arise. Again, it is important to slow things down, reassure the infant or adult with your voice and contact, and help process the forces present. The obvious preference is to avoid these issues in the first place by allowing the infant's umbilicus to stop pulsating naturally as the baby is brought into contact with the mother. There is no medical justification for the practice of immediate cord-cutting that is so prevalent today.

BONDING

Bonding is also part of Stage Four dynamics. Mother and baby need time and space to establish their new relationship and move from direct connection to separation. Successful bonding is essential to autonomic nervous system strength, and interrupted bonding can be perceived by the baby as a direct threat to survival, with potentially devastating consequences.

Changing birthing practices to actively encourage bonding may be one of the most significant reforms available in support of large-scale public wellness, because the autonomic nervous system plays such a large factor in health. Letting baby and mom rest together undisturbed and skin-to-skin for 20 minutes after delivery gives the natural bonding impulses a chance for fulfillment.

Self-attachment is a relatively new concept relating to bonding, arising from Scandinavian research. A newborn baby placed on mom's belly with a gentle supportive contact from mom will naturally move to the breast on its own, and doing this successfully seems to have repercussions for later life. Infants who can successfully self-attach have fewer medical complications and seem to be able to mobilize themselves to get what they need in later life. In contrast, babies who experienced anesthesia or shock lie passively on mom's stomach with little sense of orientation and no capacity for self-propulsion to the breast, and these babies show lower powers of motivation later in life.

Bonding is considered to occur over a month-long period, but really continues to mature for at least the first fifteen months of life. This period is called the *attachment period,* where the infant learns to moderate its needs and emotional life in relationship to its contact with mom and early caretakers. It is an important period of neural maturation.

Stage Four Head Birth, Restitution and Body Birth	
Summary of motion (Fig. 15.29)	**Cranial and whole-body impacts**
Head Birth Cranium is born through the pelvic outlet.	Cranial expansion—possible shock affects expressed in dura and fluids.
Restitution Head realigns with the body.	Cervical sprains, strains. Dural torsion.
Body Birth Body is born, anterior shoulder first.	Shoulder strain, sprain. Clavicle damage. Pseudo cervical disc syndrome. Umbilical trauma, umbilical affects generated, bonding issues.

PELVIC SHAPES AND ALTERNATIVE BIRTHING MOTIONS

The Anthropoid Pelvic Shape

The birthing dynamics within an anthropoid pelvis can be subtly different from those within a gynecoid pelvis shape. As you may remember, the anthropoid pelvis is oval shaped. It not uncommon for a baby to enter an anthropoid-shaped pelvis in a posterior position. She may remain in that position throughout the birth. Births may be slow, yet paced to the baby's needs. Cranial base patterns tend to favor extension patterns with medial compressive issues and medial intraosseous forces introduced into the dynamics of the occiput, temporal bones, and sphenoid bone. The most common intraosseous occipital distortion is the telescoping of structures described above. These relate to the anterior-posterior forces introduced throughout much of the posterior birthing process.

If the mother's pelvis is ample in size relative to baby's head, then a number of other dynamics may arise. Here, the infant may start out posterior, and begin a long slow rotation right though the end of Stage Two and there may even be some rotation in Stage Three. In other words, the rotation begins very early and can continue for much of the birth. Here, there may be a long rotational descent right from the very beginning. Other dynamics are also common. Again, if the mother's pelvis is ample, the baby may engage in almost any position. Posterior positions are common, but the infant may engage in an oblique position and begin a long slow rotation to the occiput anterior (OA) position at the beginning of Stage Three. Again there may even be rotation within Stage Three. The baby's head may even continue to rotate within the pelvic outlet in such a way that its head passes the midline in rotation. I have known one case where this confused the obstetrician, and he rotated the baby's head the wrong way as it came out of the birth canal. Strong torsional forces were introduced into the baby's system which took a number of sessions to resolve. There was much shock related to this incident, and the baby was very angry about it. This expressed itself as sleeplessness, poor feeding, and angry cries. The infant would, at the tender age of one week, hit mom's breast with its little fists in protest. It interfered with the bonding process and was a great tension for all concerned. Happily, the forces resolved, baby was able to reassociate and tell its story to mom. Contact and bonding occurred, and it was a very touching process to witness.

Let's briefly describe some typical cranial repercussions for a baby who has negotiated its way through an anthropoid pelvis. A long, slow birth with much rotation is common. Rotational forces are introduced relatively high up on the baby's cranium and descend in an arc from the parietal bone to the mandible. The rotational forces can be strong and can last longer than those of a gynecoid-pelvis birth. These forces can lead to strong rotation and torsioning within the reciprocal tension membrane, and the membranous-osseous system in general, in both baby and adult. Torsional issues within the cranial base, temporal bones, sphenoid bone, maxillae, and TMJs are common (Fig. 15.30).

The Android Pelvis Shape

The android pelvic shape can lead to very intense birthing processes. The android pelvis is triangular in shape and the pelvic yoke is very narrow. This leads to both a tight pelvic inlet and outlet within which intense forces may be generated. In Stage One, the infant may find it difficult to find an entry point into the inlet. The triangular shape can be very tight here. She may actually take a long time finding a way in. In this period, the infant's head may rotate back and forth against the pelvic inlet until engagement occurs. This can lead to rotational forces introduced high within the baby's cranium. Unlike the anthropoid pelvis, where the infant may descend in rotation right from the beginning, here the infant is not descending. Her head rotates back and forth, and a high, circular-like force is generated within the membrane. I have treated adults who had a feeling like they were wearing a very tight skull cap located relatively high up on their heads. There were strong rotational forces

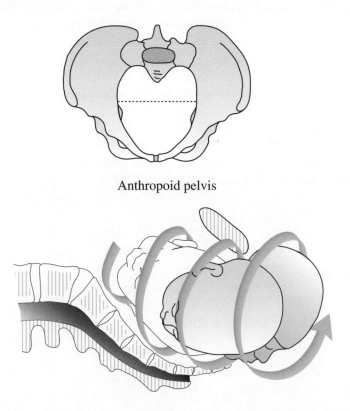

Anthropoid pelvis

15.30 The anthropoid pelvis: there is commonly much rotation through an anthropoid pelvis

within their membrane system and a sense of tor-sioning and twisting throughout the cranium. The origin of this pattern was found within Stage One of birth process as they tried to enter their mother's android-shaped pelvis. Here, unlike Stage One of a gynecoid pelvis, there is rotation right at the beginning of Stage One and it is located high up on the head in a circular pattern.

After the rotation process described above, once a way into the pelvic inlet is found, the baby commonly enters the pelvis in an oblique or transverse position. Due to the triangular pelvic shape, an oblique engagement is the most common. As the baby enters the pelvic inlet, since the android pelvis is triangular and narrow, triangular force vectors are commonly introduced into the cranium. This is because the baby's head meets three points of contact: both pelvic bones

and the sacrum. The practitioner may perceive sometimes confusing force vectors which seem to bounce off first one side of the cranium and then the other in a triangular manner. As the baby descends, it must literally lever over the sacrum to enter a synclitic position, and this can lead to very strong forces introduced into the cranium. One colleague of mine calls this a "can opener" effect. I'm not sure that I like the image, but the forces introduced by the conjunct sacrum within Stage One can be extremely intense. Strong cranial base patterns, such as side-bending, torsion, and lateral shear, can be generated here, as can intra-osseous distortions of the temporal bones, sphenoid, and occiput.

In a android pelvic shape, there is commonly not very much rotation in Stage Two. This is different from that of the gynecoid or anthropoid pelvis in which there is rotational descent in Stage Two. Here, due to the tightness of the android pelvis, the baby's head may not rotate very much, and strong medial compressive forces may be fed into the cranium. Extension patterns are commonly introduced both here and in Stage One. The baby may remain in a oblique position all the way to the pelvic floor and outlet. Its head may then very quickly rotate so that it faces the sacrum, or may remain oblique throughout Stage Three. The pelvic yoke is very narrow, and strong forces are commonly introduced in Stage Three as the infant negotiates its way under the pelvic arch. A tight android pelvis is a very difficult pelvis to be born through. This can lead to variable forces entering the cranium, depending on the position and the length of time in that position. If the infant rotates its face to the sacrum, strong vertical shear patterns are commonly generated. Intraosseous distortions of both the occiput and sphenoid bone are also commonly introduced here. Cesarean births, either planned or elected, are not uncommon due to this tight pelvic shape (Fig. 15.31).

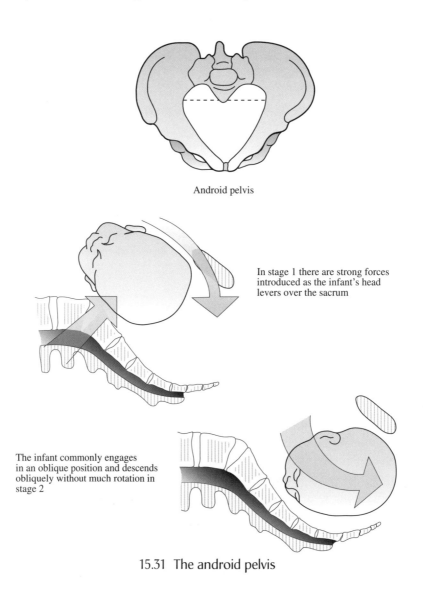

Android pelvis

In stage 1 there are strong forces introduced as the infant's head levers over the sacrum

The infant commonly engages in an oblique position and descends obliquely without much rotation in stage 2

15.31 The android pelvis

The Platypelloid Pelvic Shape

The platypelloid pelvic shape is the most difficult shape to be born through. Platypelloid means *plate-like*. This pelvic shape is transversely long and very tight. This is the kind of pelvic type in which, in earlier days, mother and baby may have died during the birthing process. Elected cesareans are the norm here. Fortunately, a pure platypelloid pelvis is relatively rare. Something like five percent of the female population has this kind of pelvic shape. If the baby births through the tightly transverse pelvis, she will enter the pelvic inlet in a transverse position and will remain in that position throughout the birth. This leads to extraordinarily strong transverse forces being introduced into the baby's head. Extension patterns are the norm. The sacrum becomes a very strong conjunct site and side-bending, torsion, and lateral shear patterns, all to the non-birth lie side, are all coupled together. Medial compressive issues in the cranial base and intraosseous distortions of the temporal bone are also common here. The adult may have a strong extension look to their face, with a "C" curve that bulges towards the non-birth lie side. I have heard this ignobly called a banana face (Fig. 15.32).

I hope that this chapter served to introduce and clarify some of the cranial issues related to the birthing process. Have patience. It may need a few read

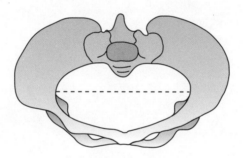

Platypelloid pelvis

The infant descends and births in a transverse position with little or rotation

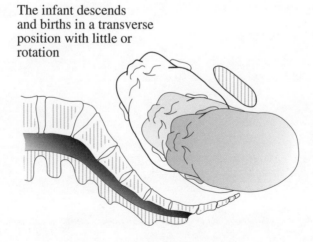

15.32 The platypelloid pelvis

throughs, as it may be difficult to imagine these motions. You may want to buy a soft pelvic model and properly scaled baby model to take the "baby" through these motions. *Childbirth Graphics* sells excellent soft models for this purpose. See the Resource section for their address.

1. Harry Oxorn, *Oxorn-Foote Human Labor and Birth,* 5th ed. (McGraw-Hill, 1986).

2. Such courses are offered at Karuna Institute, and also by Raymond Castellino, as well as Claire Dolby, D.O., and Katherine Ukleja, D.O.

3. Oxorn, op. cit., 34.

4. This is not the conventional obstetrical usage of the phrase *birth lie*.

5. Alternatively, in a synclitic engagement, there can be strong transverse forces medially compressing the infant's cranium at the parietal areas. This depends on the size of the mother's pelvis and the infant's head. If the pelvis is relatively small, both parietal eminences receive strong pressure. Sometimes the mother's pelvis is shaped in such a way that the baby has to enter in an anterior asynclitic position. This is rare and is considered abnormal. In a left birth lie with anterior asynclitism, the infant's right parietal bone is anterior and is lower than the left one in the pelvic inlet. Thus, the right parietal bone is conjunct with the pubic symphysis and will initially receive much more pressure than the left one (see Chapter 14, Fig. 14.6).

6. See Stanislov Grof, *Realms of the Human Unconscious* (Souvenir Press, 1975), and the *Holotrophic Mind* (Harper Collins, 1990).

7. From discussions with Raymond Castellino.

16

Treating Infants and Intraosseous Issues in Adults

In this chapter I would like to introduce clinical approaches to infant and adult birth issues, starting with meeting the infant and recognizing their sentience and presence and moving to working with adults' intraosseous issues that often originate in the birthing process. I always advise new practitioners, if they are interested in working with babies, to be supervised by a senior practitioner who has experience in this area. Supervised clinics are another avenue. I find that infants place me on the cutting edge of my knowledge and personal process, and a gradual approach to working with them builds confidence and allows the sessions to be a resource for all concerned, including the practitioner.

In this chapter we will discuss:

- *The treatment of infants.*
- *Special birth situations, including cesarean births and vacuum extraction.*
- *Intraosseous distortions in the adult.*

GENERAL GUIDELINES FOR TREATING INFANTS

The foundation of care for infants is recognition that they are feeling, sentient beings, as described in Chapter 14. Babies recognize the presence of the practitioner, and contact must be negotiated carefully. The theme is to wait until the baby invites us to make contact. In many hospital births, babies have experienced being handled as unfeeling objects, with little recognition of their awareness or choice. So if practitioners behave in a similar manner, we may evoke similar expectations, including fear and anger.

This is especially true for traumatized infants. With initial sessions we may not even be able to touch the cranium at all. Instead, we may have to use Emerson's *far touch* by slowly meeting their biosphere energetically with touch and presence. Until it is clear that the baby is inviting us to actually touch, we can work off the body using intention and proximity. Remote touch of this nature can be quite effective in all kinds of situations, including the processing of force vectors.

Because babies are conscious, sentient beings, do not talk over them as though they are not there. They recognize this and may become distrustful. Instead, include them in the conversations with mom and dad. They gradually can come to recognize you as a person who respects their presence and listens to their communications.

In working with infants, respect their relationship with mom. Mom is ideally their major resource. Babies' use of their mothers as a resource is usually quite evident. They will turn their heads to watch mom, follow her voice and continually monitor her presence. The baby *resources itself* by seeking the most comfortable position and most secure relationship. For most babies this means turning to the lie side and being in close visual, auditory, and physical contact with the mother. In working with babies, we try to observe how the baby resources, and then fit in or synchronize with those behaviors. Practitioners try to work within the range and nature of the baby's resources and find that they may begin to sense the practitioner as another resource over the course of a few sessions.

Infants will most clearly express the mid-tide and Long Tide rather than the CRI. The Long Tide is very much within their presence. A baby's sutures are not yet formed, the fontanels are large, and the cranium is basically a fluidic-membranous system. An appropriately light touch is used, as we patiently offer states of balance, stillness, space, direction of fluid, and disengagement of compressive forces. Access the Long Tide within states of balance. Widen your perceptual field, sense the space around and within the baby's system and be still. Babies really will orient to this most primal level of life force if given the opportunity. In other words, given the opportunity, they will orient to their ordering matrix.

Infants seem to know exactly what I am saying. They are responsive to my voice in clear ways. I know that the nervous system is immature at these early stages of life, yet I also know that they largely understand my intentions and my words. The only time this is not evident is if the infant presents dissociation and parasympathetic shock effects due to the overwhelming nature of their experience. They then cannot orient to me, my intentions, or my words. Gentle EV4s via the sacrum and ignition work are very helpful here.

Babies will directly describe their history and clinical issues through movement, sound, and orienting actions. They may direct us to sites of discomfort or focus, or reenact portions of their birth process. I have had many babies take my hand and place it over the place "where it hurts," or take my hand away if they are not ready for contact where I am touching, or if the contact is too intense or overwhelming. They will show motions relative to their traumatization and related inertial fulcrums. They may express disjointed motion and loss of orientation when they meet the edges of their motion dynamics. Notice these often-subtle expressions and respect them as valid communications as we would naturally do if they were coming from an adult. Hear their sounds, crying, gestures, and facial expressions as communications that are definitely not arbitrary.

Work within the resources of infants and respect their "No" statements. If a baby does not want you to touch in a certain place or manner, respect that. The baby may need to deal with other things first, or may not be resourced enough in your presence, or may simply need time and the space to process first. Listen for how the infant needs to resolve its trauma. Remember that trauma is not just physical. It resonates with every aspect of that baby's being. They may need to express their fear or anger, and/or they may need to resolve some sympathetic or parasympathetic shock affect. Again EV4s are helpful for parasympathetic dissociative shock affects. Stillpoints generally can help resource and slow down sympathetic arousal. Babies may need to come back from a dissociated place and really let you or mom know how bad is was. They will tell you their story. You must negotiate this contact and this work. If they say "No" by pushing your hand away, or by a traumatic activation, back off. Resource them in mom's presence; let them know that they are in control. I always talk to the infant and let them know my intentions verbally. This may seem strange since they can't talk, but I firmly believe that infants understand me. They certainly learn to understand my intentions. This can take time and patience. Be patient. Don't try to do too much in a session. It is important that you like infants and that you like to play. The infant learns that the session is resourcing and that you are fun. Then when difficult edges arise, they will look to you as a resource, not as the cause of their pain.

Various specific issues, inertial fulcrums, force vectors, and compressions will gradually present themselves to your awareness. With babies, I find that the intention of session work is less structural and more about potency. The action of potency within the fluids is very evident. Fluctuations of potency and fluid lead us to specific inertial sites as the treatment plan unfolds. Work may revolve around states of balance, direction of fluid, and the offering of space. Sometimes, simply directing potency and fluid from the sacrum superiorly, particularly during the inhalation surge, can help disengage compressive forces within the cranium. Gently offering space within compressed areas and helping a baby orient to her mother is also helpful.

Working with infants and young children[1] is different from working with adults in that we never take a baby's system into the direction of the compression or motion pattern. A baby's sutures are not yet in place. If we follow a pattern in its preferred direction, there would be no clear boundary for the expression and the infant could be shifted deeper into the pattern, intensifying the trauma. Infants do not differentiate past and present as adults do; they can experience the movement as continuous with the original trauma. Instead, the intention is always to offer space and possibility. Be patient and work slowly. Learn to follow the infant and their unfolding process, appreciating the infant skull as spacious, unformed, and fluidic (Fig. 16.1).

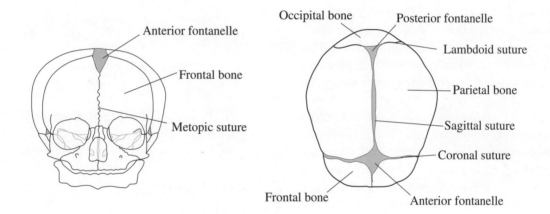

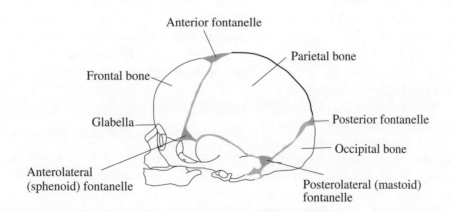

16.1 The fetal skull

Working with babies requires a slower pacing than normal. A slow-motion presence and contact is more effective. Among other factors, the birthing process is often quite a hectic scene with staff members acting quickly and efficiently. A slow deliberate contact can serve as a counterbalance for the baby's impressions of the birth experience.

THE FIELD OF ORIENTATION

I have repeatedly observed that infants have a *field of orientation* arising from unresolved traumatic issues. One direction of motion and orientation will be comforting, while another is difficult. For instance, they may orient more easily to the environment from their birth lie side, where they are familiar with contact. If mom is on this side, they may access her as a resource more easily. As mom moves to the other side and the baby's head rotates toward the midline, they may begin to lose ease of contact and express disjointed motions and distress. This is perhaps why many babies prefer feeding on one breast more than the other. By noticing the field of orientation and locating ourselves in that area, practitioners can cultivate a trusting relationship. We are making it easier for the baby to relate to us by letting them use their visual, auditory, and kinesthetic senses from their most resourced space.

Similarly, babies may have a *position of orientation*. For example, if they were born in a posterior position, (i.e., occiput posterior throughout the birth process) they may feel most oriented and prefer to lie in this position.

Look for the baby's more oriented side and/or position, or their field of orientation (Fig. 16.2), and initially work from that side or position. In early sessions I always work with the baby being held by the mother. In later sessions the baby could be placed on a mat or pillow, with the mother located nearby in the field of orientation. Gradually, the positioning of the mother becomes less significant as the baby begins to recognize the practitioner as a resource. For example, if the baby orients most easily to the left side, work from that side and have mom within their visual field on that side. Also ask mom to talk to her baby from there so that the baby can orient

to her voice as a resource. Hearing mom's voice can elicit a primal orienting response and evoke feelings of being nurtured.

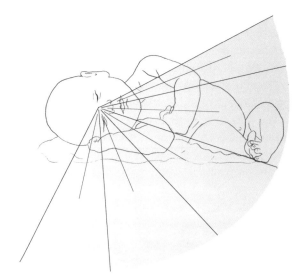

16.2 The infant has a field of orientation

COMMON INERTIAL FULCRUMS AND ISSUES IN INFANTS

A variety of patterns may be observed in babies. These generally relate to the shape of the mother's pelvis, the positioning of the birth process, and medical interventions that were used during birth. The following is a list of common cranial issues that practitioners may sense or observe in newborns and infants.

CRANIAL OVERRIDING AND MOLDING PATTERNS

Overriding refers to the slippage of one cranial bone over the other, instead of their normal abutment positioning. Almost any kind of cranial overriding or molding pattern can result from the forces experienced in birth. Common examples include overriding of parietal bones and of the two parts of the frontal bone. Overriding is not just a matter of bony relationships;

the membranes are also involved. Bones are perceived as denser places in the membranous whole, and the combination works as a unit of function. Treatment of overriding is relatively simple, involving placement of two fingers of the same hand on either side of the relationship involved. For example, if the two parietal bones have overridden at the sagittal suture, place a finger on each bone. Then very gently encourage space and disengagement across the relationship while directing fluid to the site with the other hand at the occiput. It is really a matter of engaging and directing the potency and fluids within the system.

Cranial molding issues generally relate to forces lodged within a particular bone and within the membranous-osseous system as a whole. For instance, a raised aspect within a bone such as a parietal bone may seem to be puckered-up. This is not just a structural or tissue form; it is an energetic expression of the coupling of biodynamic potency and inertial forces. Treatment of molding involves placing the fingers in a circular ring around the puckered area. Very gently spread the area with these fingers as you direct fluid to it, intending space as a means of accessing the intraosseous forces at work within the bone. Another approach is to place a finger, or fingers, directly over the puckered area, gently intending an inward direction while directing fluid to the site. Again, it is a matter of activating the potencies involved. Potency processes the inertial force and helps the membranous-osseous system reorient to natural midline phenomena.

A similar cranial molding pattern has to do with flattened areas. It is not uncommon to observe a flattened parietal or frontal bone resulting from the birthing forces placed against the membranous-osseous system. Again, we approach these with recognition that bones, membranes, and fluids are one continuous unit. For treatment of a flattened area, place the fingers in a circle around the flattened area and direct fluid toward the area as you lightly intend drawing your fingers together. This subtly gathers the tissues together and engages the intraosseous inertial forces. This is really delicate work. Meet the forces at work and access the state of balance as you direct

the fluid to the area. The potency does the work, not the practitioner's finger pressure or intention.

Compressive Issues

All sorts of compressive issues may arise from the unresolved forces of the birthing process. The following is a simple pointer to some of the more common issues, not a comprehensive list of all possibilities.

Sphenoid-Vomer Compression

It is common to find compressive issues between the vomer and the sphenoid bone. In a gynecoid pelvis shape, the forces generating this kind of compression are generally introduced in Stage Three when the baby's face is conjunct with the mother's sacrum. An inertial force between the body of the sphenoid and the vomer may be sensed in any number of ways: a membranous-osseous motion around the area, back-pressure, density and barrier below the sphenoid bone, or lateral fluctuations of fluid and potency around the area. Treatment involves placing an index finger in the infant's mouth. This must be negotiated with extra care, as babies use the mouth as a primary medium for interacting with the environment. I do not like to use finger cots with babies because they generally do not like the taste. There are several ways to work around this problem. We can wash our hands really well with antibacterial soap and then carefully rinse the soap off well, or we can wash the finger cot once it is in place. The cotted finger can also be dipped in mother's milk or a familiar-tasting formula.

An infant often accepts the finger as a sucking reflex and even as a knowing attempt to get relief from the sensation of vomer compression. Relief of vomer compression can be a factor in the impulse for thumb-sucking. Even if your finger is easily accepted, wait before doing anything. Negotiate your intention here; listen and wait for a sense of negotiated contact. When the relationship seems well-established, very gently contact the upper palate with that finger. With your other hand at the top of the infant's head, subtly direct fluid and potency to the sphenoid-vomer interface. As potency builds, gently encourage the vomer caudad with your finger, maintaining contact with the palate and maxillae. Use no force whatsoever, but rather let the fluids and potency do the work. Using force may simply enlist the baby's defensive processes and can even deepen the compression (Fig. 16.3).

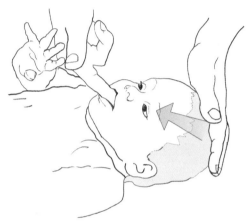

16.3 Directing fluid
to the sphenoid-vomer interface

Occipital Base Compression and Intraosseous Distortions of the Occiput

Occipital base compression and intraosseous distortions of the occiput are common issues in infants, with wide-ranging implications as described above. Patterns include rotation of occipital squama, telescoping, wedging of condylar parts, O/A compression, and a general axial compression throughout the relationships of the occiput and sphenoid.

Occipital base compression affects nearby cranial nerves and can generate many issues including digestive (sucking and feeding, colic and diarrhea) and respiratory (breathing difficulties). The occipital area

can be very sensitive to the newborn and young infant, so all our considerations about careful negotiation and slow pacing apply.

The occipital base spread is a traditional approach to this area. For infants, place the index and middle fingers of one hand at the occipital base's two condylar parts so that the foramen magnum is between them. The other hand is placed on the frontal bone ready to direct fluid. Remember that the occiput is in four parts here. See if you can sense those parts and their interrelationships as part of the whole membranous-osseous-fluid system of the cranium. Very gently spread your two fingers apart, encouraging space across the condylar parts. If a rotation of the squama is present, very subtly intend a de-rotation before the spread. Once a sense of space is accessed, hold the spread and very gently intend the occipital squama posteriorly. We are encouraging a spreading of the condylar parts and a de-telescoping of the occipital parts, the basi-occiput and the body of the sphenoid bone. Do this very subtly; it is a conversation about space, not an attempt to release anything. The intention is to help generate space within the telescoped parts. When space is accessed, let things settle into a state of balance and direct fluid to the area with the hand over the frontal bone. Again, let the potency do the work! The practitioner's role is to simply and intelligently offer space and direct potency to the area (Fig. 16.4).

Temporal-Occipital Issues

The temporal-occipital interface is another common area for inertial issues in babies. This junction will become the occipito-mastoid suture as the baby matures. The approach is similar to the one described above, with the index and middle fingers of one hand now on either side of the temporal-occipital interface. The middle finger is placed on the occipital squama while the index finger is placed on the temporal bone. The other hand is placed on the diagonally opposite frontal bone. After negotiating contact, we again very subtly intend space across the interface by lightly spreading the fingers apart. Place this intention into the baby's tissues as a conversation about space, not as a demand to release anything. Once a state of balance is attained, direct fluid toward the site with your other hand. Wait for the action of potency to take over and for the tissues to naturally spread apart as the inertial force is resolved.

Medial Compression and Intraosseous Temporal Bone Distortion

Intraosseous distortions of the temporal bone are common, as is medial compression of the cranial base. These often arise in the early stages of the birth process, especially in Stages One and Two when the baby experiences medial and rotational forces in the descent past the mother's sacrum. This can affect one side only or both sides. Again, there are a number of traditional approaches to these issues. The simplest approach is to use gentle traction to encour-

age space using the *temporal bone ear hold* described in Volume One.

In an adapted version for babies, lightly hold the baby's ear lobes. Very gently intend a subtle traction forty-five degrees posterior (toward the table if the baby is in the supine position). Do this very gently as a conversation: *no force whatsoever should be applied.* The idea is to transfer this intention of space to the tissues of the temporal bone, especially the petrous area, and to the cranial base generally. Facilitate a state of balance and let the potency do the work.

You can also work with one temporal bone at a time. This is especially useful for unilateral issues and for intraosseous issues within the temporal bone. Hold the temporal bone in the temporal bone ear hold. Place your other hand over the diagonally opposite frontal bone. Again subtly intend traction via your temporal ear hold forty-five degrees posteriorly. Do this as a conversation, a negotiation. Be gentle; the tissues are fluidic. Again the intention is to engage the inner tissues of the temporal bone, especially the petrous area, in a conversation about space. As space is accessed, direct fluid toward the area with your opposite hand on the frontal bone. Again this kind of work must be negotiated with the infant and is accomplished as much by intention as by physical engagement (Fig. 16.5).

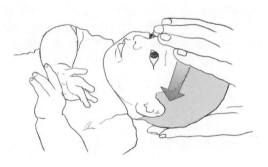

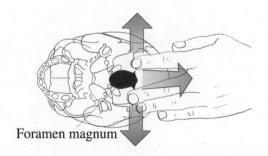

Foramen magnum

16.4 Occipital base spread and fluid direction

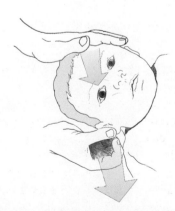

16.5 Temporal ear hold and the direction of fluid

Cranial Base Patterns

Any and all of the classic cranial base patterns may present in the infant due to prenatal and/or birthing process. I find that the most important thing for the practitioner to do is to orient to the pattern and to offer space. Generally, a simple intention to offer disengagement to the SBJ via the greater wings of the sphenoid bone is enough, using the disengagement process discussed in the previous chapter on cranial base patterns.

In a gentle *Becker's hold,* subtly intend the greater wings anterior with your thumbs (that is, toward the ceiling if the baby is supine) (Fig. 16.6). This must be done with ultimate sensitivity. Negotiate your contact and your presence. Do not grab the baby's tissues physically or mentally. Offer this intention as an inquiry into the possibility of space—a conversation about space and potency—and let the potency take over. Access the state of balance and orient to a unified potency-fluid tissue matrix and trust the unerring forces from within. Until you have had an experience of the potency from within doing the healing work, this may sound like a nice metaphor or fairy tale. It is not. It is an essential perceptual experience in this work.

SACRUM AND OCCIPUT

A simple *bipolar hold* can be excellent for babies. Holding and orienting to the two poles of the primary respiratory system can be very healing for the baby. Here we gently hold the baby's sacrum and occiput at the same time (Fig. 16.7). It may be enough to simply hold the two poles and access a state of balance. Alternately, it may be helpful to subtly intend space between the two poles. You might do this via the occiput, via the sacrum or via both structures at once. Let your palpation sense guide you. Gently intend space between the two structures and help access the state of balance. This will engage and help resolve any compressive axial force present within the baby's vertebral midline. As always, appreciate Becker's three-phase awareness and listen for expressions of Health. Let the potency resolve the forces. If an axial compression is present within the vertebral midline, a general lengthening and expansion through the midline may be perceived. Midline axial birthing forces are common in both infants and adults. An alternative approach that sometimes works is to simply intend fluids and potency cephalad from a sacral hold. This may encourage the fluid drive of the system to process the axial forces present and may even alleviate cranial compressions above.

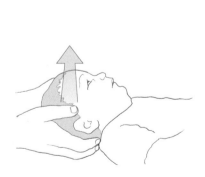

16.6 Disengagement and the SBJ

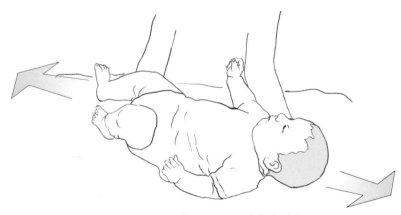

16.7 Intending space while holding
the sacrum and occiput

Other Clinical Issues:

Forceps

The use of forceps to aid delivery has a long and complex history. Forceps are commonly used in urgent situations and are not always ideally applied to the infant's cranium. Many times, too much force is used to pull the infant out, and sometimes the obstetrician simply gets the direction and motion of the infant wrong and places extra forces upon her system, against the existing direction of natural movement.

I have seen diverse baby and adult outcomes relating to the use of forceps, both positive and negative. In some cases the use of forceps undeniably helped alleviate the suffering and pain of both mother and baby. I have even seen cases where the sensitive and gentle use of forceps helped the infant and left no cranial issues whatsoever. However, these seem to be the exception rather than the rule. Common issues that derive from the use of forceps include intraosseous distortions of various bones, tissue damage, compressive forces which leave marks on the baby and generate various inertial issues in the cranium, cranial bone overriding, and the introduction of compressive force vectors into the infant's cranium. While working with adults, I have even seen forceps marks come out on their face as the forces involved were processed.

Cesarean Births

Cesarean births are becoming more and more common. If you see babies in your practice, you will certainly see many infants who have undergone this birthing process. There are two kinds of cesarean births: elective, where the baby was not engaged in the birth canal, and emergency, in which the infant was engaged and may even have been far into its birthing process. Each kind of cesarean birth may generate different issues within the baby's system.

For both kinds of cesarean, the general anesthetic given the mother is also experienced by the baby. Anesthetic shock affects may arise. Anesthesia may generate a parasympathetic response in the baby, inducing a hypoarousal state. This is basically a state of parasympathetic shock. The baby may seem listless or sleep a lot, and she may not be able to orient to her mother, or to her essential needs such as feeding. Difficulties in feeding, dissociation, fluid shock, and poor ignition are possible effects.

I have palpated many cesarean babies whose heads felt solid, almost like a cannon ball. When I first encountered this, I was surprised. What happened to the baby as a fluidic-sac pulsating with potency? Babies' heads are not supposed to feel like cannon balls! I really had to reorient to a new process here. This stasis and solidity is a direct repercussion of the fluid shock held within the core of the system. I found that I really had to orient to the Long Tide, to field phenomena, and to deeper resources. EV4s via the sacrum and gentle intentions of space throughout the system may help free up some of the inertial potency and to process some of the affects of the experience. Ignition is a real issue here, but space must be accessed in the infant's system first.

In the elective cesarean, the baby is generally removed from the mother's uterus before it has entered the pelvic inlet and birth canal. When the surgeon opens up the mother's abdomen and uterus, a very rapid pressure change is experienced by the baby. This can generate fluid shock. The potency within the fluid will become suddenly inertial in order to center the forces induced by the rapid pressure change. This may have strong repercussions for that infant. Fluid stasis results. The fluids lock up as the potency becomes suddenly inertial. This will strongly affect the ignition process at birth. The fluids may not fully ignite within the midline and the third ventricle when the umbilicus stops pulsing and the first breath is taken. See Chapter 3 on the central nervous system for ignition issues and clinical applications.

Another inevitable disadvantage of elective cesarean relates to timing. The baby has a key role to play in the birthing process in that the biochemical stimuli naturally arising to launch the whole process are a mutual product of both baby and mother's whole inner landscape. Elective cesareans are commonly done for the convenience of the mother and the doctor, overriding the baby's role. The whole situation is a reflection of the belief system that babies have little intelligence or feelings, and can be treated as medical objects. Interestingly, the educational literature describing elective cesarean, attempting to be neutral on the topic, makes no mention of the significance of consciousness in birthing, even though this whole area has been well-explored in research. It is a convenient blind spot by which the practice is perpetuated, without informed consent by the parents since the topic was never discussed. Unprepared for the birth and literally not biochemically ready, these babies often show autonomic distress indicators.

In the non-elective, or engaged, cesarean section, usually in an emergency situation, the baby has entered the birth canal. Perhaps the birth has been going on too long, or the obstetrician felt that the birth process may be dangerous to the mother and/or baby if continued much longer. In this case the baby has encountered the forces and timing of a natural birth. The doctor may need to use great force to pull the baby back out of the birth canal.

The practitioner needs to appreciate the nature of the trauma here. The baby has been through an extremely difficult experience. There was a sudden disengagement from the mother and the womb experience. This is true in both kinds of cesarean section. In the case of an engaged cesarean, this disengagement process may have been experienced as a violent wrenching away from the mother and her pelvic canal. Unusual cranial patterns will be generated by the forces of the pull. These are not forces that the system is naturally designed to meet. Natural birthing forces generally drag caudad; they do not pull violently cephalad. This will most likely be shocking to the infant. Shock affects and dissociative processes are the norm here, compounded by the anesthesia used. The baby may be left with a poor sense of boundaries as its boundaries were violated in the process. When born, the infant may not be able to orient to the space around it or to the mother, perhaps for some time after birth. Because of the emergency surgical setting, the baby may have no contact with mom at all for an extended recovery period in separate areas of the hospital. This may generate bonding and feeding issues. Either hyperarousal or hypoarousal states are common.

In emergency cesareans, the sympathetic nervous system is commonly engaged during the birthing process. But the parasympathetic nervous system may also suddenly surge to protect the infant. A coexisting parasympathetic shock response then overlays and masks the initial sympathetic response. After birth, the baby may seem dissociated and listless, yet under that, anger and fight-flight energies are still cycling. In session work, as the parasympathetic shock resolves, the underlying sympathetic cycling may come to the surface. What seemed to be a listless and dissociated baby is suddenly able to express its anger. The baby may also express pushing intentions during sessions, as these were not able to be completed naturally due to anesthesia and the cesarean section. Angry, pushing babies are thus more common in emergency cesareans, where the birth process was engaged but then interrupted. I always explain these possibilities to parents as they may blame me as practitioner, or the sessions, for their baby's anger. After all, they may have come with a placid baby who is now very angry. They need to be able to hear the anger of their infant, respond with reassurance and contact, and not take it personally.

In elected cesareans, pure parasympathetic shock is more common, as the baby's system was rapidly overwhelmed by the experience. The infant's system may be imprinted with the message that a parasympathetic response holds the best chance of survival, setting the stage for later bouts of low motivation, low energy, and chronic fatigue. As described earlier, these children are commonly not identified as needing help because they sleep a lot and are perceived as good, quiet babies. They may later have learning difficulties and poor attention spans due to the parasympathetic shock affects and dissociative processes still cycling in their systems. In these cases, I try to gently orient the infant to the possibility of movement and pushing in order to mobilize a more sympathetic nervous system response. I do this via gentle contact and upward pressure on the bottoms of their feet and the use of a reassuring and encouraging voice.

Clinical Highlight

A number of years ago, I helped set up a free clinic for infants and newborns. We called our clinic the "Whole Family Clinic," because we recognized the powerful fulcrum the baby becomes for the whole family, not just for mothers. We always had at least two practitioners present so that a mother's process could be attended to if her own birth issues arose during the session work with her baby. We also tried to have fathers attend the sessions and we worked with the family dynamics cycling around the baby. The intention of the clinic was especially to cater to young parents and young single mothers who could not afford sessions. The team included myself, a cranially trained obstetrician, and another cranial practitioner.[2] We donated one morning a week to this clinic.

A nineteen-year-old single mother came into our clinic with her two-month-old baby daughter. The father had left her and she was on her own with the infant. She was a strong and bright young woman, but had no current source of income and was on welfare. All of her energies were taken up by her new role as a mom. The baby's delivery had been an emergency cesarean section. She was pulled out after many hours of labor. It had been an exhausting and painful experience for both mother and baby. She brought the baby in because the infant was not sleeping and had a very strong case of colic. The mother also expressed her difficulty in bonding with the baby and in feeling the baby's bonding with her. This is not unusual in cesarean births. We began to see the two of them weekly.

Much was accomplished over the first two months. The colic was greatly reduced and the infant's sleeping began to enter more set patterns so that her mother had more space and more sleep for herself. Work initially revolved around a gentle negotiation of contact with the baby, as she was very traumatized by her experience. Initially it was hard to touch the infant without eliciting a fight or flight response. Her typical response was to turn her head away, cry, and go into dissociation. Babies cry for all sorts of reasons. Mostly it is to communicate something to you. I don't mind babies crying in sessions—it is part of the process—but not if they dissociate. Working while babies are dissociated can drive their trauma deeper. So initially it was a slow process of negotiating contact and short periods of hands-on clinical work. It was important for us to become a clearly felt resource for both mom and baby. This occurred over time. The infant became easy in our presence and accepted gentle contact for longer periods. It is patient work. Mom, in turn, was able to talk about her predicament. The sessions became a resource for her also. As time went on some of the traumatic vectors within the infant's system, and their related tissue affects, were processed. There were also sessions devoted to the processing of her shock affects that were expressed as fear, crying and dissociation. We had to help her slowly process all of this. Yet there was still something between mom and baby. The bonding had never really happened, and mom was acutely aware of this.

In one session, when the baby was about five months old, an extraordinary process ensued. We were attending to an intraosseous distortion of the occiput. It was a very deep pattern coupled to shock affects and fear. We were very aware of its dynamics and had worked with it in previous sessions. Mom was holding her baby upright against her body. I felt a streaming of energy out of the area and then baby focused her eyes on mom. This was something in itself, as the baby would very rarely look at her mother. Then she expressed incredible anger; rage is the best name for it. She began to beat mom with her tiny hands held in fists. She screamed in anger, and her mother was shocked. There was a deep fight or flight anger still cycling in the infant, generated at the time of the birth process. I held the baby while my co-worker supported the mother and I simply said to her, "You know mommy didn't mean to hurt you; it hurt her too." Then the mother, with tears in her eyes said, "Yes I would never hurt you; it hurt me so much too." A marvelous thing happened: the baby stopped hitting her mother and looked deeply into her eyes as the mother was looking at her with tears in her eyes, and literally melted into her arms. Her whole body softened for the first time in all these months. It was like the baby finally landed in her mother's presence and could feel her mother's heart and could finally feel safe. We all cried a bit together. After that, their relationship was completely transformed. I saw them a few years later and both were doing very well.

VACUUM EXTRACTION

Vacuum extraction, or ventouse, is becoming more and more common. In this process a suction cup is placed upon the infant's head to enable a grip for pulling the baby out. The common thinking is that suction has less potential for damage than forceps. Unfortunately, I have found this to be incorrect. If forceps are carefully and sensitively applied, repercussions can be minimized. But I have never seen minimal repercussions with ventouse. The suction applied can have highly traumatizing consequences. There is commonly a local hematoma at the site of the application of the suction, but repercussions are deeper than this. The baby's system was not designed to meet these kinds of suction forces during the birthing process. Rather than dragging forces in the cranium and body, a strong suction is introduced into the system. This is experienced as a shock, and potency becomes inertial within the fluids. Fluid stasis results. This will strongly affect the ignition of fluids with potency at birth. Ignition will be dampened

down due to systemic fluid shock.

The central nervous system is also affected by vacuum extraction births. After all, the cranial vault is made of soft bones, with large spaces between them. It is just a sheet of membrane, so the suction forces go deeply into the system and actually impact the brain. I have found in many cases that the Aqueduct of Sylvius is literally pulled up cephalad in this process and can remain in this position if not treated. If the biokinetic forces suctioning the aqueduct are not resolved, they will continue to generate a pulling force after birth. This pattern may stay with a person indefinitely, producing fluid backpressure and lowered fluid drive within the system.

The easiest way to relate to the Aqueduct of Sylvius is to place a finger, or fingertips, at the top of the baby's head. Place your other hand at the base of the occiput. In this position, form a general relationship to her fluid system. Let the fluid come to you; do not crowd or invade the infant's system. Once you have done this, see if you can sense the third and fourth ventricles. An initial visualization of these structures may help, but you must learn to actually sense the ventricles through direct perception. With the fingers at the top of the baby's head, direct fluid downward toward and through the Aqueduct of Sylvius. After a while you may sense events such as actions of potency, fluid fluctuation, a processing of the biokinetic forces present—perhaps as a streaming of energy and/or heat— a shift or settling in the aqueduct, and a settling of the nervous system as a whole. There may be a general sense of downward streaming in the body as the backpressure releases.

I have also seen cases in which the ventouse process has generated parasympathetic shock states. My sense is that the shock of the process elicits a more primitive response than fight or flight, or that the fight or flight response becomes overwhelmed very quickly and the infant enters a dissociative and withdrawn state. Sympathetic arousal may also be running under this, and after some of these issues are resolved, you may find yourself treating a very angry little person. This process can give rise to listless dissociated babies, or to very angry hyperaroused babies who do not sleep well.

INTRAOSSEOUS OCCIPITAL DISTORTIONS AND THE OCCIPITAL BASE SPREAD

In Chapter 15 we covered the many possibilities for intraosseous distortions in the cranial bones, including the many significant repercussions and the wide range of symptoms that can result from intraosseous problems. Now that we have an understanding of the clinical considerations in working with babies, let's explore treatment concepts for working with intraosseous issues in the adult. This section depends on knowing the specific anatomy of the newborn cranium as well as the specific forces at work during the process, as presented in Chapter 15. The following table summarizes the possibilities for intraosseous occipital distortions (Fig. 16.8).

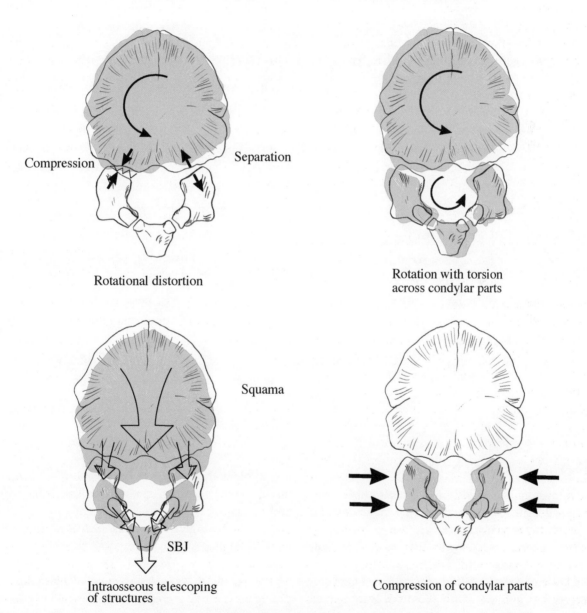

16.8 Common intraosseous distortions of the occiput

Rotational Distortions of the Occiput

During birth process, the occipital squama may be forced to rotate clockwise or counterclockwise relative to the other parts of the occiput, with the fulcrum of the rotation commonly at inion. This can lead to compression between the squamous portion and the condylar part it is rotating toward, and a spreading pattern on the other side. Intraosseous rotation of the occipital squama commonly generates cranial base torsion. In this case the fulcrum of the torsion lies not within the SBJ relationships, but within the occiput itself.

Compression Across the Condylar Parts of the Occiput

Due to the rotational distortion described above, or other medially compressive forces introduced during birth process, the condylar parts of the occiput can become medially compressed and/or torsioned in relationship to each other. Telescoping of structure as described below is a common origin of compression of the condylar parts. Compression and/or torsion across the foramen magnum will result. This will literally wedge and compress the articular surfaces of the atlas into the condylar parts of the occiput.

Telescoping of the Occiput

The squama, condylar parts, and basi-occiput may all be forced to compress together toward the SBJ. A compression across the foramen magnum may also result. This will commonly wedge the atlas between the condyles and compromise its free motion. It is very common for an intransigent SBJ compression to have its primary fulcrum within an intraosseous telescoping of occipital structure. It is no use working with the SBJ as the fulcrum of a cranial base compression if the forces at work are actually located within the occiput. The SBJ compression may be secondary to the intraosseous occipital distortion.

Working with Birth Issues in Adults

Let's now turn our intention to addressing birth issues in the adult. If the forces generated by the birthing process have not been resolved, they will continue to be organizing factors within the person's system. Intraosseous distortions represent traumatic forces that have lodged within the bony tissue and are being centered by potency within the bone. Intraosseous issues can be the fulcrum for cranial base patterns and whole body distortions. They are always of traumatic or experiential origin, often arising from pre- and perinatal birth events or early childhood. They can also be generated by trauma, such as an accident or fall, and may even be a response to severe emotional shock.

The biokinetic forces that were initially introduced during the birthing process are still present maintaining the tissue compression. The origin of the pattern is held within the present. These forces are still at work and can therefore be resolved in the present. That is why healing can occur. Clinical work is not about the past; it is about present forces at work. This reminder is especially relevant when we are encountering birth patterns in adults. The history may be compelling, drawing us out of present-time awareness, but the work depends on our being able to maintain attention with the forces at work rather than with the story of how they got there.

Birth-Related Patterns in the Occiput

Methods for addressing occipital issues in relationship to surrounding structures, along with first explorations of intraosseous patterns, were first presented in Chapters 7 and 8. The following are additional applications recognizing the special circumstances of the birth environment. Here our intraosseous work is deepened and focused in more detail.

Clinical Application: Occipital Base Spread —Disengagement and the State of Balance

The State of Balance

1. With the patient in the supine position, place your hands in the *occipital cradle hold* previously learned. In this hold, the patient's head is resting on your hands as you simply cradle their occiput with your fingers pointing inferiorly. Be sure that the heels of your hands do not place any pressure on their head. Let your hands be soft and yielding. Orient to the mid-tide. Establish a wide perceptual field and, within this field, let the occiput come to the foreground. Do not narrow your perceptual field or project your attention to the occiput. Let it come to you.

2. In this receptive state, simply listen. In this listening you are initiating a conversation with the tissues, fluids, and potencies within the occiput. Imagine/sense that the occiput is still in its four parts of infancy: squama, condyles, and basilar portion. How do these parts relate to each other?

Do you sense the squama in rotation in relationship to the condyles? Do you sense a compressive or torsional force across the foramen magnum? Do you sense a telescoping of structure anteriorly toward the SBJ? As you listen, simply let the story unfold.

3. As inertial issues within the occiput clarify, notice the dynamics that arise. The squama may rotate inferiorly in one direction, the condyles may torsion, or they may be sensed to be wedged together, and there may be an anterior drag within the squama as you sense a telescoping of occipital base parts described above. These are all expressions of unresolved biokinetic forces.

4. Follow the prominent patterns and access the state of balance. Listen for Becker's three-phase process. While holding the occiput, follow the patterns, and, as though you are holding a teeter totter, subtly slow these motions down until a state of balance is accessed. Do not hold the tissues against any sense of barrier or edge of resistance. This state of balance is not something you can impose upon the system. It is inherent within the conditions present. You are simply slowing things down. The potencies, fluids, and tissues involved will access a neutral, a state of dynamic equilibrium within their unified relationship. Listen for expressions of Health within this neutral. When the tissues again begin to move, notice how the occiput reorients to the midline and to the dynamics of Sutherland's fulcrum.

Specific Processes of Disengagement

Many times the biokinetic forces maintaining intraosseous distortions and their related tissue effects are deeply entrenched. Biodynamic potencies and inertial forces may be deeply coiled as the Intelligence of the system acts to center and contain traumatic forces in the best possible way. The compressive forces may be so deep that neutrals such as the state of balance cannot be easily accessed, or within the stillness that is accessed, there may be little initiation of forces involved. For further processing, an occipital base spread may be helpful. Here the intention will be to help access space within the inertial forces that maintain and center the tissue compression. This is an extension of the principle of disengagement. We present this in three steps for learning, but in practice these blend into each other.

Because intraosseous distortions usually represent infant patterns, we relate to the adult system as though we are holding an infant, with a focus on holding space and showing options. You would never follow an infant's pattern of inertia into its conditioned direction to a barrier or edge of resistance. This would activate the inertial forces in a way that intensifies symptoms and obstructs the process.

An effective way to work with infants is to offer space and stillness. In the process below, you will be encouraging a disengagement of the parts of the occiput in order to access the state of balance. This will help the inertial potencies express themselves beyond the forces being centered and initiate healing processes. It will also help occipital tissue express motility, or inner breath, and realign to the midline and natural functions. When inertial forces resolve, there is a natural tendency for the cellular and tissue world to reorganize and realign to the primal midline and natural fulcrums of the system. The embryological imperative and the original intention of those tissues is re-established. In all of the intra-osseous work described below, your intention must be very subtle as it comes through your hands. We are engaging the tissues, fluids, and potencies within the dynamics of the occiput and this requires great subtlety within our palpation skills.

Step One: De-Rotation of the Occipital Squama

The intention of the following process is to offer options to the tissue elements and, through the state of balance, access the inertial forces involved. If you sense a rotation of the squama relative to the rest of the parts of the occiput, you can suggest de-rotation as an option. This introduces a conversation about space and the uncoiling of the biodynamic and bio-kinetic forces within the tissues of the occiput. To do this, introduce a rotational intention within the squama in the opposite direction to the perceived rotation.

1. Orient to the mid-tide. In the occipital cradle, sense for intraosseous rotation within the occipital squama. Float on the tissues. Remember that the occiput is part of a unified tensile tissue field. Let the occiput, as part of that field, take you into its pattern of motion. See if you sense a rotational motion within the tissue of the occiput. Once you sense the boundary of this motion, subtly intend a rotation of the squama in the opposite direction. Intend this until space is accessed. Do not grab onto the tissues to do this. Maintain a wide perceptual field. If you narrow your field of attention, or if you grab onto the tissues, you will obstruct their structure and function.

2. Once space is sensed, help access the state of balance within the occipital tissues. Simply slow the motions down and notice the state of balance being attained. This is a subtle exploration into stillness at or near the boundary of the intention to de-rotate. All of this may happen naturally as you listen within the mid-tide. As you listen within a wide perceptual field with a relatively still mind, it may be sensed that the state of balance is inherent within the conditions present.

3. Within the stillness of the state of balance, listen for expressions of Health. This may be sensed as pulsations and permeations of potency and as fluid fluctuations within the occipital tissue. These are expressions of the biodynamic potency of the Breath of Life. These potencies have become inertial within the occiput to center the traumatic forces present. Within the state of balance, these are now free to express themselves beyond the compensations held. You may also sense the dissipation of biokinetic forces back to the environment. This may be sensed as a release of heat and/or a streaming of energy. Within a wide perceptual field, you may also

sense a wider permeation of potency through a much larger field of action. It may seem as though potency wells up through the whole fluid field and moves right through the fulcrum being palpated.

4. As the biokinetic forces are resolved, you may also sense an expansion within the tissues of the occiput. The biodynamic potencies at the heart of the inertial fulcrum expand and can once more move freely within their greater field of action. The tissue elements will follow and a general sense of expansion and decompression can be perceived. Give the tissues time to reorganize and to re-establish their relationship to the mid-line and to the natural fulcrums of the system.

Step Two: Condylar Spread

As we have seen, birthing forces can generate a compressive telescoping of the squama, condylar parts, and basi-occiput. A medial compression within the condylar parts and across the foramen magnum may also be generated. If you sense a medial compression of the condyles and a wedging of the atlas into the condylar parts, you can suggest a lateral spreading across the foramen magnum as we did in Chapter 7 on the Occipital Triad. In essence, you are engaging in a conversation with the tissues by the intention of traction and space across the foramen magnum. This, in turn, brings the intention of disengagement into play.

1. To intend space across the condyles, change your hand position from the occipital cradle to a condylar spread position as learned earlier. Spread the heels of your hands apart so that your fingertips point toward the occipital condyles. Make contact with the condyles by imagining that you are extending your fingers toward them. Again orient to the mid-tide level of action (see Fig. 7.6).

2. In this position, intend/suggest a spread across the foramen magnum to the boundary of the potential space accessed. This is a very subtle intention brought to the tissues as an inquiry. In this, you are engaging in a conversation with the tissues. What is possible here? Can you give yourself space? What is this really like? Once again the intention is to access enough space so that potency can express itself within the state of balance. A traditional way to intend a lateral spread across the condyles is to gently bring your elbows together. This will encourage a lateral spreading of your fingertips and this intention will be transferred to the condyles and foramen magnum.

3. At, or near, the boundary accessed listen to the tissues as they move to a state of balance. You can assist this if necessary by engaging in a very subtle exploration into the tissue motion. Slow these motions down and listen for a settling into the state of balance. Be open to the expressions of fluids and potency within this stillness. Listen for Becker's *something happens*. The condylar parts spread laterally, the foramen magnum expands, and the atlas de-wedges from the occipital condyles as the biokinetic forces are resolved.

Step Three: De-telescoping of the Occipital Base Parts

As we have seen, telescoping can involve a number of structures. Obviously the four parts of the occiput are involved, but our awareness must also include the nearby structures such as the atlas and axis, cervical ligaments, dura, and related systems because these are all one unit of function. All of these may be palpated when listening to intraosseous patterns in the occipital squama. It is also common, while palpating the occiput, to sense an anterior compressive pull, or electromagnetic-like suction, towards the SBJ. This is an expression of the biokinetic forces that are maintaining the telescoping. If you sense this kind of anterior pull, you can intend a posterior traction to engage the four parts of the occiput in a conversation about space. As you do this, you can also include an awareness of the SBJ in front, and the cervical area below, as part of the process.

1. Sit at the head of the table and hold the cranium in the occipital cradle. Again, orient to the mid-tide. With an awareness of the whole body as a tensile field, slowly and subtly engage the tissues of the occiput in a superior-posterior traction. Sense the inner tissue of the occiput as you subtly intend the occiput cephalad (toward you). This will place a posterior intention within the condylar parts and basi-occiput. Do this with a subtle suggestion within your hands. Again, when you place a subtle suggestion of traction into tissues, they will begin to communicate their history to you. No force is used. You are engaging the tissues in a conversation, asking, "Can you give yourself space here? What is possible here?" Again suggest this de-telescoping until space is accessed.

2. Help the tissues access the state of balance, and again listen for expressions of Health. Note the expansion and permeation of potency and a response within the tissues. Listen for fluid fluctuations and for the fluid drive of the system to kick in. Fluid drive is a factor of the potency within the fluids. You may sense a drive of potency and fluid toward and within the fulcrum being palpated. You may sense a gradual ratchet-like softening of structure. First one relationship may soften and then another. For instance, the squama may disengage from one condylar part, then another, and then the condylar parts from the basi-occiput, etc. This occurs as the biokinetic forces involved are dissipated back to the environment.

3. Allow the potency, fluid, and tissue elements to reorganize toward midline functions. These include Sutherland's fulcrum and the primal midline more generally. Wait for a sense of realignment and for a clear fluid tide to express itself (Fig. 16.9).

COMBINING INTENTIONS INTO AN OCCIPITAL BASE SPREAD

Once you have a sense of these relationships, you can bring the intentions together to initiate a traditional occipital base spread. To do this, first intend de-rotation of the squama. When space is accessed, add a lateral spreading of the occipital condyles via a condylar spread. Finally, once space is accessed, intend a de-telescoping of occipital base structures. The effect is a composite *stacking* of the three possibilities into one multidimensional field of perception and possibility of space. The intention is to engage in a conversation about space and potential throughout the intraosseous relationships discovered. Do not restrict the tissues against the boundaries of their motion or mentally grab the tissues to hold them in a fixed way. As you hold these relationships, see if you can then help access the state of balance within their unified dynamic. This whole process can occur more or less spontaneously as you listen within the level of the mid-tide once you have practiced it sufficiently.

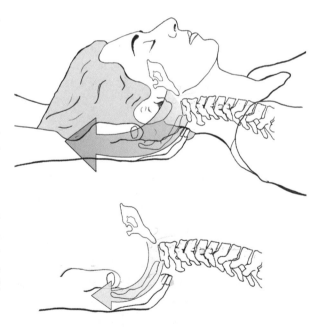

16.9 De-telescoping of structures

ENCOURAGING LATERAL FLUCTUATION WITHIN INTRAOSSEOUS RELATIONSHIPS

The fluid skill of lateral fluctuation can be very helpful in resolving intraosseous inertia. When the relationships that you are exploring have accessed their state of balance, you might sense pulsation of potency and lateral fluctuations of fluid within the intraosseous occiput. These pulsations are the expression of Health within the intraosseous patterns, expressing that health is never lost and that living bone is fluid.

1. Place your hands in an occipital cradle hold. As you sense the fluctuation of potency within the occipital tissue, subtly push against the pendulum swings of the fluctuations. These feel like lateral fluctuations of fluid even within bone. These fluctuations may be expressed as figure-eight or spiral motions of potency and fluid, and sometimes as simple back-and-forth pulsation. This is an intention, a suggestion, not a physical pressure. It is as though your fingers energetically extend to the potencies being expressed. The intention is to initiate a deeper conversation with the inertial potencies involved and to stimulate fluctuation of potency within its greater field.

2. Commonly, in adults, there is much density and inertial within intraosseous tissues. You may not sense lateral fluctuations arising at all. In these cases, you can encourage them by intentionally pushing against the fluids and potencies, first in one direction, then the other until the potency takes over and fluctuations occur on their own.

INTRAOSSEOUS DISTORTIONS OF THE TEMPORAL BONES

The temporal bone is next in our inquiry into intraosseous issues. The temporal bones are in three parts at birth: the squama, the tympanic ring, and the petrous portion. Intraosseous forces can be introduced into these tissue relationships during the birth process. Intraosseous temporal bone issues commonly arise due to medial compressive forces and rotational forces. As we have seen, during the first stage of birth strong medial forces can be placed on the baby's cranium, especially if it is in a transverse position in the pelvic inlet. Rotational and compressive biokinetic forces can then be added during the mid-pelvic descent as the baby rotates toward the pelvic floor (see Fig. 15.21).

Intraosseous distortions in the temporal bones can have profound effects on the system. In infants, compressions at the jugular foramen and hypoglossal canal may generate entrapment neuropathy in the vagus, hypoglossal, glossopharyngeal, and spinal accessory nerves, leading to digestive problems such as colic, sucking problems, and respiratory symptoms. In adults, intraosseous temporal bone issues may generate chronic cranial base patterns with resultant symptomologies, migraine headaches, digestive disorders, respiratory issues, fluid congestion, tinnitus or other hearing problems, chronic fatigue, and low potency.

Clinical Application: Intraosseous Temporal Bone Distortions

1. Begin from the *vault hold* and hold the biosphere of the patient within your perceptual field. Orient to the mid-tide. Move to the specific temporal bone that communicates an intraosseous issue to you. This may be sensed as a compressive force or pull medially and/or a rotation, or inner spiraling, within the bone. You may even sense a corkscrewing type of force within the tissue. Use the *ear canal temporal bone hold* for a more direct temporal palpation. Maintaining contact with that bone, place your other hand on the opposite frontal eminence. The frontal contact enables directing fluids and potency toward the temporal bone in question (Fig. 16.10).

2. With a relatively wide perceptual field, listen again to the dynamics within the temporal bone. Do you sense a compressive tendency within its tissues? Is there a sense of a compressive,

corkscrewing type motion? Whatever movements or patterns arise, listen and follow for a few moments. Then, with the hand at the temporal bone, subtly intend the opposite to whatever you are sensing. This is similar to your intentions at the occiput above. Intend this until space is accessed. Then, with a gentle intention, direct fluid and potency from the opposite frontal eminence toward the internal auditory meatus. Within the stillness, listen for expressions of Health, especially for the initiation and permeation of potency within the tissues of the temporal bone. You may even sense a rehydration of the tissues involved. Listen for the third stage of Becker's three-phase healing awareness. Allow the tissues to reorganize and to realign to their natural fulcrums and the midline.

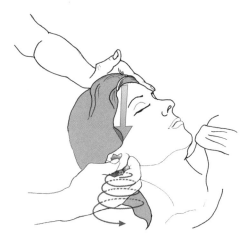

16.10 Temporal bone ear hold with other hand over opposite frontal bone to direct fluid

INTRAOSSEOUS DISTORTIONS OF THE SPHENOID BONE

As we've described, intraosseous distortions of the sphenoid bone are very common and can affect all other parts of the system. The sphenoid bone is in three parts at birth: the body-lesser wing section and the two pterygoid-greater wing sections (see Fig. 15.8). The sphenoid bone is subject to many forces during all phases of the birthing process. In the pelvic inlet it is commonly exposed to medially compressive and shearing forces. In the mid-pelvis, rotational and lateral shearing forces are often encountered. In the pelvic outlet, vertical shearing may arise (see Fig. 15.9). The effects are numerous and wide-ranging. In fact, many cranial base patterns have intraosseous issues as their fulcrum. For instance, a torsion pattern within the cranial base may be an expression of torsion between the greater wing sections of the sphenoid.

Clinical Application: Intraosseous Distortions of the Sphenoid

1. The modified *vault hold* (*Becker's hold*) is a good way to orient to the intraosseous patterns of the sphenoid. Negotiate your contact with the greater wings as you would approach an infant, thumbs gently placed at the temples. Hold a relatively wide perceptual field, bring attention to the sphenoid bone, and listen to the inner dynamics of its tissues. Almost any pattern may be expressed.

2. Follow the pattern perceived and then intend the opposite possibility. For instance, if you sense that one greater wing is relatively vertically sheared in relationship to the other, intend the wings in a de-shearing direction until space is sensed. This is a very subtle intention. It is a question, an inquiry, "Can you access an aligned potential here?" Once space is sensed, help the system access a state of balance. Listen for expressions of Health and for a sense of expansion and rehydration within the tissue of the sphenoid bone.

3. Listen for a reorganization of the tissues of the sphenoid and allow time for the whole of the cranium to reorganize and realign with natural fulcrums and the midline. This is very important. An intraosseous distortion of the sphenoid may be the fulcrum for any number of cranial patterns.

Be patient and allow the tissues, fluids, and potencies to reorganize their relationship to natural fulcrums and the primal midline.

4. If inertial potencies involved are not initiated or expressed within the state of balance, it might be useful to add another conversation here by intending lateral fluctuation of potency across the greater wings. To do this, very subtly intend a flux of potency and/or fluid, first one direction, then the other, across the greater wings. Once you perceive a fluctuation of potency within the sphenoid itself, you can stop intending the lateral fluctuation and listen for the expression of potencies within the tissues. As potencies are expressed and the inertial forces resolve, you may sense a softening and expansion within the tissues of the sphenoid itself.

5. Some people are very sensitive at the greater wings of the sphenoid. It may seem impossible to negotiate a comfortable contact via a *vault hold* or similar contact. These sensitivities are usually expressions of strong compressive forces within the tissue of the sphenoid, especially within the greater wing sections. One or both greater wing sections may be compressed into the body of the sphenoid during the birth process.

6. You can work electromagnetically to approach these situations. As you perceive the compressive forces within the greater wings, imagine that your thumbs are like magnets. Subtly intend the two greater wings laterally apart via an intention of lateral space. It is as if the potency within the sphenoid is like a pond and you are touching its surface tension. Subtly lift the surface tension laterally. You may perceive an energetic resistance to your intention. If you do, wait and listen for a state of balance. Wait for expressions of Health and for a sense of softening and expansion.

1. Age definitions: Infant—from birth to one year; young children—from one year to five years old.
2. Many thanks to Dr. Martin Hunt and Maria Harris for co-creating this free clinic.

17

Neuroendocrine Relationships and the Stress Cascade

Stress and traumatic experience is part of our everyday life experience and is a huge area of inquiry in our work. In many ways, how we manage stress and trauma shapes our personality system and our psycho-physiology. Its study has become a field in itself called psycho-neuro-immunology. Much of the suffering we see in our offices is generated by the unresolved cycling of the stress response and its neuroendocrine and autonomic nervous system processes.

In this chapter we will:

- *Introduce the physiology of the stress response.*
- *Introduce the stress cascade.*
- *Discuss the relationships of the hypothalamus, amygdala, locus ceruleus, hippocampus, and prefrontal cortex in stress responses.*

INTRODUCTION

I do not claim to be an expert in this field, but the necessity of teaching this subject in courses has led me to read research, gather relevant information, and determine what is clinically useful. I have read much research over the last ten years, some of it hard to come by or difficult to integrate from current textbooks. It is inevitable in this brief format that some areas are highlighted because they are particularly important, while other areas have to be left out. The topic of these physiological processes and their repercussions is so large that a number of books could be created without exhausting the subject.

Treatment of the topic began in Chapter 3, "The Motility of the Central Nervous System." That material is the foundation for the clinical work presented in these next three chapters. Before working with stress responses, the practitioner must clearly understand CNS motion and motility and must be comfortable palpating CNS expressions. It is amazing what we can do just by deepening into stillness and the state of balance. Also, helping set the stage for this section are Chapters 21 and 22 of Volume One, in which we explored concepts about fight or flight and related stress responses. I did not discuss physiology at that time, as practical clinical skills were initially much more important. Finally, the material presented in Volume One on verbal support for trauma resolution (also in Chapters 21 and 22) is also quite relevant here, though our focus in this section is really on cranial work and its direct links to physiology.

The term *stress cascade* denotes the whole of these processes. It includes the contents of these three chapters and more. When I get into its intricacies, it feels like spirals within spirals. The stress response is nonlinear. It is a network of interconnected and cascading processes. All the parts swirl and loop together in an integrated and intricate process of mobilization and response. As we delve into particulars, let's remember the totality of the whole system, because this is the basis for treatment.

THE STRESS RESPONSE

We inevitably find ourselves under varying levels of stress, even in ideal circumstances. Family situations, close relationships, our work and finances, challenging experiences of almost any kind, or even just the pace of modern life all present us with stress. The simple routines of going to work on the subway, driving our car, or even just walking down the street can all seem threatening. Then when we factor in life's truly overwhelming experiences such as accidents, falls, abuse, violence, crime, losing loved ones, losing our work or home, and receiving shocking news, we must readily acknowledge the huge role of stress in many health conditions.

The stress response is essentially about survival. It evolved over the course of our development to meet challenges of evading predators, finding food, and perpetuating the species. Our modern life may have factors that are only recently arrived in our experience, but the sophisticated physiological equipment that we employ in defense arises from ancient systems proven over long periods of time, all based on the survival imperative. This has been so successful that we have come to dominate the planet and ironically now threaten our own survival with this success through overpopulation. It seems we as a species have a hard time working cooperatively rather than competitively in our survival needs. This may partly be due to the very physiological mechanisms which mobilize us for action and survival. They tend to be oppositional and confrontational in nature. This is especially true in male stress responses. Women under stress tend to produce oxytocin that calms the system and orients them to cooperative processes and social contact.

The neuroendocrine-immune system is a unified system because its parts and functions are so inter-

dependent. Until recently, this complex system has not been studied to the same degree as some other biological processes, because its complexity defied attempts at research. Suffice it to say, the neuroendocrine-immune system keeps our survival machine running, monitoring both internal and external environments, helping us find food and mates, repairing damage, repelling invaders, and accomplishing a host of related functions. It is running in the background all the time. This system can be considered the command headquarters for all homeostatic and survival processes.

When we encounter stressors, the neuroendocrine system naturally shifts to special adaptive states. These can vary, but the general process is called the *general adaptation response*. The system physiologically gears up to meet the stress with almost instantaneous surges of neuroactive molecules that trigger responses throughout the body. Muscles, circulation, respiration, digestion, and other systems all respond in a symphony of complex interactions so that life can be sustained. This response generally originates in certain nuclei within the central nervous system and is mediated by their production of neuroactive chemicals. Our primary interest is in five specific areas: the amygdala, hippocampus, hypothalamus, locus ceruleus, and prefrontal cortex. Other nuclei are relevant and will be mentioned, but these five are the main players for our purposes here (Fig. 17.1). One of the great potentials for craniosacral biodynamics is the possibility of accessing and influencing these key structures to facilitate healing in dysfunctional stress responses.

The initial response to stress involves two interrelated actions. First is the activation of the sympathetic nervous system in the form of increases in norepinephrin (noradrenaline) and epinephrin (adrenaline). Concurrently we experience an up-regulation of the H-P-A (hypothalamus-pituitary-adrenal) axis with a surge in cortisol. This global response is intended to mobilize us to meet the danger, stress, or challenge successfully. Once the stress is removed, or successfully dealt with, the body physiology is designed to shift smoothly back to a baseline state of homeostatic balance (Fig. 17.2).

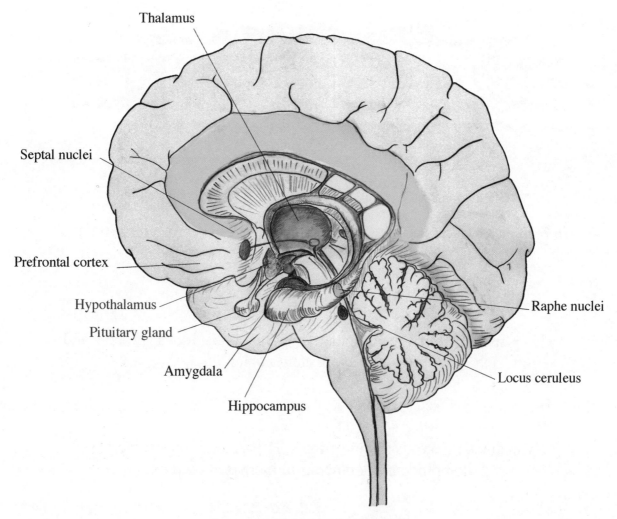

Thalamus

Septal nuclei

Prefrontal cortex

Hypothalamus

Pituitary gland

Amygdala

Hippocampus

Raphe nuclei

Locus ceruleus

17.1 Important stress–related structures

If the stress is repetitive, chronic, or prolonged, or if the traumatic incident overwhelms the system and is not able to be processed at the time, then the body physiology may not be able to shift back to a homeostatic balance. The fluidity of the system may be reduced or lost, to be replaced by a quality of fixation. The stress response may stay on even though the danger has actually passed, and we lose our ability to self-regulate in the normal way. The system may literally become fixed in this state, with an elevated set point for an indefinite period of time. This is called a *maladaptive response*. This can be disturbing, debilitating, and even crazy-making. Chronic maladaptive states can lead to physiological and psychological dysfunction. These may include immune deficiency, autoimmune states, anxiety states, hypertension, compulsive behaviors, depression, dissociative states, sociopathic behaviors, sleeping and eating disorders, somatic dys-

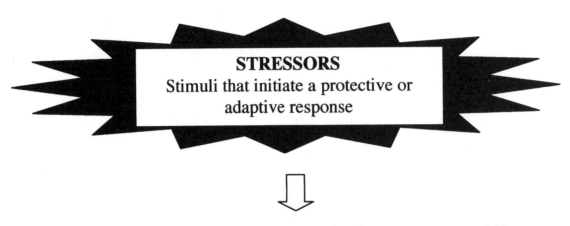

STRESSORS
Stimuli that initiate a protective or
adaptive response

In response to stressors, the neuroendocrine-immune system shifts to an
adaptive state.

This is mediated by the amygdala, hypothalamus, locus ceruleus and
other brain stem nuclei.

Sympathetic nervous system surges, H-P-A axis surges, increased
norepinephrin, epinephrin, increased cortisol.

Increased glycogen and mobilization of energy stores.

Increased arousal, vigilance, awareness, readiness for action results.
Non-adaptive pathways are suppressed, e.g. digestion and reproduction.

17.2 The General Adaptation Response

functions of all descriptions, chronic pain syndromes and psycho-emotional breakdown. Obviously, maladaptive states can have vast mind-body repercussions.

I believe that we could usefully broaden the phrase "post-traumatic stress disorder" to encompass a wide meaning. Generally, our bodies know how to survive and stay well under normal circumstances. When these natural defenses are overridden by trauma, we may experience illness in any of its forms. Craniosacral biodynamics aims to re-establish inherent resources from the inside out, in contrast to allopathic medicine's "outside-in" methods. It is useful to discuss the physiology of the stress response because experienced practitioners can perceive and specifically work with its subtle physiological interactions. The various therapeutic approaches we use, such as accessing states of balance, fluid direction, and stillness processes can be wisely and effectively employed.

There are three interrelated cycles of processing involved in stress responses. These are:

1. autonomic processes;

2. cortical processes mediating such things as memory and meaning; and

3. the H-P-A axis.

These cycles are coordinated by the interactions of the prefrontal cortex, hypothalamus, amygdala, hippocampus and brain stem (Fig. 17.3).

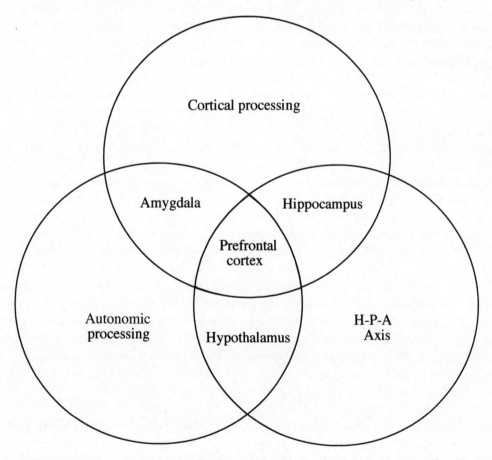

17.3 The three interconnected cycles of adaptation and emotional regulation

THE ROLE OF THE HYPOTHALAMUS

The question here for me is where to start in describing all of this. The human body and its responses are nonlinear. The stress response is a circular and holographic process. Everything is in relationship to everything else, all at once. We are really exploring an integrated and holistic neuroendocrine-immune system. Given all this, I am choosing to begin with the hypothalamus. The hypothalamus is a collection of nuclei located in the floor of the third ventricle. It is something like the conductor of an orchestra. Its main role is to help the body maintain homeostatic balance and fluidity. In order to do this it receives inputs from many areas of the body and gives regulatory outputs to many areas. It orchestrates autonomic function, skeletal muscle contraction, hormonal secretions, emotional processes, the interface between voluntary and autonomic function, behavioral drives like hunger and thirst, and body temperature. Most importantly, it orchestrates the overall nature of the stress response. It does not do this alone; it works in direct relationship to input from other brain areas such as the amygdala, hippocampus, and prefrontal cortex.

Let's first look at the major inputs to the hypothalamus. By *inputs* we mean biochemical neurotransmitter transmission (messenger molecules) as well as direct synapse connections. The hypothalamus receives input from the limbic system, especially the amygdala and hippocampus. The amygdala, located in the anterior portion of each temporal lobe, quickly assesses whether current experience is threatening or dangerous, gives emotional tone to new experience based on past experience, and mediates emotional memories related to trauma and stress.

If not down-regulated, the amygdala can keep the stress response running far beyond the time of the experience. The hippocampus, located just posterior to the amygdala, inferior and parallel to the dorsal horn of each lateral ventricle, coordinates the processing of memory. Together the amygdala and hippocampus mediate certain memory processes important in chronic stress processes and in everyday life. The hypothalamus also receives input from the cortex. The cortex provides interpretive functions and meaning to orchestrate a sophisticated set of responses. As we shall see, the long-term memory of stressful experiences and the meaning we give them, can also keep the stress response running.

In addition, the hypothalamus receives input from the special senses (the five external senses plus the internal proprioceptive sense) via the thalamus. The senses have two pathways to the hypothalamus, a "fast" path via the amygdala and a relatively slower pathway via the thalamus. The hypothalamus mobilizes the system either way, but the fast path allows for an instant reaction and is really necessary for survival. For example, we might jump when we see a curvy stick on the ground even before we have actually had the time to identify whether it is a dangerous snake or just a piece of wood, or we might jump away from a sound before we identify the oncoming car in our pathway. The hypothalamus also receives important input from the autonomic nuclei and brain stem nuclei such as those of the reticular formation. Many body activities are monitored via these connections.

Finally, the hypothalamus receives visceral and somatic input from the body itself. Much of this input relates to nociception from nerves called *nociceptors,* also known as pain receptors. Nociceptors are nerve endings that detect internal danger; there are many millions of them in the body. The topic of nociception is under-appreciated in the trauma literature, and I will devote a separate chapter to it, following this discussion. Traditionally, it was thought that the hypothalamus received somatic and visceral nociceptive input via the thalamus alone. But recent research shows that the hypothalamus also receives input *directly* from these receptors via the spinal cord.[1] Some researchers have named this the *spinohypothalamic tract* (SHT) of the spinal cord.[2] This tract has important repercussions for the stress response.

Chronic stress responses can be generated by ongoing low grade nociceptive input from somatic or visceral systems. In other words, states of anxiety, depression, and chronic fatigue are not just based on external traumatic experiences; they can also be set off by internal chronic nociceptive activity. Due to the connection of nociceptive fibers to the hypothalamus, chronic nociceptive input can directly initiate and maintain the general adaptation response and the whole of the stress cascade.[3] Chronic nociceptive input to the hypothalamus also generates a release of endorphins and signals the periaqueductal gray (PAG) cells (adjoining the cerebral aqueduct) and the raphae nuclei (in the brain stem) to attempt to down-regulate the pain response. These are parts of the natural self-balancing processes of the body, but they can be coupled with numbing, freezing, and dissociative processes. Endorphins and serotonin, a precursor to endorphins and an important neurohormone in its own right, can flood the system in this situation, further upsetting homeostasis.

Outputs from the hypothalamus that regulate homeostasis and autonomic activity are complex. Three outputs/responses are particularly important in stress responses. These are the H-P-A axis, the relationship of the hypothalamus to the locus ceruleus (a pair of brain stem reticular nuclei), and the sympathetic nervous system response (Fig. 17.4).

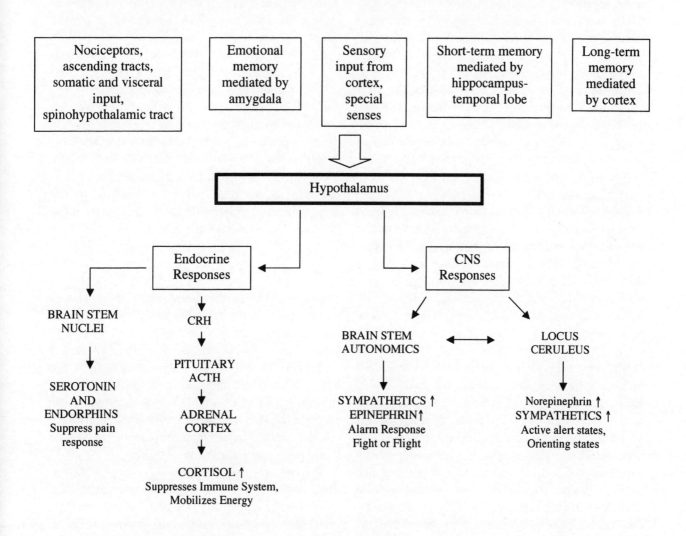

17.4 Hypothalamus: summary of major inputs and outputs in stress responses

THE H–P–A AXIS

The hypothalamus-pituitary-adrenal axis is a major relationship in the stress response. The specific area of the hypothalamus especially involved in stress responses is called the *paraventricular nucleus*. It receives input from many areas of the brain, helping it to modulate the stress response and maintain homeostatic balance within the body. When the hypothalamus receives communication that there is internal or external danger, it releases a neurohormone called corticotrophin-releasing hormone or factor (CRH or CRF). In chronic stress conditions, either the hypothalamus continually receives these inputs, or the ability to down-regulate the CRH response is lost. CRH goes to the pituitary gland which responds by producing adrenocorticotrophic hormone (ACTH). This enters the bloodstream, goes to the adrenal glands, and triggers the release of adrenal cortical steroids, especially cortisol. Cortisol stimulates the release and metabolic processing of energy needed for mobilization in the fight or flight response and also suppresses the immune system.

Baseline levels of cortisol help maintain alertness during daytime and maintain a natural brake on the immune system that peaks during the night. This braking keeps the immune system from overreacting or attacking healthy cells and tissues. In hyperarousal states with high sympathetic activation, the H-P-A axis can become overactive, leading to high levels of cortisol. High levels of cortisol inhibit the immune system, leading to immunodeficiency. This is a critical link, connecting chronic stress states with reduced immune system function, and it is one reason highly stressed or traumatized people are more vulnerable to infections. In hypoarousal states, in which there is a high parasympathetic tonus, the H-P-A axis is commonly underactive leading to low levels of cortisol. Low levels of cortisol can lead to autoimmune diseases in which an overcharged immune system becomes self-destructive of the body's normal cells. The immune system depends on the right level of cortisol, as either too much or too little causes problems.

Cortisol has a further important function. Cortisol enters the brain from the bloodstream and finds its way to the hippocampus, which has receptors for cortisol. When these receptors are filled, the hippocampus tells the hypothalamus to down-regulate the production of CRH, putting a brake on the H-P-A axis and the stress response it mediates. This is a feedback loop which down-regulates the stress response and helps the system to return to homeostasis. It has been found that chronically high levels of cortisol can overwhelm the cortisol receptors in the hippocampus, and they can then lose their ability to down-regulate the stress response. This alone can lead to chronic cascading of stress responses and the general adaptation response.

Fig. 17.5 outlines the H-P-A axis. The locus ceruleus is included in this figure even though it is not technically part of this axis. It has an important role to play and is discussed below. I also include the amygdala, as its input is critical in setting the axis into play when danger is perceived. It is important to remember, however, that many factors can set the axis into motion, such as images and traumatic memories held within the cortex, emotional memories mediated by the amygdala and hippocampus, and nociceptive input via the SHT spinal tract mentioned above (Fig. 17.5).

THE LOCUS CERULEUS

The locus ceruleus is composed of two bilateral nuclei and is located at the superior floor of the fourth ventricle in the posterior aspect of the brain stem. The locus ceruleus has projections to just about every part of the nervous system. It has ascending fibers to the hypothalamus and amygdala and to virtually all of the brain and its cortex. It has descending fibers through the spinal cord, its interomediolateral cell column, to the preganglionic sympathetics, and to the sacral preganglionic parasympathetics.

The locus ceruleus produces norepinephrin (noradrenaline), a key arousal system neurotransmitter. Norepinephrin has wide ranging effects within the mind-body system. Norepinephrin is what wakes us up in the morning. In stress response it leads to heightened awareness, increased cortical activity, and an active-alert, hyperaroused state. In the flight or flight process, the locus ceruleus surges during the orienting response and facilitates an actively alert state. In maladaptive states, the locus ceruleus may be chronically turned on, creating hypersensitivity to sensory input. This is called hypervigilance and is a classic aspect of post-traumatic stress disorder, chronic anxiety, and depressive states.

A further important consideration relates to how the locus ceruleus and hypothalamus communicate with each other. When activated, the locus ceruleus sends norepinephrin to the hypothalamus. This induces the hypothalamus to produce CRH and activates the H-P-A axis. The hypothalamus also sends CRH to the locus ceruleus, which induces it to send out more norepinephrin, creating a two-way, positive feedback loop that augments the stress response. If this loop does not down-regulate, the stress response keeps cycling. As we shall see, the locus ceruleus can be chronically stimulated by the amygdala and by chronic nociceptive input from the visceral and somatic systems (see Figs. 17.4 and 17.5).

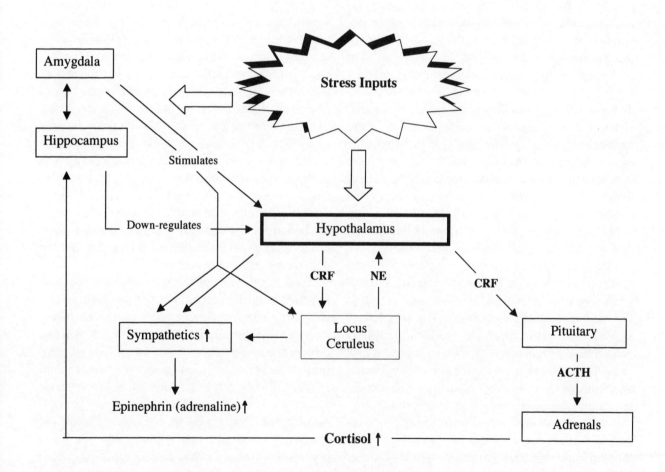

17.5 The H–P–A Axis

The Sympathetic Nervous System

The sympathetic nervous system prepares and mobilizes the musculoskeletal system for action. It surges strongly during fight or flight processes. The sympathetic nervous system keeps surging until the danger is passed and the mobilization response is down-regulated. This process is largely mediated by the hypothalamus. The sympathetic nervous system, among other effects, accelerates the heart rate and flow of blood to skeletal muscles and to the brain, while generally restricting the flow of blood to the digestive organs. It stimulates the release of glycogen from the liver for energy. It also has fibers that directly connect to the adrenal glands, signaling the adrenals to release epinephrin (adrenaline) into the system. Epinephrin reinforces the action of the sympathetic nervous system in many ways. It constricts the smooth muscle of the skin and the blood vessels in the core of the body, such as digestive organs, and generally inhibits nonessential activities not directly needed for immediate survival. It dilates the smooth muscle in the arterioles of skeletal muscles to enhance their ability to contract in response to the fight or flight impulse. It excites cardiac muscle, increasing the rate and force of contraction. It also mobilizes the glycogen reserves in the body and increases the amount of energy that is available for action. Chronically high levels of epinephrin can help maintain anxiety states, exhaust the system, and lead to all kinds of symptomology.

Finally, the sympathetic nervous system has fibers that end in the immune system. All primary and secondary immune glands and lymph nodes, as well as the immune tissue lining the digestive tract, have a sympathetic nerve supply. The sympathetic system helps modulate immune responses. In general, a high level of sympathetic signals to the immune system has an inhibitive effect. In other words, chronic stimulation of the sympathetic nervous system tends to inhibit the immune system. Coupled with the high levels of cortisol present in stress states, this can have a devastating effect on the body's defensive systems. Chronic stimulation of the sympathetic nervous system can lead to all sorts of mind-body issues, including anxiety states, depression, cardiac problems, respiratory problems, muscle tension, sleeplessness, under-eating, immune suppression, and physical breakdown.

The Amygdala

The amygdala is a key nucleus in the initiation of arousal responses, active alert states, and of the fight or flight response. The role of the amygdala in the stress process is elegantly and fully described by Joseph LeDoux in *The Emotional Brain*.[4] I highly recommend this book, as it goes into much more detail than I am able to do here.

The amygdala has direct connections to both the hippocampus and the hypothalamus. One of its roles is to signal the hypothalamus that danger is present. The amygdala also signals the locus ceruleus, along with other brain stem nuclei, to quickly activate a systemic sympathetic nervous system mobilization. Signs of external danger are taken into the brain by the special senses. These include seeing, hearing, touch, and smell. These signals first go to the thalamus before processing the information. The signals can then take two routes to the amygdala. The first is a relatively slow route. Signals go from the special senses to the thalamus and then to the cortex for processing. The cortex makes appraisals of the input, and, if the signals are registered as danger, or challenging to the system, a signal is then sent to the amygdala to initiate the stress response. By the time this all occurs, however, the snake would have bitten you and the damage would have been done.

There is a shorter and faster route to the amygdala in which cortical processing is not involved. In this route, the sensory signals go from the thalamus directly to the amygdala. LeDoux calls it a "quick and dirty processing pathway."[5] The internal representation of the object or situation is crude compared to cortical processing, but allows for a much faster response to danger or threat. Thus, you find yourself running from the tiger before you actually see it, and jumping away from a snake only to find that it is a branch of a tree. If you had to wait for the cortex to process the sensory information, you might have been bitten by the time you realized there really was a snake. Cortical processing can override this quick response so that you realize that the curving figure is a branch and not a snake. Then your stress response would not be set off. This quick response is important in sudden, dangerous situations. However, if this fast route is sensitized or facilitated, as in chronic stress states, we may find ourselves jumping and running from every sound or every twisted branch. Indeed, in conditioned fear states this is exactly what happens (Fig. 17.6).

Once the amygdala is aroused by internal or external danger signals, a cascade of processes ensues. It signals the hypothalamus to stimulate the H-P-A axis to produce cortisol, it stimulates the locus ceruleus to flood the system with norepinephrin, and it mobilizes the sympathetic nervous system surge. The amygdala, like the hippocampus, also has receptors for cortisol.

In the presence of high levels of cortisol, the amygdala intensifies its signal to the hypothalamus, which, in turn, produces more CRH. This will keep the stress response running. Once again, the cortisol receptors on the hippocampus are critical in the down-regulation of the stress cascade.

Finally, the amygdala stimulates the nucleus basalis to release acetylcholine (ACh). This neurohormone generally arouses the cells of the cortex and makes them more receptive to incoming signals. It focuses the mind, so to speak. Norepinephrin generally places the person into a hyper-alert state and ACh makes the brain more responsive to the signals coming in. However, like norepinephrin, if this neurohormone is present in chronically high levels, hyperarousal and anxiety states will result (Fig. 17.7).

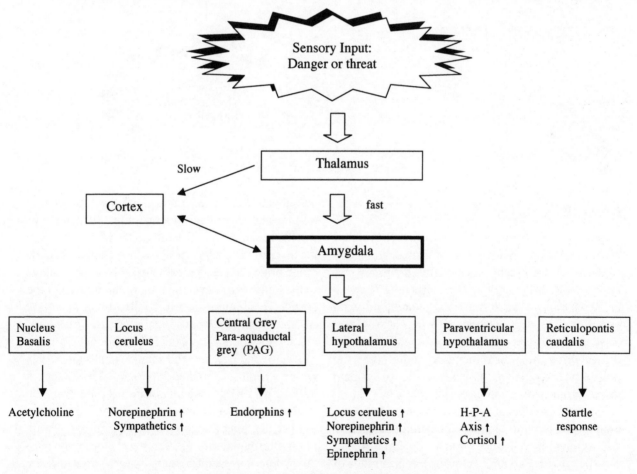

17.6 Sensory Fast Track to the Amygdala

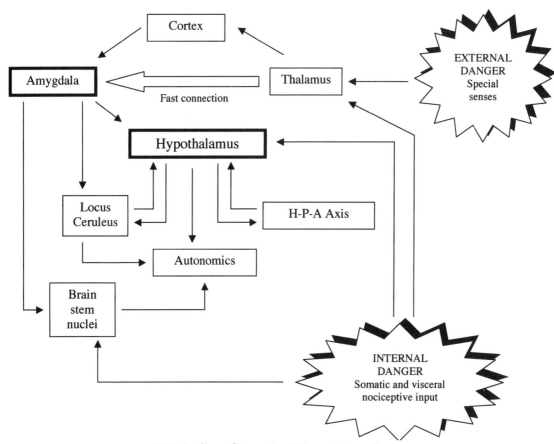

17.7 Outline of Important Stress Interactions

MEMORY CYCLES

Experience is internalized via several interrelated processes. Memory is not a singular process; it is mediated by several different systems. There are four memory processes to consider in stress responses. They are (1) *explicit memories* about stressful and emotional experiences, (2) *implicit emotional memories,* (3) *long-term memory* mediated by the cortex, and (4) *working memory,* short-term memory mediated by the prefrontal cortex. All of these memory loops can help drive chronic stress responses (Fig. 17.8).

Explicit memories are short-term memories mediated by the temporal lobe-hippocampus system, as well as long-term memories that are spread throughout the cortex. The hippocampus has a number of roles to play both in how we perceive our experience

and how we remember that experience. The sensory inputs of an experience (sound, sight, touch, taste, or smell) are sent by the thalamus to the parts of the cortex that process each particular sense. Then these parts of the brain send their representations of these inputs to the hippocampus via the temporal lobe area of the cortex. This temporal area is called the *transitional cortex.* The hippocampus then integrates these various sensory inputs into a unified experience. Thus, we can sense and perceive the sounds, smells and sights within a room as a unified experience. Experience is initially held within the hippocampus-temporal lobe system as short-term memory, and, over time, these explicit memories are stored in other parts of the brain as long-term memory. The temporal lobe-hippocampus system stores explicit memory for up to two years; then the sensory components are transferred to other

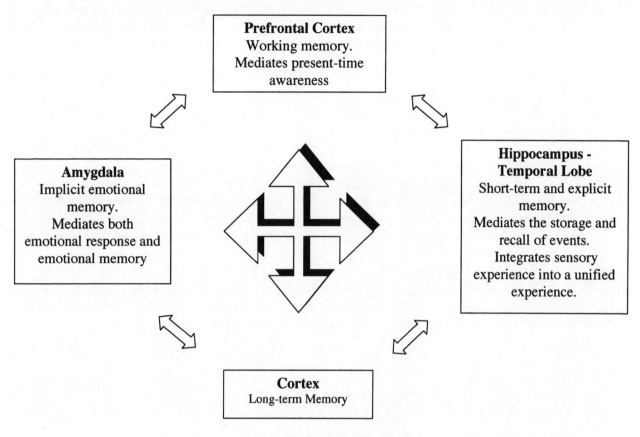

Prefrontal Cortex
Working memory.
Mediates present-time
awareness

Amygdala
Implicit emotional
memory.
Mediates both
emotional response and
emotional memory

**Hippocampus -
Temporal Lobe**
Short-term and explicit
memory.
Mediates the storage and
recall of events.
Integrates sensory
experience into a unified
experience.

Cortex
Long-term Memory

17.8 Memory Loop Relationships

parts of the cortex for storage. In either case, it is the hippocampus which integrates the different aspects of memory into an integrated total experience.

Implicit emotional memories are mediated by the amygdala. These are memories of the emotional component of a stressful or challenging experience. It is the amygdala that both initiates an emotional response to an experience and maintains an emotional memory of it. These are the charged, defensive emotions of fight or flight and may be expressed in a spectrum from fear and anger to terror and rage.

These memory cycles all have connections to the amygdala and hypothalamus. Thus, a memory of a trauma can set off the stress cascade and related dissociative processes. Let's say I had an accident that involved a bright flash of light. In the future, if I again encounter a bright flash of light, the amygdala interprets the flash as threatening based on its prior experience. Instantly, the memory of the accident arises along with the stress response related to the original event. I begin to sweat, my heart pounds, and I can hardly breathe. The physiological responses are all coupled with the light. Even more confusingly, I may not consciously remember the flash of light from the original accident. It may not be held as an explicit memory. This time, when I encounter a flash of light, no direct memory of the accident arises, but the emotional memory does. So I end up sweating and afraid, but do not know why. I may feel anxious and become fearful, yet have no recognition of an event and no sense of what my fear is about. An experience of this kind can be really crazy-making and confusing.

Interpretive meaning provides another factor in memory processing. Human beings give *meaning* to experience. These are called *life statements* in psychotherapy, and they can have a great impact. For instance, perhaps we experienced early childhood trauma of some kind in relationship to a close caretaker. We might be left with a felt-sense of despair coupled with a meaning such as "I will be destroyed by intimacy." This may become transferred onto close relationships. The closer the relationship, and the closer the sense of intimacy, then the more engaged the life statement and its felt-sense becomes, and the more the stress response is activated. We may find intimate relationships hard to maintain as we become more and more anxious, fearful, and angry without ever really knowing why. Fight or flight processes kick in and we run away from the relationship or become angry and confrontational. This is a maddening loop. The very thing that is wanted—intimacy—is sensed

as dangerous and suffocating. This is a simple example of how meaning, mediated by the cortex, will keep the stress response running. The amygdala again plays a role in this scenario, since some sensory experience of intimacy that was once associated with real threat can be perpetually interpreted as new danger, erroneously subverting or amplifying the whole interpretive meaning process. (Fig. 17.9)

The cortical processes that give meaning to an event also have connections to the amygdala. The meaning we give to traumatic experience can keep the amygdala running and prevent the processing of the experience. We have to somehow recognize and let go of the given meaning and process the experience, but this is very difficult to accomplish via any rational process. There is a way out of this loop, however, and that has to do with present time. Healing is only accessed in present time, and present time awareness is mediated by the prefrontal cortex.

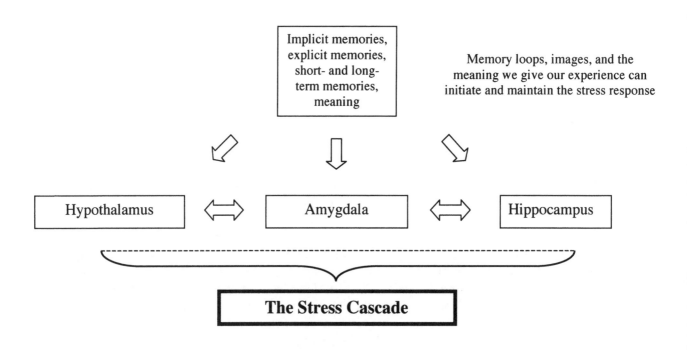

17.9 Cortical Stress Connections

THE PREFRONTAL CORTEX

The prefrontal cortex (especially its orbito-frontal area) plays a major role in mediating the stress response. The prefrontal cortex is where our present experience is integrated. This is called *working memory*. Working memory is an extremely short-term memory system. It holds the present-time awareness of experience. All sensory areas of the cortex have inputs to the prefrontal cortex, as do the hippocampus and amygdala, so this area receives all short- and long-term memories and their emotional tone or charge. The prefrontal cortex can also send signals back into these areas. Therefore we have a fluid interface with our past within the true here-and-now. Emotional memories mediated by the amygdala and explicit memories mediated by the hippocampus can be recalled within our present experience, and present experience can then be incorporated into both (Fig. 17.10).

The prefrontal cortex sends the amygdala information about the present nature of experience, about present time. It has the ability to say to the amygdala, "Hey, that experience is not happening now, cool it!" In other words, present-time awareness can help down-regulate the emotional cycling of the amygdala and thus down-regulate the stress response running in the system. I believe that Peter Levine's very effective "Somatic Experiencing" method derives some of

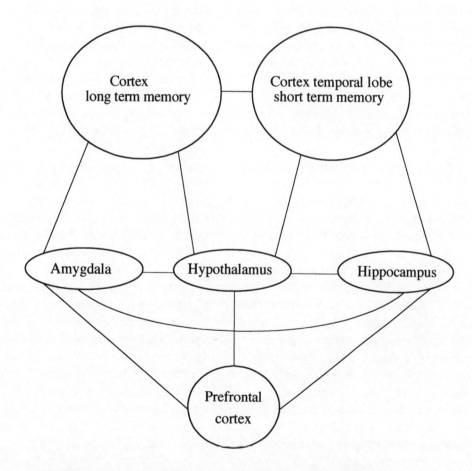

17.10 Interconnections for stress and emotion affect regulation

its effectiveness from this prefrontal cortex role.[6] The emphasis on present-time awareness in some psychotherapy forms, such as Gestalt and Core Process Psychotherapy, also keys into the regulatory role of the prefrontal cortex. Similarly, Eugene Gendlin's Focusing process is very helpful in accessing the felt experience of an arising process within present time. This alone can help down-regulate the stress response.

Likewise, therapeutic processes that work through the body in present time, mediated by the prefrontal cortex, give access to real healing. Simply paying attention to sensation in the body can have this effect. Practitioners working with trauma should work to help patients come into a present-time relationship with their experience. This means helping a person to be present in a non-dissociative way, through all of their senses in the immediacy of present experience. Awareness of inner sensations and feeling tones is especially useful as they give access to the nature of our inner experience. Present-time awareness helps down-regulate sympathetic activation and related stress hormones. As the prefrontal cortex communicates to the amygdala the present nature of experience, the amygdala has the opportunity to down-shift its emotional response.

This is not as easy as it might sound. It takes repeated journeys into the present to let go of the past. Negotiating the stress responses as they arise in the present needs sensitive management and accurate practitioner recognition of the stages of processing, or the responses can become overwhelming and even retraumatizing. The patient's process may need to be moderated for the safe discharge of the sympathetic arousal and down-regulation of the stress response. We explored a number of approaches in Volume One that can help moderate the patient's experience, largely based on Levine's work. Some key points are: accessing and developing resources, accessing a present-time awareness, orienting to sensation and embodied experience, accessing the felt-sense to help negotiate the felt meanings of experience, uncoupling memories and meanings from the sensations of the immediate experience, and slowing down emotional processes. We have to develop a resourced state

within which the sympathetic cycling can safely discharge and the system can return to homeostatic balance (Fig. 17.11).

SUMMARY OF THE STRESS CASCADE

Signs of external danger come in through the special senses and go to the thalamus. From here signals reach the amygdala by the two routes outlined above. The amygdala initiates the stress cascade and the system is mobilized for action. Signals about internal danger can also reach the hypothalamus, amygdala and locus ceruleus from nociceptors. Chronic nociceptive input can elicit both a chronic pain response and the general adaptation response.[7] Once the amygdala and hypothalamus are alerted to danger, the sympathetic nervous system is engaged, the adrenal glands release epinephrin into the blood system, the H-P-A axis produces cortisol, and the locus ceruleus pumps norepinephrin into the system. The system is flooded with norepinephrin, epinephrin, and cortisol.

The norepinephrin released by the locus ceruleus also goes to the hypothalamus and augments its release of CRH, which, in turn, also loops back to the locus ceruleus to facilitate its release of norepinephrin. Both the hypothalamus and locus ceruleus thus reinforce each other's action, and both receive input from the amygdala. The amygdala continues to signal danger in the presence of implicit and explicit memories, high levels of cortisol, and chronic nociceptive input. This keeps the stress response running until it is down-regulated.

Cortisol within the blood stream goes to the hippocampus, which has receptors for it, and the hippocampus then down-regulates the production of CRH. This down-regulates the whole stress cascade. These receptors can become overwhelmed, and the feedback loop to the hypothalamus is then compromised. The stress cascade can also be down-regulated via present time awareness mediated by the prefrontal cortex. The prefrontal cortex maintains overall control over stress responses and emotional regulation in general. The prefrontal cortex sends information to the amygdala and hypothalamus about present

> **Prefrontal Cortex**
> **Working memory**
> **Mediates present awareness,**
> **self-consciousness.**

 Emotional input

 Present-time awareness

> **Amygdala**
> **Mediates stress responses, emotional**
> **memory with stress components**

The amygdala gives the prefrontal cortex an emotional context for present experience, while the prefrontal cortex gives the amygdala the context of present time. Present time awareness can help down-regulate the stress cascade.

> **Stress Cascade**
> **H-P-A axis – CRH, ACTH, cortisol,**
> **Locus ceruleus - norepinephrin**
> **Sympathetic nervous system – mobilization, epinephrin**

17.11 The Prefrontal Cortex and Present Time

experience and can tell them "there is no tiger here" (Figs. 17.12 and 17.7).

All of this is not about the rational mind; it is physiologically driven and body oriented. That is why craniosacral biodynamics, with its emphasis on embodied forces and the manifestation of these in form and motion, is so effective in the healing process. Within a cranial context, states of balance within the nervous system, and the direction of potency and fluid to areas of facilitation and hypersensitivity, can dramatically help in the down-regulation and healing process.

CLINICAL PRESENTATIONS

Repercussions of chronic stress-related activation can present as active hyperarousal states within which everything seems to speed up, or as hypoarousal states within which everything seems to freeze or become immobilized. A patient in a hyperarousal state will be cycling norepinephrin, epinephrin, cortisol, and CRH. They may appear to be tense, excitable, and nervous. They may present with anxiety states, anxiety depression (exogenous depression), depressed

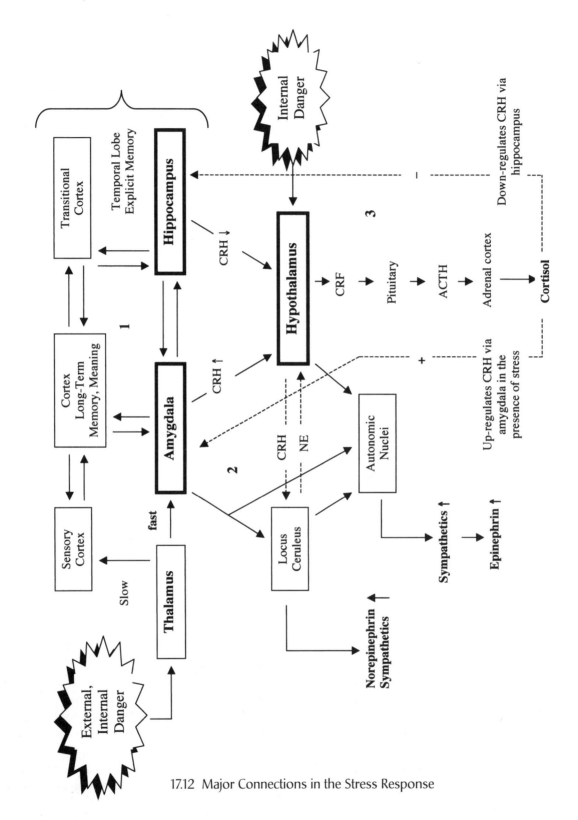

17.12 Major Connections in the Stress Response

immune function, poor appetite, and sleeplessness. These are all clinical indicators of chronic stress states such as post-traumatic stress disorder.

The opposite of these states, hypoarousal, is equally common. The patient may exhibit listlessness, lethargy, sleep a lot, eat a lot, and be constantly tired or exhausted, with low energy, autoimmune issues, and true depression (atypical or endogenous depression), with low energy and low motivation. Each of these states has a particular physiology.

PALPATION OF STRESS PROCESSES

Sympathetic cycling may be perceived as perturbation within the cerebrospinal fluid and tissue activation such as subtle trembling or more obvious shaking. It may be difficult to access the deeper, slower tides, and the CRI may be all that is apparent. This is an indication that much potency is bound systemically in an attempt to center the stress conditions. A chronically activated stress cascade is a systemic process and tends to be globally centered by the potency through the fluid system. Hence, the fluid tide may seem sluggish or dense, the fluid drive of the system may be low, the availability of potency will be lowered, and the motility of the CNS will be affected. There will be a sense of a depressed state at the core of the system, with bound resources, yet there is activation and perturbation cycling though the system at the same time.

Sympathetic activation may also be palpated as an electric-like discharge through the fluids and tissues. For instance, you may be palpating the sacrum and sense an electric-like streaming coming from the sympathetic ganglia. This streaming may be perceived to move through the buttocks and stream down the legs. This kind of discharge may be sensed when working with any tissue or tissue system. For instance, you may sense a sympathetic discharge when working with a vertebra, the cranial base, or an organ. This is commonly an indication that potency is processing the sympathetic cycling and its energy is being cleared. The patient may sense heat, tingling sensations, or muscular trembling. If the patient becomes overacti-

vated in a sympathetic discharge, (for example, the person may express an emotional flooding, or enter a frozen and immobilized state), it may be important to supply supportive verbal contact and slow pacing for the process as described in chapter 22 in Volume One.

In hypoarousal states you may perceive opposite kinds of processes. Little or no sympathetic discharge may be sensed. You may instead sense immobilized, depleted states with a density of potency throughout. The patient may experience coldness, numbness or a seeming paralysis. There may be dissociative processes involved. The patient may seem entirely non-expressive. Dissociation may be sensed as a vacancy in the patient's system, as if "no one is home," or as a sense that the patient is very distant and unable to verbally communicate. They may seem to be split off from their sense of embodiment and disconnected from sensations. However, with these hypostates, be aware that they may be overriding and concealing a hyperstate underneath, so the treatment may show a progression through hypo- to hyper- processing, reflecting the sequential deployment of autonomic strategies. Pure parasympathetic states, in which there is no underlying sympathetic charge, are also common.

CLINICAL APPROACHES

Craniosacral biodynamics offers very effective processes to down-regulate and moderate chronic stress responses. Systemic neutrals are great starting points because accessing these initiates autonomic clearing and a return to homeostasis. The CV4 process is a traditional way to help lower the hypertonicity of the system and restore access to resources. If dissociative states are coupled with the stress process, EV4s can be used to help reintegrate the psyche with the soma and to help access potency. Simply slowing a hyperarousal process down by subtly shifting pacing may also be useful. In the case of frozen and immobilized states, lateral fluctuation processes can stimulate potency and initiate a clearing of the cycling energies.

It is easy to get lost in complex physiology. Among all of these neuro-endocrine interactions, it is crucial to remember that it is the potency of the Breath of Life that is centering the process. As we work with the stress cascade, we are helping to resolve cycling energies being centered by the potency. As you help slow down or moderate the arising process, space is generated that allows potency to manifest. Lateral fluctuation processes also stimulate the potency to act beyond the conditions present. Rather than an inward spiral of reduced options and closed loops, an outward spiral opens as cycling forces resolve and potency becomes more available to mediate the process. The Health does the processing, not our interventions. Our interventions may orient the system to states of dynamic equilibrium and generate the space for this to occur, but the answer is already enfolded in the cycling forces.

Clinical Applications

Almost every patient I see begins to express some of these states during session work. Over the course of sessions, as the Inherent Treatment Plan is expressed, these stress cycles naturally come to the forefront. Orienting to primary respiration, the holistic shift, and systemic neutrals can all help to down-regulate stress cycles. Working with the motility of the central nervous system is also very helpful. The key is the state of balance and the accessing of dynamic equilibrium within the forces present. As the fulcrums organizing the central nervous system are resolved, potency is liberated and more resources become available for processing stress cycles.

This clinical application offers options in relating to the central nervous system, particularly the brain stem and the structures within the diencephalon. Again, it is essential to know the anatomy of the central nervous system. Look at the brain stem's relationships to the diencephalon (composed largely of the thalamus and hypothalamus), the limbic structures, especially the location of the amygdala and hippocampus, the temporal lobe area, and the cortex in general. Then put these images aside and let the living anatomy speak to you.

Accessing a Neutral

1. Use either Sutherland's or Becker's vault hold. Negotiate your contact with the patient's system and orient to the mid-tide. Listen to the motion and motility of the CNS as described in Chapter 3. Ideally the whole CNS moves as a unit of function with the lamina terminalis (anterior wall of the third ventricle) as its natural fulcrum. Give the system space. Orient to the ventricles and their motion and include an awareness of neural tissue. Let the motion of the central nervous system come into your awareness. Don't look for anything; let it come to you. Do not immediately engage inertial patterns. Simply orient to the inhalation and exhalation phases of primary respiration.

2. Wait for a holistic shift to resources to occur. When this happens, it will truly feel like you are palpating a unified potency-fluid-tissue field. You may also sense a clarity arising in the expression of primary respiration. Have patience here and give this time. Once the holistic shift occurs, continue to orient to primary respiration. Maintain an awareness of the ventricles and CNS motility and listen for the action of potency, either within the fluids or the field around the person.

3. As you are listening, over time, an inertial pattern may clarify. It may be sensed as an eccentric motion, a point of restriction, or as a density within the neural tissue. You may even sense a quality of agitation, or perturbation in areas that are running a chronic stress response. Alternatively, you may sense density and inertia in particular areas. Do not look for anything; let the tissues and fluids take you into their patterns. Wait and listen. Give the system time to express its priorities.

4. As an inertial pattern clarifies, follow its expression. Again give space to the potency, fluids, and tissue. Listen for the organizing fulcrum. Do you sense a locus of stillness around which the motion

is organized? Remember your anatomy. Is there a fulcrum within the brain stem? The diencephalon? The limbic structures? Do you sense activation or density within the hypothalamus, amygdala, or hippocampus? Follow the motion present and listen for Becker's three-phase healing process to arise. If needed, very subtly help the tissue and/or fluid elements to settle into a state of balance. Very gently and subtly slow things down. As you sense the motion within the inertial pattern, slow the fluid and tissue motion down until there is a settling into a state of balance. Do not mentally or physically grab onto any of the three fields of potency, fluids, and tissues as you intend this. If you do, you may obstruct the system. Maintain your wide perceptual field. Do not lose a sense of the whole as you do this. Listen for the unfolding of the healing process and for expressions of Health as previously explored in Volume One.

5. When motion is again re-established, listen for the third stage of Becker's process—the reorganization of the potency, fluid, and tissue fields. Does the motion of the CNS seem to be more aligned with its natural fulcrum at the lamina terminalis? Does the motion of the ventricles seem more balanced in inhalation and exhalation? Wait for the period of reorganization to complete. You may sense a surge within the fluid tide as this occurs and/or a consistent expression of a new pattern of organization in relationship to the midline and the lamina terminalis.

This general treatment can be effective in resolving stress response problems. In addition, we can use other approaches as described below.

Fluid Applications

In the above application, you may sense a fulcrum in a particular area of the central nervous system, presenting as a density or as an area of activation. Sometimes you can actually sense a buzz coming from a specific facilitated nuclei. An area of density may be a manifestation of an entrapped force vector. Directing potency within the cerebrospinal fluid to a specific fulcrum can be very effective.

1. Using the work above, a fulcrum may be sensed within some of the structures we have been discussing. For instance, there may be an eccentric pattern of motion around an area within the brain stem, or the right amygdala may become highlighted. Let these structures come into your field of awareness. Do not narrow your perceptual field as you do this.

2. A number of options are available here. You can direct fluid and potency via the thumbs or index fingers from the vault hold in the work above. This could be used within a state of balance if there is a flatness to the state, or more directly as the fulcrum is sensed in order to liberate potency and access the state of balance.

3. Simply direct fluid toward the fulcrum and sense the response. For example, you may sense a density, motion, or activation related to the left amygdala (located at the anterior aspect of the floor of the left lateral ventricle). Direct fluid toward that area with your right thumb or index finger. You may sense fluid fluctuations or echoing of fluid and potency. Wait for a sense of softening and processing of the stress cycle and related biokinetic forces involved. This may be sensed as a streaming of a force vector, as expansion and softening, and/or as a clearing of perturbation within the cerebrospinal fluid.

4. Alternatively, you may change the hand position. Working from the occipital cradle can be very useful when the intention is to direct fluid toward the brain stem or limbic structures. It can be especially useful when relating to the hypothalamus, amygdala, and hippocampus.

States of Balance and Directing Fluid from the Occipital Cradle

1. Using the occipital cradle hold, again listen to the motility and motion dynamics of the central nervous system. As you sense its motility, orient

to the brain stem, diencephalon, hippocampus, and amygdala. Orienting to the third ventricle can give you a way into the hypothalamus, which is located in the floor of the ventricle. Similarly, orienting to the lateral ventricles can give access to the hippocampus, which is the floor of the lateral ventricle, and to the amygdala, located just anterior to the hippocampus.

2. Sense the motility of the central nervous system and see if you perceive any motion dynamics oriented around these structures. Alternatively, you may sense density or activation, like an electric charge or buzzing, coming from any of these.

3. If you sense anything which draws you to an area as a fulcrum, direct fluid and potency toward it. This can be done directly, or within a state of balance. Listen for the response from the area. Let's take the example of the amygdala. As in the example above, you may sense a motion or activation related to the left amygdala. Orient to the left lateral ventricle and sense the amygdala as the front wall of the lateral ventricle. From your cradle hold, access a state of balance relative to the amygdala as an inertial fulcrum. Then direct fluid with the heels of your hands toward the amygdala. You may sense fluid fluctuations, echoing of fluid and potency, etc. Wait for a sense of softening and processing of the stress cycle and related biokinetic forces involved. This may be sensed as expansion and softening and/or as a clearing of activation.

CV4 AND EV4 IN ACTIVATION STATES

In hyperarousal states, CV4 can help slow things down, down-regulate the central nervous system, and affect the entire neuro-endocrine axis. It can help shift the set point of the autonomic system from fixity to a more fluid response to the environment. It can also help the system discharge the shock affects of trauma within a resourced state, as potency within the fluids acts to resolve the traumatization. As this occurs, the practitioner may sense perturbations and electric-like clearing within the fluids as the shock affects disperse.

In hypoarousal states, where the system is running a different physiology, EV4s can help the system come out of freezing and immobilization. EV4s can also help manifest the resources of the system from the center out and help in the reassociative process. In this expression of potency from the core to the periphery, the dissociated psyche is helped to find its way back to embodiment. CV4 and EV4 are specific in their effects. An EV4 can exacerbate an activated state, and a CV4 can do the same for a hypo- or dissociative state. Let the system guide you to the appropriate strategy, with CV4 as the general approach for hyper- and EV4 as the general approach for hypo- and dissociative conditions.

The *sacral-ethmoid hold* described in Chapter 2 can be used to good effect in hypoarousal and dissociative states. With the patient side-lying, place one hand over the sacrum, pointing caudad with the middle finger over the coccyx. Place the index and middle fingers of the other hand in a "V" over glabella anterior to the ethmoid bone. This hold can help the patient feel contained and held. Tune into the patient's primal midline and ordering field. Very gently initiate an EV4 via the sacrum. Listen for the action of potency within the fluid midline.

Clinical Highlight

A young woman had low-back pain, sciatic pain, and anxiety states that manifested as a general tension in her everyday experience, sleeplessness, and constant worry. In the first few sessions, the most pressing clinical intention was to find a way into contact and relationship because she initially experienced touch as painful. Contact literally intensified her discomfort. I began with resourcing processes and was able to help her find some sense of resource in her body sensations after a number of sessions. Her system was in a very activated and seemingly confused state. Pain tended to shift around and her system moved quickly from fulcrum to fulcrum without any healing processes being engaged. There was a high sympathetic tonus present and a sense of density in the fluids and tautness and dryness in her membrane system. After a number of sessions oriented to establishing safety and contact, we began to work with CV4s via the fluid system. It took about seven sessions for her system to be able to access systemic neutrals. Once this happened, the Inherent Treatment Plan could begin to unfold.

In one session, potency shifted toward her pelvis and there was a clarification of patterning around her right sacroiliac joint. She shared how the feeling tones seemed to be coupled to an old car accident. This was an extremely frightening experience for her. She was in the hospital for nearly a month after the accident. Some sympathetic shock affect was cleared, and I was able to help her stay with a coupled fear response. Both seemed to move through her body and dissipate, and a more settled state arose. Over the next sessions, her system shifted to vertebral issues, cranial base patterns, and central nervous system activation. The cranial patterns which presented seemed to relate to birth trauma and early childhood issues. The main intention in this phase was to help generate space within the structural and primal midlines. I also introduced her to the focusing process, which she found very helpful. She managed to process some very deep cranial base patterns in a resourced and paced manner.

In one session in particular, her potency shifted deeply within her ventricle system, and the motility of the central nervous system came to the forefront. Here, I worked largely as described above, first from a vault hold and then from an occipital cradle. The session work oriented to deepening states of balance, stillness, and Long Tide phenomena. Again, there were periods of sympathetic clearing, especially from the brain stem. In one session I more actively directed potency towards the right amygdala-hippocampus area, which seemed to be highlighted and activated by the action of potency within the cerebrospinal fluid. This seemed to help clear the cycling within those relationships and led to a deepening into a state of balance.

Her low-back issues were alleviated after the first eight sessions, and after fifteen sessions, her sleep patterns normalized and her anxiety levels were lowered. We continued to work with focusing sessions, neutrals, and stillness over a number of further sessions. Her system seemed to be moving to a more fluid and homeostatic state. Her autonomic tonus was regularized and seemed much less prone to activation. In the twenty-fourth session she stated that she felt empowered enough to hold her process in ways that were not possible before, and sessions were terminated at that point. We had a follow-up session a number of months later, and her system had indeed maintained autonomic balance, and she was able to hold her personal process with much more space and equanimity.

1. Glenn J. Giesler, *Nociception and the Neuroendocrine-immune Connection, Studies of Spinal Cord Neurons That Project Directly to the Hypothalamus,* ed. F. H. Williard and M.M. Patterson (American Academy of Osteopathy, 1994).

2. Ibid.

3. Ibid.

4. Joseph Ledoux, *The Emotional Brain* (Touchstone Books, 1998).

5. Ibid.

6. Peter Levine, *Waking the Tiger* (North Atlantic Books, 1997).

7. F. H. Willard and M.M. Patterson, eds., *Nociception and the Neuroendocrine-immune Connection* (American Academy of Osteopathy, 1994).

18

The Polyvagal Concept
and the Triune Nervous System

The *polyvagal concept* is an important new understanding of the autonomic nervous system, developed by Stephen Porges, Ph.D., and introduced in Chapter 14. I think that Porges' work holds tremendous implications for the health fields because it refines our recognition of the processes at work in stress response beyond the currently prevailing model. This field is changing rapidly, but in the several years since I first encountered these new concepts, their validity has been repeatedly confirmed.

Venturing into such a new field, I invariably must rely on Porges' written articles, and therefore I would like to express a caution. This concept is still developing and is not yet widely distributed. I would like to apologize in advance for any misconceptions, in the sincere hope that inclusion of this material furthers the collective development of effective therapeutic methods for stress and trauma sufferers.

In this chapter we will:

- *Describe the polyvagal concept.*

- *Describe the fight or flight process in terms of the polyvagal concept.*

- *Present a new approach to autonomic nervous system support.*

As a final preliminary, this chapter assumes the reader has a basic understanding of the autonomic nervous system as presented earlier. If necessary, please review your basic physiology and the material already presented in Volume One and also in this volume in chapters 3, 14, and 17.

AUTONOMIC NERVOUS SYSTEM

The autonomic nervous system is the underlying control system regulating survival functions. Its importance cannot be overstated. There are few health problems that are not a factor in some way of the autonomic nervous system, directly or indirectly. Certainly the entire field of post-traumatic stress disorder falls within its scope, along with most degenerative diseases, all stress-related situations, autoimmune diseases, and many others. The odd fact of public health awareness is that many people are largely uninformed of this most critical part of their own anatomy, and are surprised to learn that their symptoms have a clear basis in physiology.

Traditionally the autonomic nervous system is considered to have two branches, parasympathetic and sympathetic, and these are thought to operate in a generally reciprocal manner: when one is up, the other is down. These two are thought to work synergistically to operate the key functions starting with the heart/lungs supplying nutrient- and oxygen- rich blood to the brain. In addition, all other essential functions are coordinated through autonomic action, including digestion, reproduction, and elimination.

Trauma theorists have naturally focused on autonomic functions in understanding the stress response.

Great interest has been placed on the *fight or flight* response of the sympathetic, and the *freeze* response of the parasympathetic. Similarly, the control centers of autonomic function have been studied deeply. The hypothalamus provides higher-level control and regulation, and the amygdala initiates fight or flight processes via connections to the hypothalamus, locus ceruleus, and sympathetic system. Porges has developed some important clarifications in relationship to the autonomic nervous system, mammalian defensive responses, and social activities which have to do both with how the autonomic system has evolved and how its anatomy is organized.[1]

Triune Autonomic Nervous System

Porges proposes a new model of a *triune autonomic nervous system* based on a hierarchy of phylogenic relationship. Phylogeny is the study of the evolution of life forms' functions, from ancient simplicity to modern complexity. The Porges' three-part system includes:

1. The first layer is an evolutionarily more primitive unmyelinated *parasympathetic nervous system* that sets a metabolic baseline for survival. Originating in the distant past when creatures were passive feeders in a liquid environment, the parasympathetic has a small range of responses to novelty and stress, in the form of adjustments in metabolic rate including death feigning or freezing via down-regulation of heart rate. Examples of parasympathetic-dominant animals are invertebrates and worms. The anatomy of this system consists of the nerves that operate heart/ lung, digestive, and reproductive organs, particularly the vagus nerve and the cervical and sacral plexuses. Some authors also place the enteric nervous system (the *gut brain*) in the parasympathetic category although the enteric operates with significant independence and has also been described as separate from the central nervous system.

2. The second component is a more recently developed *sympathetic nervous system* that adds mobility and therefore a much more robust set of survival options. These later animals, including vertebrates all the way up the evolutionary ladder to mammals, have much wider survival options for finding food, finding mates, and escaping from predators by virtue of their striated muscle-driven appendages. The anatomy of this system consists of nerves that modify the parasympathetic system and operate muscles involved in mobilization activities and fight or flight. Particularly notable are the double chain of sympathetic ganglia running along either side of the spine, connecting with the spinal cord at thoracic and upper lumbar levels.

3. The third layer in this new scheme is a most recently developed myelinated system called the *social nervous system* that advances survival repertoires even further by enabling sophisticated information-processing and group behaviors. This new capability, exhibited in mammals and highly developed in primates, tremendously increases survival chances. The anatomy of this part includes nerves that operate facial expression, voice, hearing, mouth and head-turning, particularly cranial nerves V, VII, IX, and part of X and XI. The social nervous system enables many important social behaviors, but perhaps none is more important for survival than the mechanisms that generate maternal bonding. As brain size increases, babies need enough time to mature and become independent. Structures and functions to secure this protected time are not a luxury; they are essential. The responses involved are not voluntary; they are too important for that, so they are hard-wired into autonomic-level functioning. The solution is a complex set of structures and functions that together create a neurophysiologic-biochemical phenomenon whereby the newborn baby can find the mother, get her attention, find the breast, nurse, coordinate sucking, breathing, and swallowing and elicit profound care-giving motivations that endure for decades or even a whole lifetime. With this set of functions, ample time for sophisticated cortex development is secured and the ultimate survival machine, the human being, is enabled.

These three systems are highly interactive and overlap substantially. Most organs are directly innervated by at least two of the three, and indirectly affected by all three. But within that interdependent complexity, they generally operate in sequence. The newer systems operate by inhibiting and modifying the older, so the parasympathetic sets a baseline, the sympathetic acts on the parasympathetic, and the social acts on the sympathetic. In the presence of threat or novelty, this sequential scheme unfolds. We use our most sophisticated equipment first (social), then we try the older strategy (sympathetic), and if that fails we try the oldest (parasympathetic).

For babies, the social strategy is really the only viable option, since they are too small and dependent to fight or flee. The archetypal defeat of the social nervous system is betrayal by a caregiver, whether intentionally or just as a by-product of modern hospital practices. If the social tools are ineffective, the baby devolves to its next most primitive option, a sympathetic fight or flight response. Then if the sympathetic is not successful, the system will revert to the more primitive parasympathetic responses of immobilization and dissociation. Indeed, the primal defensive strategy of a baby is dissociation and withdrawal. Fight or flight has little use if you cannot move or protect yourself, so infants tend to readily move to their most primitive strategy.

The Triune Autonomic Nervous System and Survival Mechanisms

- *Social Nervous System*

  Social communication, orienting, self-calming.

- *Sympathetic Nervous system*

  Mobilization, fight or flight.

- *Parasympathetic Nervous System*

  Immobilization, freezing, death feigning.

THE VAGUS NERVE AND ITS NUCLEI

The term Polyvagal Theory originated with Porges' finding that the traditional understanding of the parasympathetic system's key pathway, the vagus nerve, did not account for some anatomical subtleties. Rather than being a single system, the vagus nerve has been clearly demonstrated to have multiple nuclei (dorsal motor nucleus, nucleus ambiguus, and nucleus solitarius, all long bilateral brain stem fibers at the level of the foramen magnum) and variations in structure and function that do not conform to conventional parasympathetic classification rules.

The ventral or pharyngeal branch of the vagus (ventral vagal complex) arises from the nucleus ambiguus (NA). These fibers do not meet the normal criteria for classification as part of the parasympathetic branch of the autonomic nervous system. This system does have inputs to the heart and bronchi, appropriate for parasympathetic function, but it also is myelinated, not unmyelinated as is the norm for parasympathetic. Similarly, the ventral vagal's association (via the corticobulbar tract) with the nerves and structures controlling the face, neck, and throat also disqualifies it from classification as purely parasympathetic, because these are voluntary muscles. Nonconformance of these fibers serves as Porges' basic evidence that the vagus is not all parasympathetic, as previously assumed.

The dorsal branch of the vagus (dorsal vagal complex) arises from the dorsal motor nucleus, descends to the torso, and innervates the heart/lungs and the viscera below the diaphragm. These are classic unmyelinated parasympathetic fibers. The dorsal motor nucleus (DMN) operates the heart/lungs and viscera in their baseline and "rest/repose" night-time mode under the parasympathetic system. Under stress, the DMN mainly slows the heart down and lowers oxygen consumption to generate an immobility state. This system is associated with freezing and dissociative states in humans. In prey animals, this down-regulated state ("playing possum") has great survival value in that a predator may lose interest due to evolutionary programming against eating old meat that may be spoiled or infected. In human babies, the down-regulated state can make the baby less conspicuous, but may be dangerous as lowered heart rate and oxygen levels can compromise autonomic func-

tion and baseline metabolism. Extreme parasympathetic down-regulation can be fatal (Fig. 18.1).

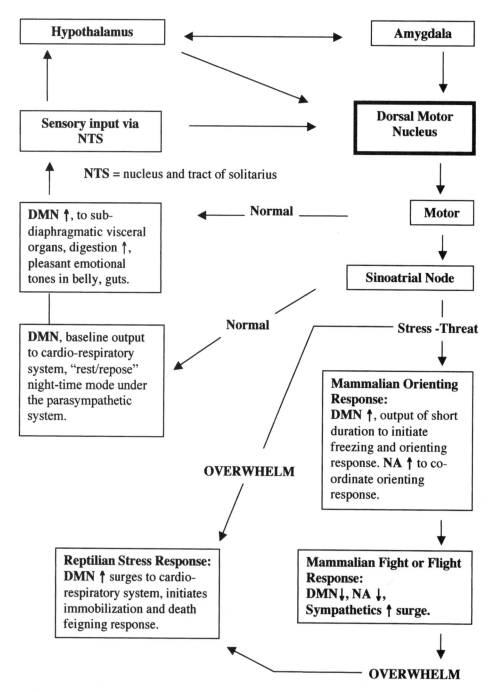

18.1 Polyvagal Responses: Dorsal Vagus Complex and Dorsal Motor Nucleus

The nucleus ambiguus has a significantly different job description involving all three branches of the autonomic system. It projects to the heart and bronchi, but it also goes to the muscles of the face, scalp, and neck. The projections to the heart and bronchi coordinate breathing with heart rate, allowing the heart and breath to speed up and remain in synchronization as we walk faster. It provides a vagal brake on the sympathetics to the cardiovascular system and is involved in self-calming processes. As the vagal brake is reduced, the sympathetics take over, and heart rate and breathing increase. When this NA-vagal brake is removed in threatening situations, a rapid response to danger is allowed as the sympathetics can take over without having to engage the sympathetic-adrenal system first. This is a typical mammalian response.

In its social nervous system function, the NA coordinates head and neck motion in the orienting response, and in conjunction with its cardiovascular supply, mediates the relationship between chewing, swallowing, sucking, and breathing, controls the intonation of vocalizations, and is involved in the communication of emotional states and needs. All of these have direct bearing on infants' survival engagement with their mothers. Thus, infants can orient toward the sight and sounds of mother, vocalize their needs, and show their related emotional states through facial expression. They can make sounds of joy, smile at their mothers, nurse, and breathe all at the same time in an integrated and coordinated way. In terms of defensive strategies, the NA coordinates the orienting response and allows the animal to calmly scan the environment for danger (Fig. 18.2).

We have covered autonomic stress phenomena in this book and in Volume One. All the material presented on working with trauma, working with the central nervous system through states of balance, resolving pre- and perinatal issues, and (in the next chapter) working with nerve facilitation, can all be combined into one body of knowledge within craniosacral biodynamics.

For this chapter, our practical focus is on exercises and applications to support the triune autonomic nervous system, in light of the work done by Porges.

CRANIAL APPROACHES TO THE TRIUNE HIERARCHY OF DEFENSIVE STRATEGIES

The following section explores some very interesting work being developed by John Chitty, RCST. I have experienced this work first-hand and see great potential in its becoming a useful part of a cranial approach to activation and unresolved autonomic cycling within the system. I offer the following as my own extrapolation of the new methods being developed based on the Porges model.

The work is described in four stages:

1. Recognizing signs of autonomic activation.
2. Resolution of parasympathetic activation.
3. Resolution of sympathetic activation.
4. Re-establishment of the social nervous system.

In working with each of the three autonomic systems, session work will include palpation skills and patient interaction.

SIGNS OF AUTONOMIC ACTIVATION

The following is meant to be an adjunct to general session work. It is perhaps best used when sympathetic or parasympathetic activation is sensed or expressed during sessions. Various signs of sympathetic arousal can be sensed via palpation as perturbation within the fluids, especially cerebrospinal fluid. This is an expression of the discharge of autonomic energies into the fluids. It is commonly a sign of the processing of these forces by the potency within the fluids. You might also sense an electrical streaming through the body. It is not uncommon to sense this kind of discharge from the center of the body to the periphery. An example might be a discharge of energy inferiorly through the sympathetic ganglia chain, through the sacrococcygeal ganglion, and down the legs. It is common to sense this kind of discharge as you palpate the sacrum. You may sense this as a contained and resourced clearing within a state of balance.

Alternatively, you may sense a more parasympathetic state within the body. There may be a sense of

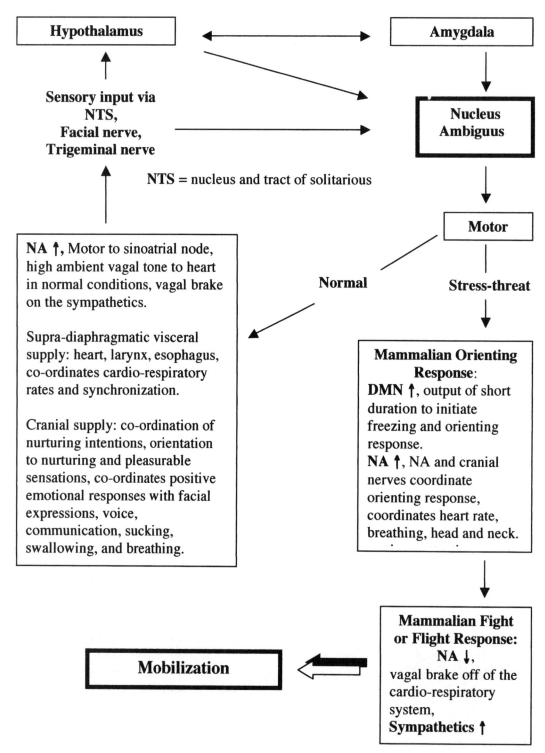

18.2 Polyvagal Responses: Ventral Vagal Complex and the Nucleus Ambiguus

density, coldness, numbness, and fluid stagnation as you palpate a particular area. This all indicates the presence of inertial potencies centering and containing some kind of force within the system. Common cranial approaches to these more frozen states might include EV4s and the use of fluid skills such as lateral fluctuation and fluid drive processes.

Other, more overt signs of autonomic activation may include tissue fibrillation and body trembling and shaking, skin color changes such as redness and red blotches, sweating, and increased breathing and cardiac rates. These are common sings of sympathetic arousal. Also included in this kind of sympathetic activation are states of emotional flooding and processes which suddenly and dramatically speed up. The person may be flooded with alternating memories, images, and related emotional couplings. Cranial approaches classically include CV4s, slowing motion down and states of balance. The practitioner must appreciate that the emotions being expressed are manifestations of past traumatization. Acknowledgement of the power of the emotional process, slowing that process down, and helping to resource the patient in the midst of the experience are key points here. Please see Chapters 21 and 22 in Volume One for trauma skills related to these states.

Parasympathetic activation may be sensed as coldness and numbing. The patient will commonly relate that they are cold, or that a part of their body is cold or numb. Experiences of numbed areas of the body, and even of immobilization and seeming paralysis, are possible. For instance, a patient may report that their legs have gone numb and they cannot move them. This can be a frightening experience for both patient and practitioner. The practitioner must understand that this is an opportunity to resolve the forces cycling within the system. A verbal acknowledgement of the power of the process and verbal reassurance to the patient may be very important here. Traditional cranial approaches might include the state of balance and the use of lateral fluctuation to stimulate the expression of potency. Again, please see Chapters 21 and 22, Volume One, for trauma skills related to these states.

Clinical Application:
The Triune Nervous System

The following process consciously works with the hierarchy of nervous system response and activation and can be repeated a number of times within a session to help down-regulate the cycling stress cascade. In each phase, there is a particular hand position, an anatomical visualization, and a component of patient participation. Getting the patient's participation helps to clearly engage the particular system and empowers the patient to experience their own process in present time. Under stress, the organism will first try to respond via the social nervous system and orienting response. When this is overwhelmed, the system will default to a sympathetic response and, if this is further overwhelmed, to a parasympathetic one. Here we will follow the hierarchy back up from the parasympathetic, to the sympathetic and finally to the social nervous system response.

Parasympathetic Activation

1. Start with an *occipital cradle hold*. Shift this hold more caudad (inferior) to place your index fingers on either side of the anterior-lateral aspect of the neck, over the pathway of the vagus nerve as it exits the jugular foramen on each side. Check your anatomy here. Visualize the torso of the person as an elongated tube, banded in the middle by the diaphragm. This promotes access to the parasympathetic unit of function, a visceral tube and the ancient worm-like nature of a primitive digestive tube (Fig. 18.3).

2. Now visualize both visceral vagus nerves and form a relationship to their dual pathway from the jugular foramen, innervating the heart and lungs, through the diaphragm and over the organs below the diaphragm. This need not be an exact anatomical image. Simply visualize its branching, tree-like nature. Combine this with your visualization of the tube-like shape as one whole unit of primitive function. Orient to the mid-tide and its 2.5 cycles per minute rhythm.

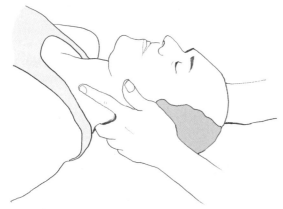

18.3 Parasympathetic nervous system hold

Hold a wide perceptual field and orient to this tube and the vagus nerves within it as a whole.

3. When the relationship is well established, ask the patient to actively participate in the process by bringing attention to the sensations generated in their belly by the movement of their own breath. Let this continue this as a focus of their attention for a minute or so until they seem to settle into their breathing and a parasympathetic level of functioning. Some clients may have a hard time staying with this attention to breath process, either falling asleep or spacing out as the parasympathetic state becomes established. If this happens, simply carry on with the work; it is not necessary to make them try to stay focused for an extended time period.

4. Settle into your relationship. Orient to the fluid tide and then include tissue motion. See if you can allow the motion of this visceral tube-vagus unit of function to come into your hands within the phases of primary respiration. As an inertial pattern is expressed within the total combined unit of function, listen for Becker's three-phase awareness. Seek a state of balance and listen for expressions of Health.

5. Within this context, also listen for signs of the processing and discharge of shock affects and a shift in the system. The patient may cycle from numb, frozen, and immobilized states to more active sympathetic processes. The patient may sense their body literally "coming alive." They may sense themselves reassociating and "coming back" into their body. You may notice movements of their body, perturbations within the fluids, discharges of energy, etc. The patient may sense trembling, streamings of sensations in their arms and/or legs, tingling, feelings of fight or flight impulses like the urge to move and emotions arising. They may also begin to move their head and neck in orienting types of motions. Allow this to settle. These are all indications that the system is shifting out of a frozen parasympathetic state to a wider autonomic repertoire. These are cues to move to the next phase of the process. All this can occur in a relatively short period of time, even after just a few minutes.

Sympathetic Activation

1. When the time feels right, shift your orientation from the parasympathetic nervous system to the sympathetic nervous system. The placement of your hands stays roughly the same, with your index fingers shifting slightly posterior over the superior cervical sympathetic ganglion at the superior aspect of the sympathetic chain on both sides. This ganglion is immediately adjoining the vagus nerve in the sides of the neck that we used in the previous part of the process. The fingers are pointing inferior from just below the head towards the feet.

2. Now visualize and sense the pathway of the sympathetic ganglion chain down either side of the vertebral column. See if you can hold a recognition of its overall form including its connections to the spinal cord and its termination in a single ganglion just anterior to the coccyx. Each chain also has a filament supplying sympathetic innervation to the cranium. Orient to the whole of the sympathetic chain at once. Again hold this within a holistic awareness of the body and biosphere.

You are not "tracking" the chain from top-to-bottom; you are holding *all of it at once as a single unit of function* within your wide, biosphere-midtide perceptual field. Again, review your anatomy of this area. When you "have" the sympathetic chain in your hands, you will have a sense of its continuity (Fig. 18.4).

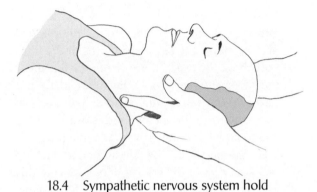

18.4   Sympathetic nervous system hold

3. When your relationship to the sympathetics seems well established, enlist patient participation again. Ask the patient to very slowly and briefly flex their arms and clench their fists. As they do this, also ask them to slowly tighten their pelvic and leg muscles, flex their feet back and push through the heels of their feet. This engages the musculoskeletal echoes of the fight or flight response within their body. Have them briefly do this and then instruct them to soften and relax. Have them track the sensations that may arise within their body. You can have them repeat this a number of times if appropriate.

4. As they stay with sensations and feeling tones that may have been elicited in the process, orient to the whole of the sympathetic pathway-ganglion chain. Again, if an inertial pattern of form and motion is expressed through the whole of the sympathetic pathway, follow this and help access a state of balance. Pay particular attention to patterns at the level of the respiratory diaphragm, as these seem to be especially prevalent and powerful. Again orient to expressions of Health and to any sympathetic nervous system clearing. This may be sensed as a streaming of electric-like energies, as perturbations within the fluids, and as the clearing of the inertial forces and force vectors involved.

5. The cue to the transition to the social nervous system is a resolution of the sympathetic activation, a resolution of the inertial shape palpated, and a settling of the sympathetic nervous system into a stillness with a concomitant rise in the sense of potency within the system. You may even sense the orienting response being elicited as the person begins to rotate or move their head, or the face becomes animated. This sympathetic process seems to often take more time than the parasympathetic, and it can be more dramatic in terms of discharge. Trauma resolution skills presented in Volume One may be useful here as well.

Social Nervous System Re-establishment

1. In this next part of the process, we shift our orientation to the social nervous system. The visualization component is based on the anatomy. To access the social nervous system as a unit of function, change your hand position to a contact spreading across the sides of the face and upper sides of the throat. This position approximates the *pharyngeal arch* structure that contains the original fibers of cranial nerves V, VII, IX, and part of X. With your thumb lightly in the ear canal, spread your other fingers over the mandible and upper anterior neck.

2. Once you negotiate and settle into this new hold, visualize the inner ear structures, especially the inner ear muscles (the stapedius and tensor tympani) and cranial nerves V and VII. Visualize the relationship of these nerves to the inner ear. You can also include an awareness of the nucleus ambiguus in the brain stem at the level of the foramen magnum. Your main orientation will be to the petrous temporal bone and its inner ear structures. Once again, review your anatomy so that these structures are clear to you. Settle into

a mid-tide orientation and perceptual field. Let these structures come to you. Do not narrow your perceptual field in order to do this (Fig. 18.5).

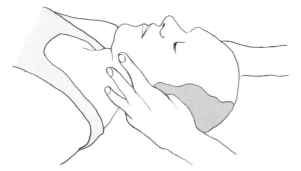

18.5 Social nervous system hold

3. You will now again enlist the patient's active participation in the process. Ask the patient to visualize a person from their early childhood whose "eyes would light up" in appreciative greeting if they met. This should be a person with whom they had a simple, mutually warm and friendly relationship. Friends, pets, and relatives all qualify here, or even an archetypal image of some kind, such as a baby. Be creative and negotiate with the patient to identify a good visualized encounter with a truly non-threatening person. The relationship with close family members (especially parents) is too complex; an aunt or uncle, friend, or pet is more likely to be effective for invoking the appreciative greeting felt-sense experience. The key here is the ability to access the *feeling tone* of the bright, affectionate, and smiling facial expression of that person, to hear their warm greeting in the imagination. To encourage this access, it may be helpful to have the patient imagine an encounter with this resourcing person from their early childhood, complete with recalling the likely setting of the encounter in some detail, including visual, auditory, and/or kinesthetic components.[2] The intention of this is to generate a sense of an early nurturing encounter that elicits the social nervous system and its orienting processes.

4. Sometimes the patient cannot relate to early childhood, or the question brings up upsetting memories. If this occurs, have them first orient to any person, pet, or relationship from any phase of their life, with whom they had a fully resourcing connection. Sometimes orienting to a place they feel safe in, like a particular place in the natural world, can help.

5. Once this imagined encounter is established, orient, via your hand contact, to the pharyngeal arches and/or the inner structures of the temporal bone. Be especially aware of the fine inner muscles that relate to orienting to sound. Do not narrow your perceptual field as you do this; remember to hold an awareness of the whole and to let these inner structures come to you. If your anatomy knowledge is sufficient, include an awareness of the cranial nerves serving this area, especially cranial nerves V and VII. Follow any inertial patterns that come into your awareness and allow any processing of stress responses which arise here. It is common for the patient to begin to express orienting motions, such as head rotation and eye movements. Similarly, warmth and tingling may spread through the face, and memories of loving contact may arise. Brief waves of feelings, positive and/or negative, may wash over the lower face, including the throat area. Allow these to occur, slowing the process down if necessary. Acknowledge to the patient anything that seems important.

6. Work with Becker's three-phase process and orient to expressions of Health, potency, fluid, and tissue processes. Wait for any processes of reorganization and realignment to occur.

An optional extra component for this application is to work with the amygdala using the process described in the previous chapter. This seems to "reset" the system, ready for a fresh, present-time experience of life instead of constantly interpreting experiences based on past history.

These three phases of hierarchical work may cycle through relatively quickly, and the whole process can be repeated within a session to gradually arrive at a sense of real completion. It may also take a number of sessions to resolve a particular level of stress response in the system. I think that this process has great potential and would like to hear from practitioners who have experience over a number of sessions with many patients.

As a final note for this application, EV4 can be a very beneficial strategy to integrate the above work. It is excellent for patients who are set in dissociative and low-energy parasympathetic states without an underlying sympathetic response. The EV4 seems to gradually help the patient re-associate and mobilize potency for healing processes.

Fight or Flight Reviewed

I introduced the flight or flight process in Volume One, and it is now appropriate to fill out its basic physiology in the light of Porges' work. The above processes will help to down-regulate the fight or flight response, integrate early childhood experience, and re-establish normal autonomic baselines.

As described in Volume One, there are four basic stages to this response. They are the (1) *ideal state,* (2) *active alert,* (3) *fight* or *flight* and (4) *overwhelm-shock.* The ideal state is a fully resourced, relaxed, and present-time state. It is a largely parasympathetic state in which we are relaxed, our minds are quiet, and the vegetative processes, such as digestion and reproduction, are in the forefront.

When novelty or danger is sensed, we very rapidly shift into active alert. It is sometimes called the alarm state. In this state we momentarily freeze and orient to the environment. This is a calm state where there is heightened awareness and a sense of mental clarity.

If danger is present we engage in fight or flight. This is a highly charged state. The sympathetic nervous system surges. Energies move to the periphery, and our body is mobilized for action. Vegetative activities like digestion and reproduction are down-regulated, and the parasympathetic brake on the cardiovascular system is removed. Ideally, when the danger passes, this state is naturally and fluidly down-regulated and we return to a more baseline state.

If the fight or flight process is thwarted, if our intentions to protect are overwhelmed, then we may enter another kind of state. This is a state of overwhelm and shock. Here we may experience freezing, immobilization, and dissociation. In this state, the parasympathetic nervous system surges and overlays the sympathetic charge. During this state of immobilization, there are still powerful sympathetic energies cycling. This is important to understand. These energies have to be discharged and resolved in some way. Ideally, as we come out of shock states, we have the opportunity to resolve the sympathetic charge. We may tremble, shake, and express strong emotions. The attempt is to discharge the energies within the immediacy of the experience.

This process of resolution is commonly thwarted. Our minds, the meaning we give the experience, and our past traumatization may all get in the way. The upshot of it all is that we may be left with some of these energies still cycling within us. As we have seen, this can lead directly to chronic autonomic arousal, the initiation of the general adaptation response and the stress cascade, anxiety and depressive states, immune disorders, and, over time, the loss of our ability to fluidly respond to life (Fig. 18.6).

The Fight or Flight Response and the Polyvagal Concept

In threatening or novel situations, the parts of the triune autonomic nervous system act communally to meet the arising experience, and the dorsal motor nucleus and nucleus ambiguus work cooperatively. The following is my interpretation of these relationships.

The ideal state is largely one of rest, repose, and vegetative functions. There is high NA vagal tone to the heart and bronchi, and high DMN vagal tone to the digestive organs.

During the active alert stage, the amygdala and hypothalamus signal the dorsal motor nucleus, the nucleus ambiguus, and the locus ceruleus that danger is present. The DMN *momentarily* surges to stop us so that we can orient to the environment. Along with this, the locus ceruleus acts to release norepinephrin,

Ideal State
Fully resourced
Relaxed, resourced and present.

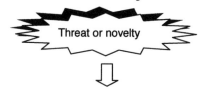

Threat or novelty

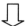

Active Alert State
Freezing, orienting response, heightened alertness, orienting to danger.

Fight or Flight Response
Highly aroused state, highly charged mobilization of defensive energies.

Overwhelm
Resources overwhelmed.

Shock response
Freezing, immobilization and dissociation.

18.6 Fight or Flight

and we enter the active alert state. During this stage, the NA acts to coordinate the overall orienting response. Head and neck motions are co-coordinated with breathing, heart rate, and active attention to scan the environment for danger. Here the dorsal motor nucleus and the nucleus ambiguus act cooperatively. As we shall see, this cooperative process can break down.

In fight or flight, a present danger is sensed and physiology rapidly changes. The nucleus ambiguus and dorsal motor nucleus are down-regulated and the sympathetics surge. The system is flooded with epinephrin and norepinephrin, nonessential activities are down-regulated, energy reserves are accessed, and the musculoskeletal system is mobilized for action.

If this process is thwarted or overwhelmed in any way, the person may go into shock, immobilization,

and dissociation. In overwhelm, a strong surge of the DMN generates a frozen and immobilized state. This is different from the surge that occurred during the orienting response. It is both more intense and of longer duration. There is a concurrent flooding of the system with endorphins and dopamine. This places the person in a dissociated and euphoric state. This is why a patient who manifests frozen and immobilized states generally also experiences dissociation.

Ideally this shock state only lasts for ten minutes or so. As the person comes out of overwhelm, the parasympathetics surge, and the release of dopamine and endorphins, subsides. The person may then tremble, shake, express anger, or even run to discharge the cycling sympathetic energies. If this happens, a resolution of cycling energies and a return to homeostatic balance is more likely to occur (Fig. 18.7).

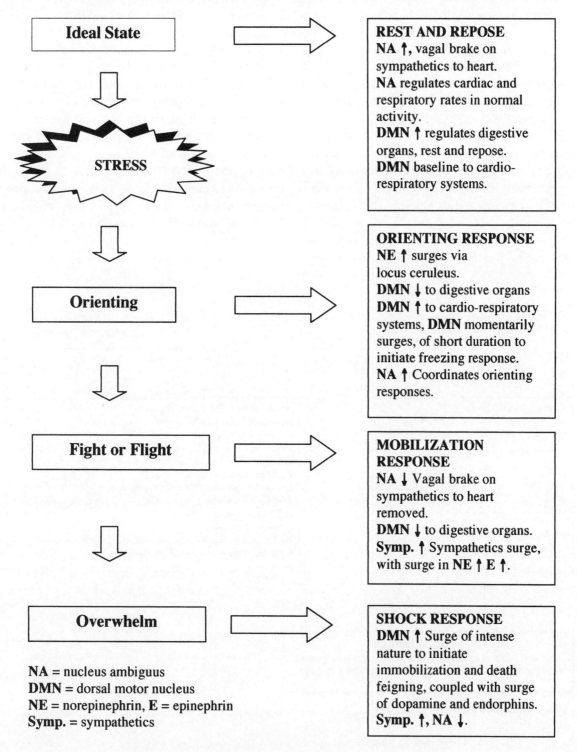

Ideal State

REST AND REPOSE
NA ↑, vagal brake on sympathetics to heart.
NA regulates cardiac and respiratory rates in normal activity.
DMN ↑ regulates digestive organs, rest and repose.
DMN baseline to cardio-respiratory systems.

STRESS

Orienting

ORIENTING RESPONSE
NE ↑ surges via locus ceruleus.
DMN ↓ to digestive organs
DMN ↑ to cardio-respiratory systems, **DMN** momentarily surges, of short duration to initiate freezing response.
NA ↑ Coordinates orienting responses.

Fight or Flight

MOBILIZATION RESPONSE
NA ↓ Vagal brake on sympathetics to heart removed.
DMN ↓ to digestive organs.
Symp. ↑ Sympathetics surge, with surge in **NE ↑ E ↑**.

Overwhelm

SHOCK RESPONSE
DMN ↑ Surge of intense nature to initiate immobilization and death feigning, coupled with surge of dopamine and endorphins.
Symp. ↑, NA ↓.

NA = nucleus ambiguus
DMN = dorsal motor nucleus
NE = norepinephrin, **E** = epinephrin
Symp. = sympathetics

18.7 Fight or Flight Cascade and NA/DMN Responses

However, this resolution process may not go so smoothly. As we saw in our last chapter, cortical loops of memory and meaning can intercede and keep the process running. These can be memories of past trauma, psychological life statements, or even cultural injunctions such as, "big boys don't cry," or "emotions shouldn't be shown in public." So thoughts and meaning can signal the amygdala and hypothalamus either that the event is not yet over, or can literally get in the way of the discharge and clearing process. The amygdala also mediates emotional memory. The amygdala itself may be cycling the emotional memories of past trauma and these too can get in the way of resolving the present trauma.

Due to all of these possibilities, confusion may set in. The parasympathetic surge of the dorsal motor nucleus may not be down-regulated, the person may be left in a dissociative state, and the sympathetic energies may not be fully cleared. The next time that person meets stress or feels threatened in any way, when the DMN surges in the orienting response, it may not turn off. It may respond as though the current situation is totally overwhelming. It may start to work in opposition to the NA and the orienting response. Furthermore, the dissociative process is commonly coupled with the freezing response mediated by the DMN. The person may thus become immobilized and dissociated. They cannot orient to the present situation. Have you ever experienced this? Your boss or friend says something challenging to you, or they jump at you emotionally. You can't find the words to respond, you feel frozen and spacey.

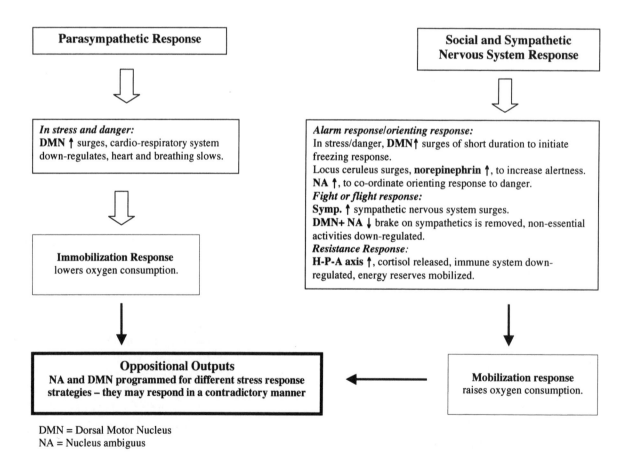

18.8 Polyvagal Responses to Stress and Oppositional Outputs

You're rooted to the spot, frozen and immobilized. Alternatively, the underlying sympathetic energies break through, and you get inappropriately angry or even express rage (Fig. 18.8).

EARLY CHILDHOOD TRAUMA

It became obvious in my clinical practice that the hypoarousal physiology at work in many young children is very different from the classic fight or flight process described above. There seemed to be no underlying sympathetic cycling involved. Some discussions I had with Emerson in the mid-1980s were very helpful. In his huge experience with infants and their prenatal and birth patterning, he had clearly seen that a large proportion of infants, if overwhelmed by their experience, default to the most primitive protective response, the parasympathetic. The infant cannot protect itself either by fighting or fleeing; hence, their primal defensive strategy is withdrawal and dissociation. You see this in even small ways in young infants. If they do not like something—a sound, sight or person—they simply turn away from it. In other words, they withdraw.

Porges' polyvagal concept has helped clarify some of what is happening in such cases and how to orient to it clinically. If an infant is rapidly overwhelmed, the DMN surges, coupled with a flooding of serotonin, endorphins, and dopamine, and the infant enters a frozen and dissociated state. This may occur before any sympathetic cycling can be generated. These infants are not generally seen to have problems. They sleep a lot, are "good" babies, and do not give the parents any trouble. They may have some feeding and attention difficulties, but these are not generally picked up or considered to be a problem. Some recent research seems to bear this out.[3]

There is evidence that this kind of early childhood experience can generate a *parasympathetic setpoint*. The person becomes set in a parasympathetic response to stress. They cannot mobilize sympathetic energies. In later childhood, attention deficit states may occur, with an inability to concentrate or to mobilize to achieve success. In later life, the person may collapse into parasympathetic states of listlessness, tiredness, oversleeping, poor motivation, and even immobility. Chronic fatigue syndrome may have its roots here. It is a chronically exhausted, low sympathetic, low cortisol, low norepinephrin state in which the person enters dissociation easily and has problems focusing attention and maintaining awareness. They may withdraw from stressful situations, avoid challenges, become very tired easily, collapse into sleep states, etc.

The immune system is greatly affected by all this. The sympathetic supply to lymph nodes tends to generate a sympathetic brake on the immune system. It down-regulates immune responses and helps keep the immune system from eating us alive. Furthermore, cortisol also functions as a brake on the immune system. Because the system has shifted to a chronic parasympathetic state, the H-P-A axis is down-regulated and cortisol levels are lower than normal. As people set in parasympathetic mode have low cortisol levels, this brake on the immune system is also not functioning. These people are thus prone to autoimmune conditions, inflammatory responses, muscular and connective tissue breakdown. Arthritic and rheumatic conditions may be generated. Syndromes such as chronic fatigue syndrome and autoimmune states are common (Fig. 18.9).

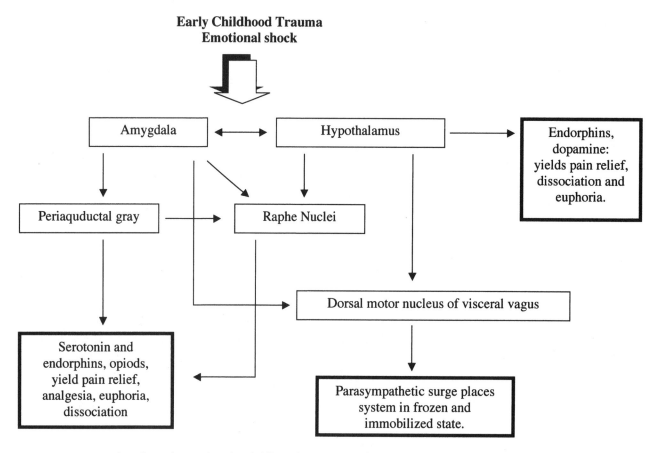

18.9 The Physiology of Early Childhood Trauma and the Parasympathetic Stress Response

Clinical Application: Orienting Exercise

This final application, based on Levine's work, is a simple exercise to help re-establish the orienting response and the natural balance between the nucleus ambiguus and the dorsal motor nucleus.

A traumatized person has difficulty in being present and in orienting to present experience. Experience is sensed and seen through the veils of past trauma and unresolved experience. There is also a feedback loop between neck area and the brain stem. The locus ceruleus receives proprioceptive input from neck muscles. This gives the stress system feedback about danger through the orienting response. When neck muscles tense, the locus ceruleus reads this as possible environmental danger. The sympathetics are up-regulated, and the active alert stage intensifies. If the system is in a chronic hyperarousal state, a feedback loop can ensue in which the neck muscles are signaled to tense and the tension is read by the locus ceruleus as an orienting response to danger. The person is caught in a chronic orienting-active alert feedback loop.

In this process, we will work with these orienting issues and ask our patients to really come into present time as they look and hear. Then we will have them very slowly rotate the head from one side to the other as they scan the environment, actively listening and seeing as they scan the room. As they do this, we will also ask them to be aware of the sensations and feeling tones that arise in their bodies, and help them track those sensations and work appropriately with them.

As the patients come into present time, they are using their working memory within the prefrontal cortex. This conveys information about the current nature of experience to the amygdala. If the relationship with the practitioner is sensed as a resource and there is trust present, this will be communicated to the amygdala and to the deepest recesses of the psyche. As the person comes into seeing and hearing, as they rotate their head, they are also entering the sphere of the nucleus ambiguus and the social nervous system. The dorsal motor nucleus and its freezing response may be down-regulated as the orienting response comes to the forefront.

This application assumes that the client has developed sufficient resources to orient to sensations and feeling tones in the body without immediately dissociating. It also assumes that a safe therapeutic environment has been established. There must be a sense of trust and safety both in the environment and in the relationship for any of this to be helpful. For these prerequisites, please review the trauma concepts and skills outlined in Volume One.

1. Have the patient sit comfortably in a chair or on a cushion. Locate yourself in a position nearby that they feel comfortable with. They may want you to sit a certain distance away, or in a certain position, such as diagonally instead of directly opposite. Find an appropriate viewing distance and location.

2. As in the focusing process,[4] first help them orient to their embodied space. Help them form a relationship to sensations and feeling tones in their body. Sometimes following their breath into their inner body space can help. Do not, however, force a person to be in sensation or within their body; simply orient them to sensation and feeling tones. Respect where they need to be.

3. Then instruct the person to really pay attention to their seeing and hearing experiences. Help them look at the objects in the room, the light, the colors, the forms, and help them hear the sounds, the tones, the pitches in the environment. Then ask them to very, very slowly and gently rotate their head, first in the direction it seems to want to go and then in the other direction. As they do this, also again help them perceive the sensations and feeling tones in their body.

4. As they slowly rotate their head, they may find a subtle barrier to their rotation; this may be a sense of tension in the muscles, or a sense of strain. Have them stay near this edge and explore the sensations that arise. This subtle boundary indicates the "edges" of their field of orientation in everyday life. Traumatization tends to literally narrow this field. This is physically expressed by restriction to allowable head motions, neck tension, and strain. Again remind them to orient to seeing and hearing and the outer environment.

5. As in the focusing process, also help orient them to the felt-sense of what arises, as this also brings the felt meaning of the activation into play and may help down-regulate cortical involvement. In other words, it may help them let go of coupled meanings and memories and generate space in mental-emotional couplings. Simply explore and see what arises without any need for anything particular to happen.

6. Gently work with these intentions and notice any activation that arises as they explore this process. Help them work with the activation processes that arise (see Chapters 21 and 22 in Volume One). This may occur within any pole of the sympathetic-parasympathetic spectrum. It may even rapidly shift from one to the other. Slow things down and help them be with one process at a time. This is an exploration with the only intention being to explore present time within the context of the orienting response.

This simple process can be very powerful, useful when the patient has built resources and trust and can be with their arising process. In my experience it does help the person re-orient and come into present time. It allows the parasympathetic-sympathetic poles of cycling to arise in their own time and to process and resolve trauma patterns. It seems to re-establish the natural balance between the DMN and NA.

In a cranial approach, the practitioner can make contact with the neck/cervical area with the cervical hold learned in Chapter 7, "The Occipital Triad." The practitioner's fingers line up vertically along either side of the midline over the cervical articular masses. While making a firm yet negotiated contact, the motility and motion dynamics are explored and states of balance are accessed. This can help down-regulate the feedback loop from the cervical area to the locus ceruleus.

1. Stephen Porges, "Orienting in a defensive world: Mammalian modifications of our evolutionary heritage. A Polyvagal Theory," *Psychophysiology,* 32 (1995); Stephen Porges, "The polyvagal theory: phylogenetic substrates of a social nervous system," *International Journal of Psychophysiology* 42 (2001) 123–146. A full listing of Porges' writings in this area can be found at www.trauma-pages.com.

2. See John Chitty, "The Triune Nervous System" (unpublished paper, 2001) available at www.energyschool.com/writings.

3. See Bruce Perry, MD, Ph.D., Ronnie Pollard, MD, "Homeostasis, Stress, Trauma, and Adaptation, A neurodevelopmental View of Childhood Trauma," *Child and Adolescent Psychiatric Clinics of North America* 7(1), January 1998.

4. See Chapter 22, Volume One, for a description of the focusing process.

19

Nociception and the Stress Response

Internal stressors can be just as powerful as external stressors in setting off the general adaptation response and its stress cascade, an important point often missed or overlooked by the trauma therapy community. This chapter focuses on internal stress response mechanisms and the under-appreciated role of nociceptors.[1] These ubiquitous nerve endings sense for danger, tissue damage, and toxicity within the body. Internal stressors, such as inflammatory processes, fluid congestion, tissue damage, and pathologies of various kinds can engage the general adaptation response and its stress cascade just like external stressors do. Many of the complaints we see in our offices can be traced to nociceptive activity, including chronic pain, injuries that don't get better, and ongoing disorders that have no direct apparent cause or external etiology. A cranial approach to these internal stressors can be direct, precise, and effective.

THE SPINAL SEGMENT

Understanding spinal segments and the simple reflex arc forms a basis for our subsequent exploration of internal stress responses. A basic spinal segment is composed of (1) a sensory nerve, (2) a dorsal horn neuron within the spinal cord, (3) a connecting intermediary or secondary neuron, and (4) a motor nerve. This simple segment also sends information, via the secondary neurons, to higher level processors in the brain and also receives higher level input from these.

In this chapter we will discuss:

- *The spinal nerve segment.*
- *The concept of facilitation.*
- *The four stages of facilitation.*
- *Nociception and the sensitization of peripheral nerves and neurons.*
- *Hypersensitive or facilitated spinal nerve segments.*
- *The transduction of dorsal horn neurons.*
- *Higher level facilitation and the sensitization of the general adaptation response.*
- *Clinical approaches to facilitated states.*

Information is sent to the spinal cord by sensory (afferent) peripheral nerves. These are in contact with either visceral or somatic tissues and the fluids around these tissues. The neurons or cell bodies of these nerves are located in the dorsal root ganglia near the spinal cord. Both visceral and somatic sensory nerves travel within a spinal nerve and have their neurons located there. From here they enter the spinal cord and synapse with multiple dorsal horn neurons. The dorsal horn cells form what has been described as an *interneuronal pool*. This is a three-dimensional pool of connected neurons. These cells form a matrix that is more like the multiple nonlinear interconnections of servers on the internet than like the linear connections of a telegraph system. Input to one neuron can take many routes and affect many others, and many neurons may be affected by incoming information.

The dorsal horn cells function as local processors of information. From here a reflex motor (efferent) response may be sent back to the particular somatic or visceral tissue from which the input originated, forming a complete-circle information loop by which a peripheral area reports to the spine and the spine responds with command messages. This simple input-local processing-output loop is called a *reflex arc* (Fig. 19.1). At this stage, no higher processing is needed, and homeostasis can be maintained without overwhelming the higher level processes with information.

The system is adaptable in that sensory input meets the interneuronal pool and is received in up to three spine segments, for redundancy and fast response. The spine is not horizontally segmented for this purpose, but rather the dorsal horn cells directly interconnect to several vertebral levels. Information also travels up and down the spinal cord and can stimulate response in many areas. The spinal cord itself is thus vertically, not horizontally, oriented (Fig. 19.2).

In addition, signals may be sent to the head via secondary neurons from the dorsal horn interneuronal pool to brain stem nuclei, the amygdala, the thalamus, the hypothalamus, and the cortex for higher level processing. If the signals are intense enough, the dorsal horn cells tell these higher-level processors that something serious is happening below.

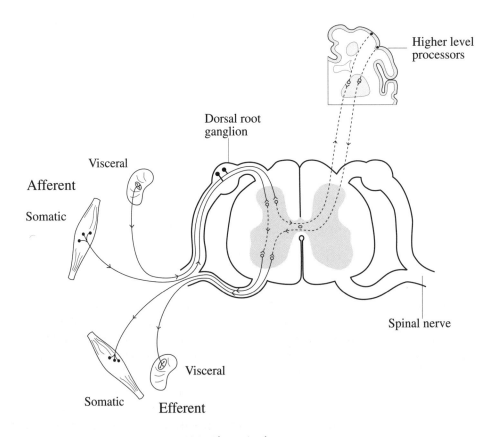

19.1 The spinal segment

Composition of the Spinal Nonsegmented Neuronal Web

- Visceral or somatic sensory afferent nerves with their neurons in the dorsal root ganglion.
- Multiple connections (up to three segments) from these nerves to the dorsal horn neurons.
- The dorsal horn neurons and the interneuronal pool they are part of.
- Efferent motor nerve or nerves.

FACILITATION AND THE FACILITATED SEGMENT

The term *facilitation* means that something has been made easier. In this case, it indicates that a nerve has become hypersensitive or hyperexcitable. The nerve's threshold of firing has been lowered and it fires with

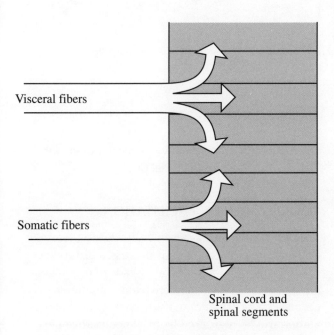

Visceral fibers

Somatic fibers

Spinal cord and spinal segments

19.2 Multi-segmental sensory input to spinal cord

less than normal sensory stimulation. Facilitation commonly occurs when there is ongoing and chronic input to a nerve. The nerve becomes overwhelmed by the input and becomes hypersensitive, and its firing is made easier due to some chronic pathological process in the body. The spinal segment described above or the larger multisegmental neuronal web can become facilitated and hypersensitized.

This has important repercussions throughout the system. Spinal nerve segments that serve both the visceral and somatic components of the body may become hypersensitive and fire inappropriately, generating somatic and visceral pathologies. Tense or flaccid muscles, loss of joint mobility, joint pathologies, and visceral dysfunctions can all arise due to these facilitated, chronic nociceptive inputs. Most importantly, chronic nociceptive input to the higher order nuclei of the brain stem, diencephalon, and cortex can set off the general adaptation response and its stress cascade.

In osteopathic practice, a sensitized spinal segment is called a *facilitated segment,* and it is seen to have a number of possible origins. One is a vertebral fixation that impinges on a nerve root leaving or entering the spinal cord, as nociceptive input floods the sensory nerves and spinal cord. Other common origins of facilitation are chronic inflammation within the musculoskeletal system and visceral inflammation and pathology.

Constant nociceptive input into sensory neurons can cause what is known as *transduction.* In transduction, the nature of the nucleus and cell membrane of neurons changes. The nerve becomes more easily stimulated, and the output from the cell nucleus may change. Nerves that normally produce particular hormones or proteins may begin to produce others in response to the ongoing nociceptive input and hypersensitivity. In some respects, it is a local version of what happens under constant stress in the body at large. Cells become overwhelmed, and physiology changes.[2]

Transduction has major repercussions for sensory, nociceptive nerves. Nociceptors monitor for danger, tissue damage, and inflammation. They are sometimes called *pain receptors*. They are *high threshold, small caliber* nerves; it takes relatively intense inputs to set them off. Other sensory nerves, such as touch receptors, proprioceptors, and mechano-receptors, are *low threshold, large caliber* nerves; they are faster nerves, and less stimulation is needed to set them off. This allows for sensitive feedback in relatively subtle processes like touch and pressure reception and body position and motion. Under chronic sensory input, nociceptors can transduce and become sensitized to lower levels of input. They then begin to act as though they are low threshold nerves, and ordinary stimuli, such as moving an arm or pressure against the skin, can then be erroneously interpreted as danger.

VISCERAL–SOMATIC CONVERGENCE AND THE SPINAL SEGMENT

Another complication arises because the various nerve cells in the dorsal horn intercommunicate by sharing synapses in the dorsal root ganglia. Nociceptors, proprioceptors, mechano-receptors, chemo-receptors, and nerves from somatic and visceral sources all are linked. When the neurons of nociceptors transduce and act like high caliber fibers, they can signal other sensory neurons within the dorsal root ganglia that danger is present. Localized responses can be generated in other parts of the body without spinal cord processors even being involved! Remote sensory nerve endings may then release a chemical called *substance P* into their areas, setting off inflammatory processes. Thus, even before input is sent to the dorsal horn cells within the spinal cord, whole-body referred inflammatory processes can be initiated. Within the dorsal root ganglia a somatic-visceral convergence can also occur. Somatic sensory nerves can begin to signal visceral sensory nerves that danger is present, and likewise, visceral sensory nerves can signal somatic nerves.

There is also visceral-somatic convergence within the spinal cord. Both visceral and somatic nerves can synapse with multiple spinal cord segments and multiple dorsal horn neurons. Their sensory inputs converge on the dorsal horn interneuronal pool, and multiple motor outputs result. Thus, input from a visceral sensory nerve may stimulate somatic efferent output and vice-versa. A sensitized spinal segment may therefore affect many areas of the body and many systems, both somatic and visceral. Thus, we are really talking about a *facilitated non-segmental neuronal web* with wide repercussions in the body.

Lastly, there is also visceral-somatic convergence with the secondary neurons that carry information from the dorsal horn area to higher centers above. The convergence within the dorsal horn area can also lead to interlinked output to higher centers such as the hypothalamus, thalamus, amygdala, locus ceruleus, and autonomic nuclei (Fig. 19.3).

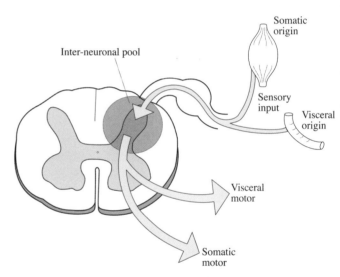

19.3 Visceral–somatic convergence in dorsal horn interneuronal pool

FOUR STAGES OF FACILITATION

The facilitation process can enter the deepest recesses of the nervous system. In this process, a disturbance of some kind generates a local cascade of pro-inflammatory, neuro-endocrine-active and immune-active chemicals. The presence of tissue damage and inflammation will be registered by local nociceptive nerve endings, and these nerves will send input into the dorsal horn of the spinal cord. If the disturbance is chronic, the nociceptive nerve will transduce and become sensitized to further input. This sensitized input goes to the dorsal horn neurons, and motor output is sent back to the area of disturbance. A sensitized spinal segment begins to form.

In the next stage, the dorsal horn neurons also transduce, and the sensitized reflex arc is even more intensified. The transduced dorsal horn cells, whose interneuronal pool receives input from all sorts of sensory processes, begins to read all sensory inputs as though they are nociceptive. Inputs that warn of danger flood the higher centers of the brain, and the stress cascade can be set off. The nuclei and neurons of higher level processors, such as autonomic nuclei, the amygdala, and the hypothalamus, may also become overwhelmed by the amount of input arising, and become sensitized. A vicious circle results in which inputs and outputs keep the sensitized cycles running, in what I call the four stages of facilitation.

Stages of Facilitation:

- The sensitization of a peripheral nerve.

- The sensitization of a spinal segment or segments.

- The transduction of the dorsal horn neurons.

- The sensitization and transduction of higher level nuclei in the brain stem, diencephalon and cortex, and the generation of a general adaptation stress response in the body that can enter the deepest recesses of the nervous system (Fig. 19.4).

Stage One

In the first stage, a disturbance of some kind, typically some kind of tissue fixation, pathology, or damage, generates an inflammatory process. When cells are damaged, their cell membranes release a cascade of chemical messengers. This includes neuro-endocrine-active and immune-active chemicals. The intention of this cascade is both to warn the system that damage and danger is present and to initiate healing responses. Nociceptors respond to these pro-inflammatory chemicals by releasing a chemical called substance P into the area that further stimulates the inflammatory

response. Substance P stimulates a further cascade of histamines, prostaglandins, bradykinins, norepinephrin, serotonin, and cytokines, to name just a few. This becomes a *sensitizing soup* of neuroactive chemicals. This soup further stimulates nociceptive nerve endings. A vicious cycle can occur in which these chemicals stimulate the nerves endings of nociceptors to produce more substance P, thus initiating the release of more pro-inflammatory chemicals (Fig. 19.5).[3] The presence of tissue damage and inflammation is detected by local nociceptive nerve endings, and these nerves report the situation to the dorsal horn of the spinal cord.

If the disturbance continues and becomes chronic, the nociceptive nerve involved may become overwhelmed, its neuron may transduce and become sensitized, and the nerve—a high threshold, small caliber nerve—now acts as though it is a low threshold, large caliber nerve.[4] Inputs which do not normally cause it to fire, now will. Motion, pressure, and proprioceptive inputs will cause a firing of the nociceptor. Moving a knee, putting pressure on a leg, or just walking may all be registered as pain. What's more, if a nociceptor transduces, it may remain sensitized even when the initial disturbance has healed. Nociceptive input may still be sent to the spinal cord, even when the disturbance is over[5] (Fig. 19.6).

Stage Two

In the second stage, a sensitized spinal segment begins to form. The transduced nociceptive nerves alert the lower order processors (dorsal horn cells) within the spinal cord that something is up. The dorsal horn cells trigger firing of motor neurons related to the area, initiating a spinal segment (also known as a *sensory-motor reflex arc*), intensifying the whole situation. As more input floods the dorsal horn area, more motor output is produced and more sensory input is stimulated. A vicious circle is set up.

Stage Three

In the third stage, the dorsal horn neurons, flooded with information, also transduce. The sensitized reflex arc is then even more intensified. The transduced dorsal

1. Sensitized peripheral nerve

Cell neuron

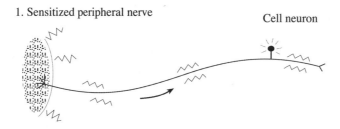

2. Hypersensitive spinal segment

Dorsal horn neuron

Sensory

Motor

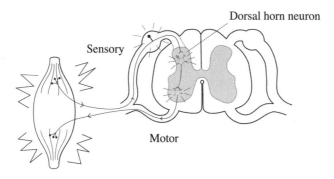

3. Transduction in dorsal horn cells

Brain

4. Higher level sensitization

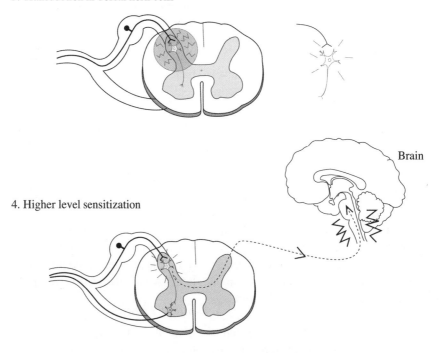

19.4 The four stages of facilitation

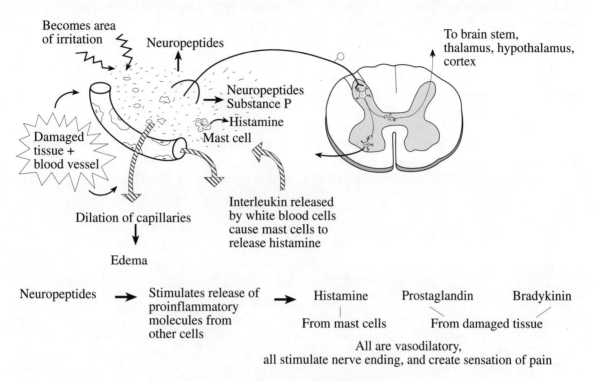

Becomes area
of irritation

Neuropeptides

To brain stem,
thalamus, hypothalamus,
cortex

Neuropeptides
Substance P

Histamine
Mast cell

Damaged
tissue +
blood vessel

Dilation of capillaries

Interleukin released
by white blood cells
cause mast cells to
release histamine

Edema

Neuropeptides → Stimulates release of → Histamine   Prostaglandin   Bradykinin
                   proinflammatory
                   molecules from   From mast cells   From damaged tissue
                   other cells

All are vasodilatory,
all stimulate nerve ending, and create sensation of pain

19.5 Sensitization of peripheral neurons

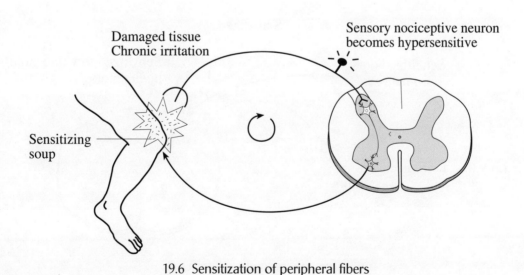

Damaged tissue
Chronic irritation

Sensory nociceptive neuron
becomes hypersensitive

Sensitizing
soup

19.6 Sensitization of peripheral fibers

horn cells, whose interneuronal pool receives input from all sorts of sensory processes, begins to read all sensory inputs as though they are nociceptive. The multilevel spinal segment will be kept cycling by this misinterpretation of sensory input. The somatic or visceral tissues that the reflex arc serves now also become sensitized, leading to joint dysfunction, muscle tension or spasms, and functional degeneration. There is some evidence that arthritis in joints may be generated by this process.[6] Similarly, facilitation of nerves supplying viscera can produce increased sym-

pathetic tonus, changes in organ function, changes in vasomotor tone, and changes in fluid balance. I have treated cases of chronic hyperacidity which had their roots in this process (Fig. 19.7).

Stage Four

This leads to the fourth stage, in which inputs warning of danger flood the higher centers, and the general adaptation response and its stress cascade is set off. The transduced dorsal horn cells, misinterpreting

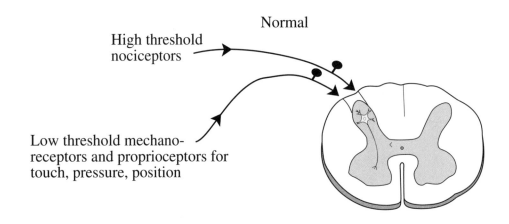

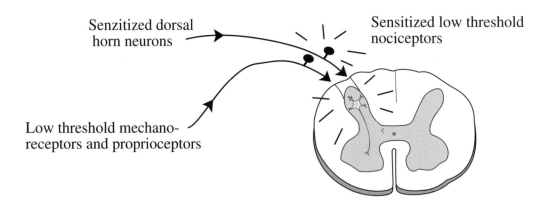

19.7 Sensitization of dorsal horn cells

sensory information, begin to signal higher order processors that there is danger below. These inputs to higher centers travel via secondary nerves in the spinothalamic tract, the spinohypothalamic tract[7] and the spinoreticular tract. When nociceptive inputs reach the cortex via the thalamus, they are registered as pain. However, low level inflammatory processes may not be intense enough to initiate a cortex mediated perception of pain, yet may still impinge upon brain stem, limbic system, and diencephalon neurons. The nuclei and neurons of higher-level processors, including autonomic nuclei, the amygdala, and the hypothalamus, may also be overwhelmed by the input

arising and become sensitized to further input. A vicious circle results in which inputs and outputs keep the sensitized cycles running. It becomes self-perpetuating, beyond the original disturbance, which by this time may have already healed. This is a physical parallel to the amygdala's misinterpreting current-time events as threatening based on past history. What emerges is a system-wide alarm state that is internally generated, self-perpetuating and is perhaps unrelated to any continuing real threat. A state of anxiety comparable to post-traumatic stress disorder symptoms may ensue that originates in a seemingly simple, low-grade inflammatory process! (Fig. 19.8)

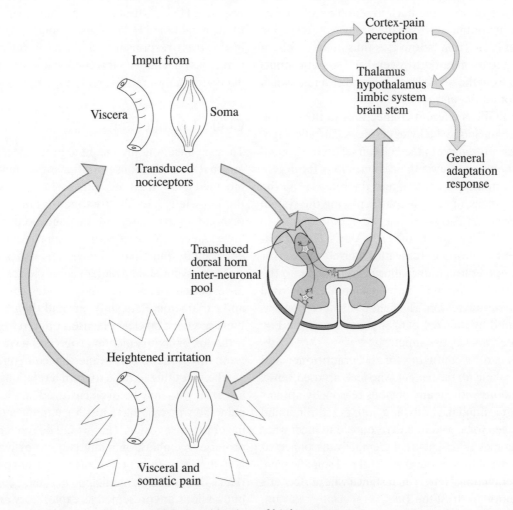

19.8 Sensitization of higher centers

We can understand facilitation in the high processing centers more specifically. Nociceptive input, real or false, converge on a number of important interrelated nuclei. The nucleus paragigantocellularius, abbreviated as PGi, is a bilateral nucleus in the brain stem with multiple afferent and efferent connections, including connections with the stress cascade. It receives input from both visceral and somatic nociceptors, the hypothalamus, the amygdala, and the nucleus and tract of solitarius and other sources. It has important connections both to the sympathetic chain and to the locus ceruleus. It receives direct visceral and somatic nociceptive input from the dorsal horn interneuronal pool via secondary nerves. It also receives input from the nucleus and tract of solitarius, the major nuclei within the brain stem receiving visceral input from below. It is thus in an excellent position to monitor both visceral and somatic inputs coming from the whole body. It becomes a real switch point for autonomic activation.

The PGi has efferent connections to the sympathetic chain and to the locus ceruleus. Chronic ongoing nociceptive input to the PGi can set off the general adaptation response via these connections. It can generate sympathetic arousal and the release, via the locus ceruleus, of norepinephrin, placing the system in active alert and signaling the hypothalamus to release CRH to activate the H-P-A axis. The sympathetic stress response cascades, muscles tense for action, epinephrin (adrenaline) is released into the system and the person is now on a mobilization road for no external reason. The fight or flight response is generated by internal danger signals mediated by facilitated nociceptive input.

This can be confusing for the practitioner and crazy-making for the patient, who feels aroused, tense, and anxious without any obvious reason. Symptoms can shift around the body, and both practitioner and client need to be patient and resourced to meet what is sometimes an onslaught of seemingly disconnected symptoms of hyperarousal, visceral and somatic pain, and dysfunction. Here is an instance where Becker's admonition to "trust the Tide" is especially relevant.

Nociceptive input also travels directly to the hypothalamus via the spinohypothalamic tract. The stress response may also be activated via this route. Direct, facilitated nociceptive input alerts the hypothalamus to internal danger and signals the sympathetics and the locus ceruleus to place the system in active alert and mobilization, launching the whole now-familiar sympathetic cascade.

The amygdala also receives nociceptive input from below, further complicating the situation. Nociceptive input arrives at the amygdala via the PGi and other brain stem nuclei. The amygdala can thus respond directly to internal danger in much the same way that it responds external danger. Nociceptive input causes the amygdala to set off the stress response. High cortisol levels may also be cycling due to the heightened H-P-A axis, keeping the amygdala in its stress response. I have successfully treated numerous patients with this condition, which was making their life miserable (Fig. 19.9).

Clinical Applications

These applications are meant to give a clear sense of internal stress response relationships; they are not intended to be "treatment protocols." Once you have the knowledge, let the treatment plan unfold and respond appropriately to the conditions present. I have had good success with this approach in peripheral joint dysfunction and in visceral issues.

Let's assume that a patient comes to see you having experienced ongoing anxiety states, chronic pain, and exhaustion. Pain shifts around their body, and there has been no clear diagnosis offered from either orthodox or complementary sources. I have encountered this scenario many times, haven't you?

The first thing to do is to form a relationship with a person who may be oversensitized and in chronic pain and who may have lost hope in the situation. I never promise results. That would be foolhardy. I do promise to embark on a mutual journey which may help their situation. I can usually say from past experience that the work has helped in similar conditions, but sessions are presented as exploratory and open. I commonly ask a patient to commit to at least ten

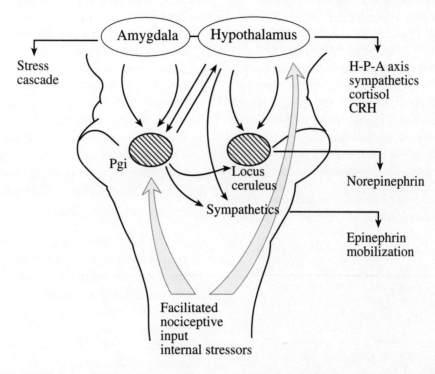

19.9 Facilitation of higher centers driven by sensitized nociceptive input from below

sessions. Work may unfold in a helpful way in a shorter time, but it can take me anywhere from six to ten sessions to get through to a person's system at a level deeper than the physiology and pain that is cycling. My intention generally is to help initiate resources within their system, to access the deeper tidal rhythms, and to resource them in the session process. States of balance, stillness, and holding a wide and open perceptual field are all important. A relationship must be generated in which they begin to feel resourced and held in their pain. This is a humbling experience for both me and the patient. When potency begins to become available within a patient's system, particular fulcrums will be highlighted and particular stress patterns will come to the forefront. As sessions continue, the potency will move to process the stress responses cycling in the system. Activation may occur, and related biokinetic forces will come to the surface. Again, you must have the sensitivity to track this and to relate appropriately to the activation present.

Facilitation Stages One and Two: The Sensitizing Soup and Peripheral Nerve Facilitation

In the following exploration, we are working with peripheral fulcrums that can generate chronic nociceptive signals and nerve sensitization. Our focus is on somatic (muscular) or visceral (organ) fulcrums, to lower hypertonis of the peripheral nociceptors and help to reset the CNS. We want to relate the peripheral area to its related spinal segments.

1. Start by choosing one fulcrum of either visceral or somatic origin and place both hands there. This might be a somatic tissue area, such as a joint or connective tissue relationship, or a visceral structure such as the liver or heart. If you are palpating an organ, simply listen for a sense of its motility, especially for a sense of inner primary respiration, expansion and settling within the mid-tide. You may encounter the sensitizing soup discussed above. This may have an activated quality with lots of fluid perturbation, electrical discharges and a feeling of density.

2. Within the cycles of primary respiration, orient to inhalation and exhalation until an inertial pattern seems to clarify from within. Follow the pattern of motion and fluid fluctuations or perturbations to a state of balance. Listen for Becker's three-phase awareness. Bring in any appropriate skill, such as fluid direction, lateral fluctuation, and disengagement. All skills orient to the state of balance and stillness. Sense for resolution and reorganization within the local area and reorientation to the midline.

3. Now connect that area to the related area of the spinal cord. Keep one hand on the peripheral area (organ, joint, etc.) and move your other hand to the area of the spinal cord which relates to the somatic or visceral relationship. The general guide for finding the spinal area is based on embryology and spinal nerve pathways. For lower limbs and lower organs, place your upper hand under T10-L1. For the upper limbs, look to the C7-T2 area. For locations in the torso, place your hand more or less transversely to the site of interest. When the right spinal point is contacted it may seem to "light up" with a pulsatory recognition or felt-sense of energetic connectedness. The spinal contact is relating to long fibers spanning multiple vertebrae, not narrow horizontal bands.

4. Holding both the spinal segment area (visualizing its dorsal horn) and the peripheral fulcrum, access the mutual state of balance. Listen for expressions of Health. Listen for any release of neural charge such as the peripheral nerve discharging its cycling energies. This indicates that the sensitized peripheral nerve is clearing its facilitation. Wait for a setting of all of this into stillness. Listen for a reorganization and realignment of whole tissue field from the spinal segment to the peripheral area. See how these tissues now orient to the primal midline. Finish with a CV4 if appropriate.

Facilitation Stage Three: Dorsal Horn Facilitation and Brain Stem Nuclei

1. Place your caudad hand under the dorsal horn area of the spinal cord level being palpated. Follow the motion expressed within the phases of primary respiration. Wait for a pattern to clarify, for the action of potency, and the state of balance. Listen for expressions of Health (such as expressions of potency and fluid within and around the fulcrum).

2. You can also direct fluid to the spinal cord area by placing your cephalad hand over the top of the patient's cranium. Orient to the fluid field and direct potency and fluid through the foramen magnum towards the dorsal horn area. Let any discharge of neural energy clear. It is important to sense a clearing from the dorsal horn area and some kind of change in its dynamic. You may sense easier motility, better fluid motion, and a down-regulation of the charge that seemed to be cycling from that area.

3. Once you sense a clearing from the dorsal horn area, place your other hand under the occiput and orient to the brain stem area. Holding both the dorsal horn area and the brain stem, follow motility within the phases of primary respiration. Wait for a pattern to clarify and help access the state of balance. Again be aware of any neural clear-

ing and dissipation of the facilitation. You may sense electrical clearing, fluid perturbation, etc.

4. CV4s may also help to restore equilibrium to dorsal horn cells. Becker wrote that repeated CV4s can process the "memory traces" within the spinal cord.[8]

Stage Four: Brain Stem Motility

As we have seen, the brain stem is a major focus for stress and flight and fight responses. Its nuclei are switch points for information and responses to stress and traumatic situations. There are neural connections from below bringing information about visceral and somatic homeostasis to its nuclei, and from the hypothalamus and amygdala above. The hypothalamus can be thought of as the maestro of an orchestra who gets information from all of the instruments and who gives direction and maintains balance and harmony within all of its functions. The brain stem contains nuclei that act as switch points for the sounds the hypothalamus hears from below and for giving, receiving, and responding to its directions.

In this exercise we specifically orient to the motility of the brain stem and access states of balance by using the occipital cradle hold. Be aware of the release of shock affects from the central nervous system as you listen to the response of the CNS.

1. In the occipital cradle, orient to the patient's system as a whole and sense the motility of the central nervous system. First orient to the ventricle system and let the motion within the phases of primary respiration come to you. Within this, orient to the brain stem. Let the motion of the brain stem come into your awareness. Allow it to come to you. Don't look, but listen. The brain stem will ideally rise towards the lamina terminalis and slightly widen in inhalation. Follow this in the cycles of surge and settling within primary respiration.

2. As you do this, see if a pattern clarifies. Access the state of balance. Facilitation within brain stem

nuclei manifest as a palpable electric-like "buzz" or "hum" or as a sense of density within a particular area. Motion may be organized around these fulcrums. Sense and help access states of balance within tissues, fluids, and potency of this area.

3. Within the state of balance, listen for expressions of Health and for any manifestation of the discharge of shock affects. These may be perceived as streaming electrical discharge, perturbations within fluids, or as tissue tremblings and shaking. Allow these to occur and clear; do not rush the process. Use your verbal trauma skills if appropriate. Listen for the expression of potency as forces are processed. Remember that it is the potency that is doing the work, not your machinations. Wait for reorganization of tissues, fluids, and potency.

Clinical Application: The Brain Stem-Limbic-Hypothalamus-Adrenal Axis

In this application, we will be extending the work with the brain stem above to other important higher centers. As above, you will first relate to the brain stem and its nuclei, then to the brain stem-limbic-axis and finally to the brain stem-hypothalamus-adrenal axis. The intention is to again access states of balance within their dynamics. Fluid direction and CV4 can also be used to lower hypertonis and to initiate inertial potencies within the dynamics.

1. In the vault hold, tune into the fluid tide and its potency and sense the motility of the central nervous system. Work with any inertial patterns that clarify via neutrals and states of balance. Shifting to an occipital cradle, again sense the motility of neural tissue. In the application above, we oriented to the brain stem. Here we will orient to a larger area, including the brain stem, the floor of the third ventricle (for the hypothalamus) and the floor of the lateral ventricle (for the hippocampus and amygdala). Visualize this brain stem-limbic-hypothalamus axis, reviewing

anatomy as needed. See what clarifies within the phases of primary respiration.

2. Note any inertial patterns and areas of facilitation. Again these may be sensed as activated areas that seem to "buzz," as areas of density, and as areas with unusual fluid fluctuations. Help access the state of balance. Be aware of any expressions of shock affect. Let the neural energy discharge until a state of stillness is sensed. Wait within this stillness and widen your perceptual field towards the horizon. Settle into an even deeper stillness. Do not expect anything. See what arises from within.

3. You can also direct fluid toward any activated nuclei or dense areas perceived using the heels of your hands via the cisterna magna. You can also direct fluid toward the hippocampus, amygdala and hypothalamus from the cisterna magna. This can sometimes help to down-regulate the brain stem-limbic-hypothalamus axis and the H-P-A axis at least temporarily.

THE KNEE AS AN EXAMPLE

Now we can put these parts together to get a sense of the combined treatment. To illustrate this method, let's say a person injured a knee playing football, and it has not resolved. Within a session, we sense that the knee joint is an organizing site for segmental and dorsal horn facilitation within the spinal cord.

1. First hold the knee with both hands in any comfortable position that provides a good perception of its condition. Establish your practitioner fulcrums and negotiate your relationship with the patient's system as usual. Hold a wide perceptual field and orient to the biosphere and mid-tide.

2. Within the phases of primary respiration, follow whatever motion patterns arise to a state of balance. If the area is very inertial, use lateral fluctuation processes to stimulate the potency within the fulcrums involved. Work to a state of balance and listen for expressions of Health. Within the stillness, you may sense the processing of the sensitization in the area. There may be electric-like discharges from nerve endings and fluid fluctuations as the potency acts to increase circulation and clear the sensitizing soup that may be present. Wait for a sense of settling and realignment to the midline.

3. When you sense a local resolution, connect the knee to the related dorsal horn-spinal cord level. One hand stays under or over the knee, and the other hand is at T10-L1. Orient to the whole fluid-tissue field as you hold both poles of the sensory-motor nerve loop. Orient to the whole fluid-tissue field you are holding. Do not narrow your perceptual field as you do this. Wait for a pattern to clarify and for a settling into a state of balance and orient to Becker's three-phase awareness. Be especially aware of the processing of neural cycling and the discharge of neural energy through the relationships being palpated. You may literally sense the whole sensitized nerve loop clearing.

4. If you sense that the facilitation extends to the higher centers, proceed up the body. One hand can hold the spinal segment while the other goes to the brain stem, listening for the motion expressed and gently listening for discharge and states of balance. Finally, moving to the head, use the occipital cradle and/or vault to encourage reorientation to the midline, full CNS mobility within the mid-tide, and discharge of forces held in the relevant brain areas.

5. With all of these hand positions, let the Inherent Treatment Plan guide the sequence and pacing. You may feel called to repeat one step or omit a step, or to cycle back and forth between two hand positions.

1. For an excellent introduction to the world of nociception and neuro-endocrine issues, I refer you again to: F. H. Willard and M.M. Patterson, eds., *Nociception and the Neuroendocrine-immune Connection* (American Academy of Osteopathy, 1994).

2. Ibid.

3. Thanks to Katherine Ukleja, D.O., for this diagram relating to lectures by Dr. Frank Willard.

4. Op. cit., Willard and Patterson.

5. Ibid.

6. Ibid.

7. New research has discovered that there are direct connections from nociceptors below to the hypothalamus above. In other words, input can go directly to the hypothalamus without going through the thalamus first.

8. R. E. Becker, *Diagnostic Touch: Its Principles and Application I, II, III, IV* (Academy of Applied Osteopathy Yearbooks, 1963, 1964, 1965).

Index